GRAPHIC DISCOVERIES

MEDICAL
BREAKTHROUGHS

by Gary Jeffrey

illustrated by Terry Riley

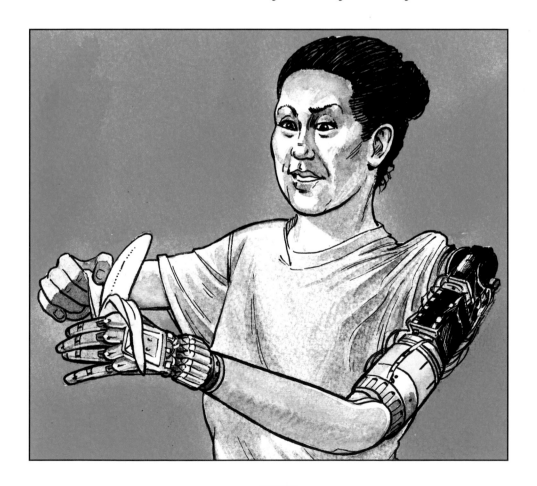

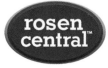

rosen
central

The Rosen Publishing Group, Inc., New York

Published in 2008 by The Rosen Publishing Group, Inc.
29 East 21st Street, New York, NY 10010

Designed and produced by
David West Books

Editor: Gail Bushnell

Photo credits:
4b, National Library of Medicine; 6b, Library of Congress Prints and Photographs Division Washington, D.C.; 7tr, Corbis; 7tl, Public Health Image Library; 44tl&r, Corbis.

Library of Congress Cataloging-in-Publication Data

Library of Congress Cataloging-in-Publication Data

Jeffrey, Gary.
  Medical breakthroughs / Gary Jeffrey ; illustrated by Terry Riley. -- 1st ed.
     p. cm. -- (Graphic discoveries)
  Includes bibliographical references and index.
  ISBN-13: 978-1-4042-1086-8 (hardcover)
  ISBN-13: 978-1-4042-9588-9 (6 pack)
  ISBN-13: 978-1-4042-9587-2 (pbk.)
 1. Medicine--History--Juvenile literature. 2. Medical innovations--History--Juvenile literature. I. Title.
  R133.5.J44 2008
  610--dc22

                                        2007007689

Manufactured in China

CONTENTS

EARLY MEDICINE

In ancient times illness was seen as the result of witchcraft or the will of the gods. Often, patients would pray and make offerings to a god. The rise of scientific medicine in the last two centuries has replaced these historical practices.

ANCIENT MEDICINE

Although little was known about the workings of the human body, early medicine provided some effective cures. Plants were being used as herbal medicines as early as 25,000 B.C. Drilling teeth was practiced over 5,000 years ago in India, while in ancient Egypt, the earliest known surgery was performed around 2,750 B.C. In ancient Greece, the first known medical school was set up in 700 B.C. Later, Hippocrates founded a school in Kos, Greece, in around 400 B.C. Hippocrates is called "the father of medicine." He and his followers were the first to describe many diseases and medical conditions.

Imhotep was the first known doctor. He lived in ancient Egypt over 4,500 years ago.

Hippocrates (460–370 B.C.).

MIDDLE AGES

After the fall of the Roman Empire, around A.D. 400, medical knowledge in Europe was based mainly on Greek and Roman writings. Ideas about diseases and cures were a mixture of ancient knowledge, spiritual beliefs, and astrology! Understanding how the body worked through anatomical studies was held back by religious laws. It wasn't until the 16th century that anatomy studies were revived and important discoveries were made about the human body. Despite the religious views, anatomy schools in universities sprang up all around Europe. By the middle of the 19th century the anatomy of the human body was available to doctors as the printed *Gray's Anatomy*.

Leonardo da Vinci (1452–1519) was a brilliant artist and anatomist, among many other things, and made anatomical drawings (right). One of these inspired a British heart surgeon to find a new way to repair damaged hearts in 2005.
The study of anatomy flourished in the 17th and 18th centuries, as seen in this typical scene, Anatomy Lesson of Dr. Nicolaes Tulp, by Rembrandt van Rijn, 1632 (below).

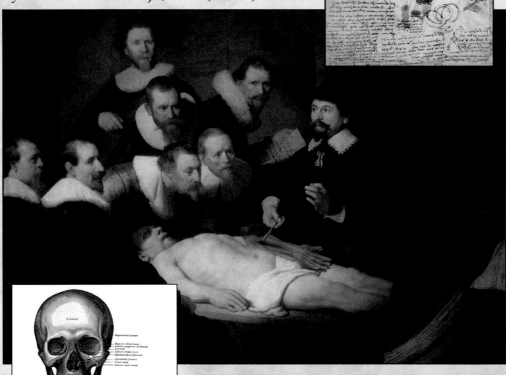

Even when using Gray's Anatomy (above), doctors of the 18th and 19th centuries were often ignorant about the human body. They gave cure-all potions and bled patients, which often did more harm than good, as illustrated in William Hogarth's The Visit to the Doctor, 1743 (right).

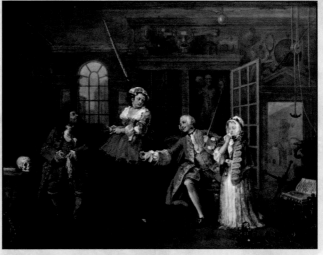

A BRIEF HISTORY OF MEDICAL SCIENCE

The search to understand how the human body works has taken many centuries. Along the way, medical inventions and discoveries have improved our understanding, and our ability to treat illnesses and infections.

A scholar with glasses in Das Narrenschiff *(1494).*

INVENTIONS AND DISCOVERIES

- **Artificial limbs** have been around since ancient times. Around 500 B.C., Herodotus wrote of a prisoner who escaped his chains by cutting off his foot, which he replaced later with a wooden one. In 1529, French surgeon Ambroise Paré used amputation to save lives. Soon after, he started developing artificial limbs.
- **Glasses** first appeared in common use during the late 13th century. Marco Polo first reported seeing them in China in 1275.
- **Vaccination** was discovered by the English doctor Edward Jenner, who successfully immunized a young boy against smallpox in 1796. Louis Pasteur, a French chemist, confirmed that germs cause disease, and invented **pasteurization** to kill germs in liquids in 1862. He also created the first vaccine for rabies.

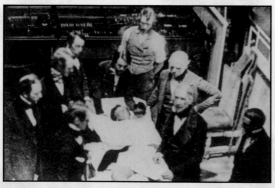

Reenactment of the first operation under anesthesia (ether) by W. Morton.

- **Anesthetics** were used in a crude form by the Incas, who caused numbness by chewing coca leaves and spitting the mixture into the wound they were operating on. Nitrous oxide (laughing gas) was used in the 1790s on a small scale, usually by dentists. In 1846, an American dentist performed the first public showing of a new anesthetic called ether. Chloroform was also used at this time, but many patients died if it was not given properly.

- **Antiseptics,** substances that prevent infection, were first introduced to modern surgery by an English surgeon, Joseph Lister, in 1867. He used carbolic acid to clean wounds and surgical instruments.
- **X-rays** were discovered by the German scientist Wilhelm Roentgen in 1895. He realized their medical use when he made an image of his wife's hand using X-rays.

A medical X-ray reveals the unseen.

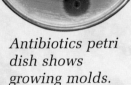

Antibiotics petri dish shows growing molds.

- **Antibiotics,** in the form of molds and plants, were used by many ancient civilizations to treat infections. Modern antibiotics began with the discovery of penicillin in 1928, by Scottish biologist Alexander Fleming. During World War II, 15 percent of lives were saved by penicillin preventing infection of wounds.
- The structure of **DNA**, the molecule that carries our genetic information, was discovered by Crick and Watson in 1953.
- In 1957, an American engineer, Earl Bakken, made the first wearable, external **artificial heart pacemaker**. It had controls to change the heart's pace and was connected through wires to the heart.

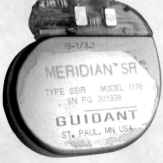

A heart pacemaker.

- The first human **heart transplant** was successfully made by South African, Christiaan Barnard, in 1967.
- **The CAT scanner** can make 3D images of the inside of the human body. It was invented by an English engineer, Godfrey Hounsfield, and the first scans were made in 1971.
- **Ultrasound scanning** uses sound to produce moving images of internal organs of the human body. One of its many uses is to check the growth of a baby inside a pregnant woman. It was refined from industrial ultrasound equipment by a Scottish doctor, Ian Donald, in 1958.

Images from a CAT scan.

THE DISCOVERY OF DNA

IN 1859 BRITISH NATURALIST CHARLES DARWIN PUBLISHES "THE ORIGIN OF SPECIES," IN WHICH HE SETS FORTH HIS THEORIES OF EVOLUTION.

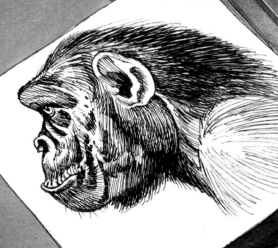

IN 1868 HE VISITS THE POET ALFRED LORD TENNYSON...

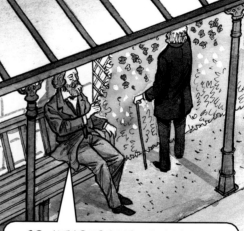

...SO, ALTHOUGH WE UNDERSTAND THE *THEORY* OF EVOLUTION, WE DON'T KNOW THE WORKINGS OF IT.

EXACTLY—*HOW* DO LIFE FORMS, LIKE THESE SWEET PEAS, CHANGE OVER MILLIONS OF YEARS?

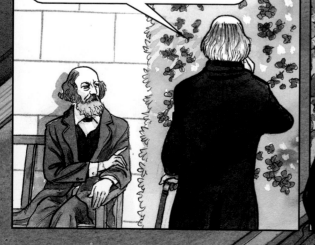

WHOEVER UNCOVERS THE SECRET OF THE MECHANISM WILL HAVE SOLVED THE BIGGEST PUZZLE OF ALL!

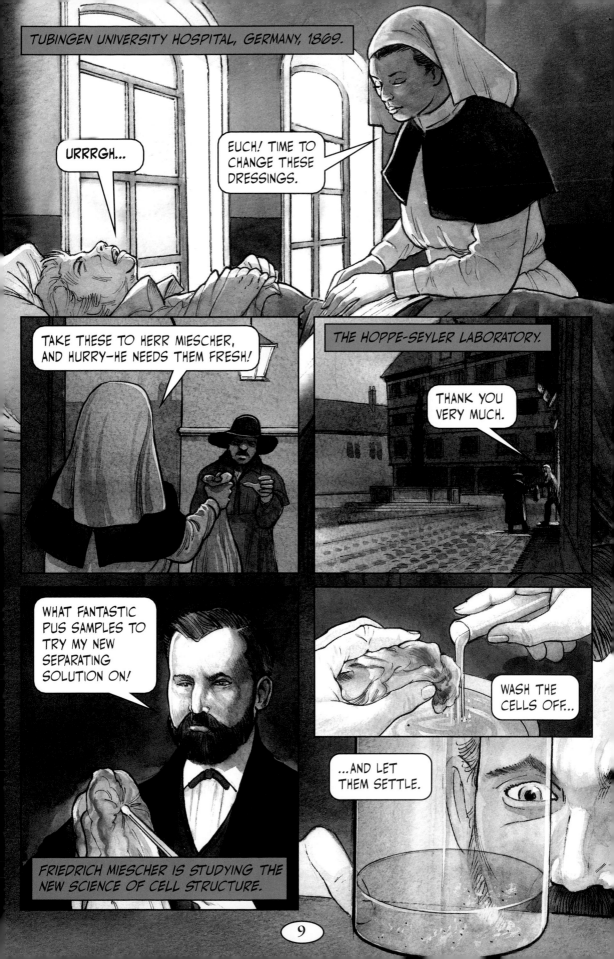

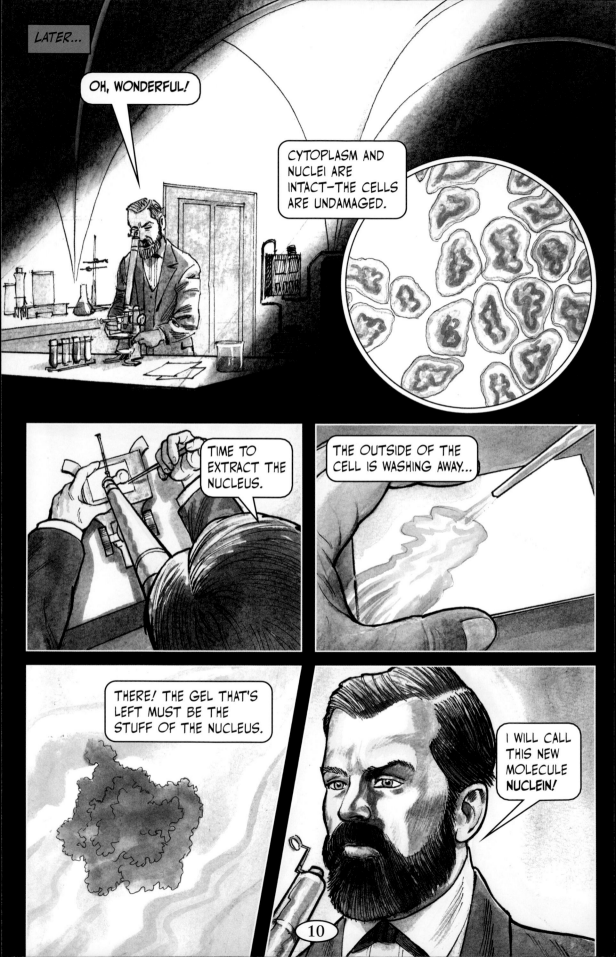

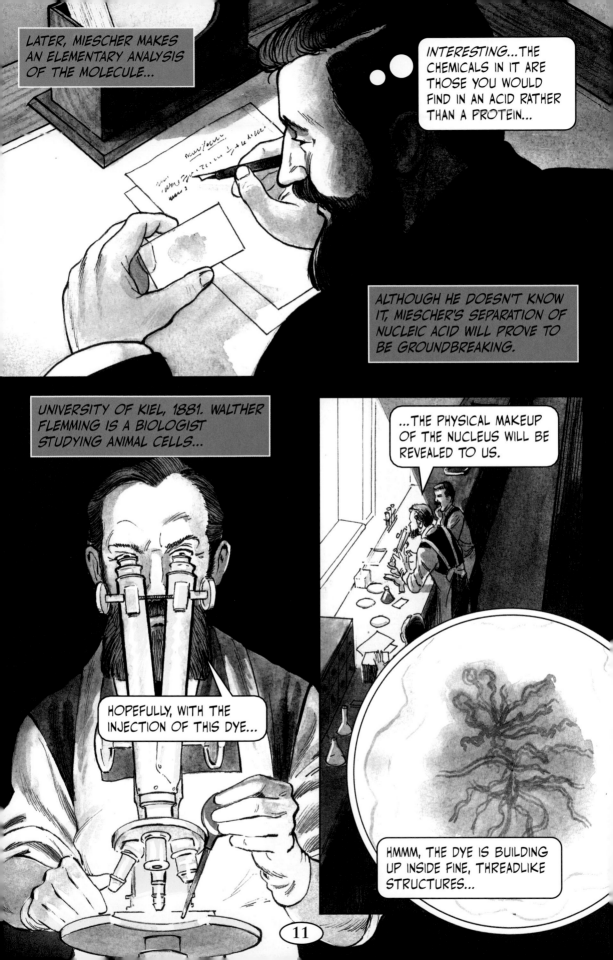

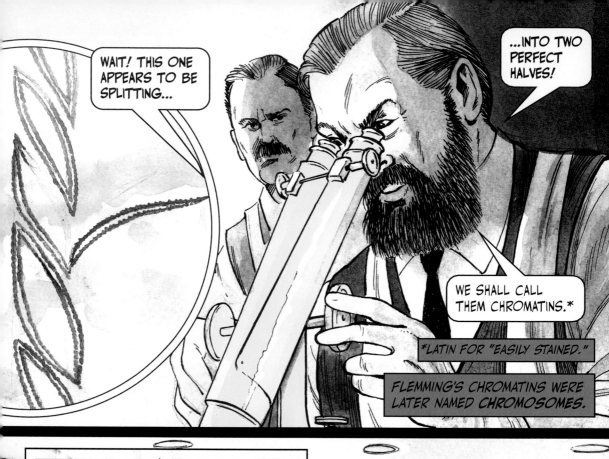

WAIT! THIS ONE APPEARS TO BE SPLITTING...

...INTO TWO PERFECT HALVES!

WE SHALL CALL THEM CHROMATINS.*

*LATIN FOR "EASILY STAINED."

FLEMMING'S CHROMATINS WERE LATER NAMED **CHROMOSOMES.**

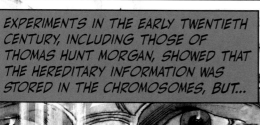

EXPERIMENTS IN THE EARLY TWENTIETH CENTURY, INCLUDING THOSE OF THOMAS HUNT MORGAN, SHOWED THAT THE HEREDITARY INFORMATION WAS STORED IN THE CHROMOSOMES, BUT...

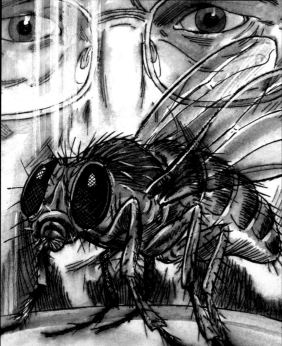

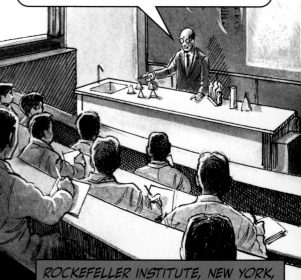

...WE STILL DON'T KNOW EXACTLY HOW THE CHROMOSOMAL CODE IS PASSED ON, AND WHICH CHEMICALS CARRY IT.

ROCKEFELLER INSTITUTE, NEW YORK, 1944. BACTERIOLOGIST OSWALD AVERY IS GIVING A LECTURE...

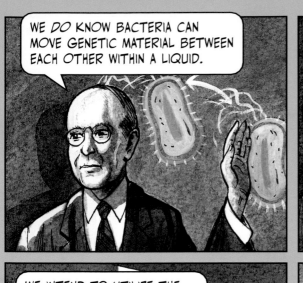

WE *DO* KNOW BACTERIA CAN MOVE GENETIC MATERIAL BETWEEN EACH OTHER WITHIN A LIQUID.

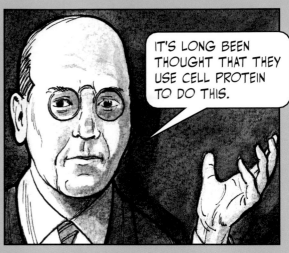

IT'S LONG BEEN THOUGHT THAT THEY USE CELL PROTEIN TO DO THIS.

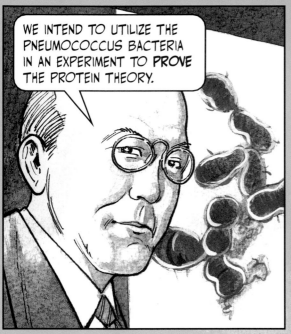

WE INTEND TO UTILIZE THE PNEUMOCOCCUS BACTERIA IN AN EXPERIMENT TO **PROVE** THE PROTEIN THEORY.

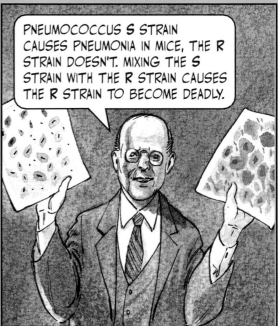

PNEUMOCOCCUS **S** STRAIN CAUSES PNEUMONIA IN MICE, THE **R** STRAIN DOESN'T. MIXING THE **S** STRAIN WITH THE **R** STRAIN CAUSES THE **R** STRAIN TO BECOME DEADLY.

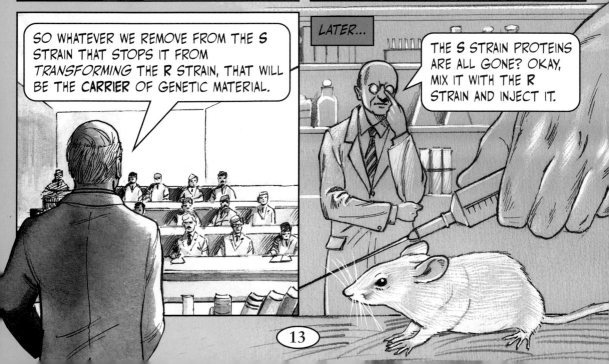

SO WHATEVER WE REMOVE FROM THE **S** STRAIN THAT STOPS IT FROM *TRANSFORMING* THE **R** STRAIN, THAT WILL BE THE **CARRIER** OF GENETIC MATERIAL.

LATER...

THE **S** STRAIN PROTEINS ARE ALL GONE? OKAY, MIX IT WITH THE **R** STRAIN AND INJECT IT.

13

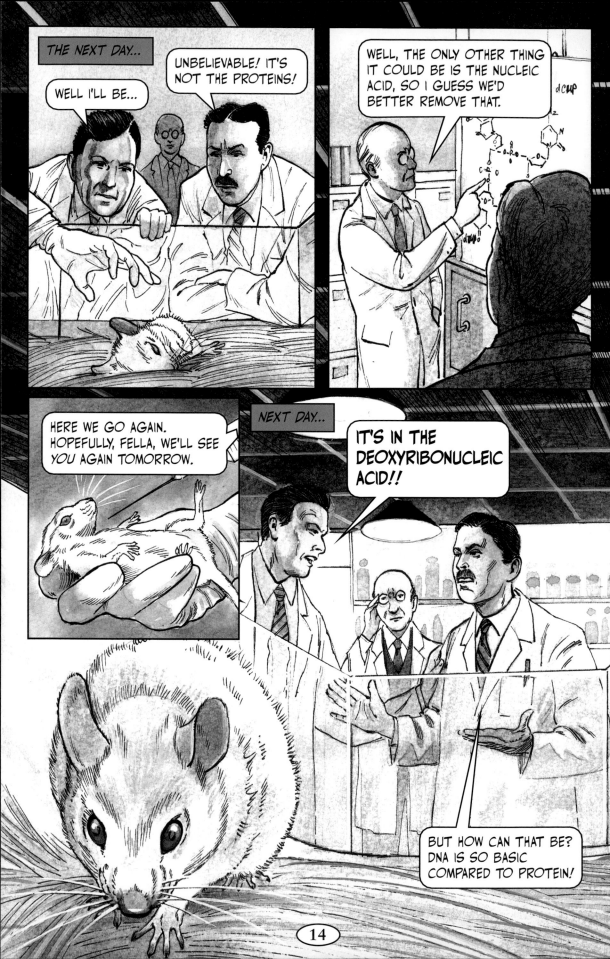

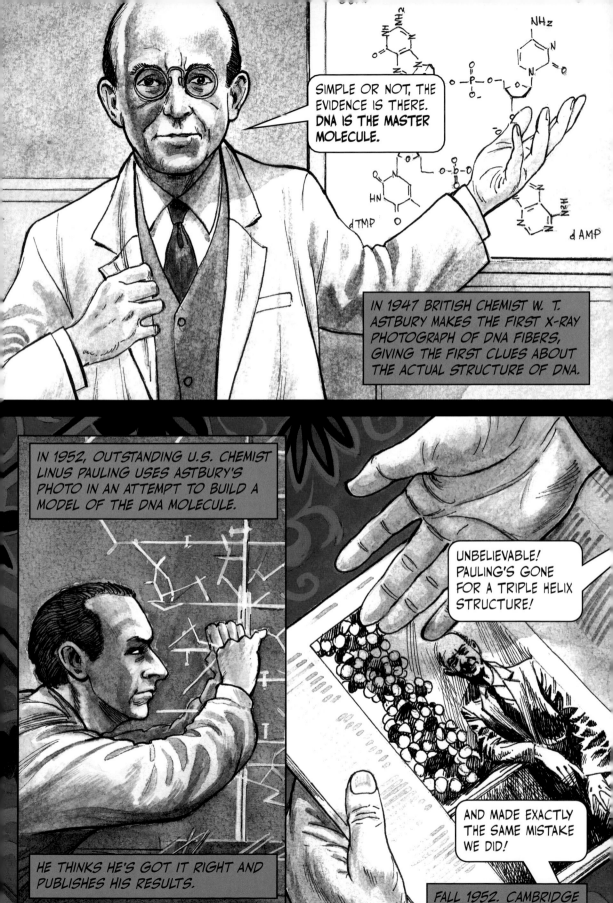

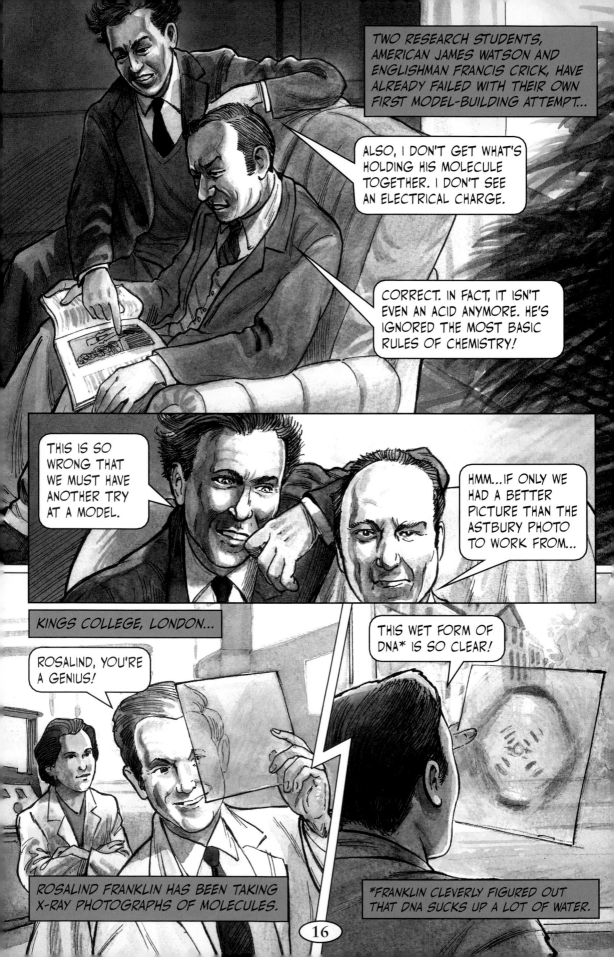

TWO RESEARCH STUDENTS, AMERICAN JAMES WATSON AND ENGLISHMAN FRANCIS CRICK, HAVE ALREADY FAILED WITH THEIR OWN FIRST MODEL-BUILDING ATTEMPT...

ALSO, I DON'T GET WHAT'S HOLDING HIS MOLECULE TOGETHER. I DON'T SEE AN ELECTRICAL CHARGE.

CORRECT. IN FACT, IT ISN'T EVEN AN ACID ANYMORE. HE'S IGNORED THE MOST BASIC RULES OF CHEMISTRY!

THIS IS SO WRONG THAT WE MUST HAVE ANOTHER TRY AT A MODEL.

HMM...IF ONLY WE HAD A BETTER PICTURE THAN THE ASTBURY PHOTO TO WORK FROM...

KINGS COLLEGE, LONDON...

ROSALIND, YOU'RE A GENIUS!

THIS WET FORM OF DNA* IS SO CLEAR!

ROSALIND FRANKLIN HAS BEEN TAKING X-RAY PHOTOGRAPHS OF MOLECULES.

*FRANKLIN CLEVERLY FIGURED OUT THAT DNA SUCKS UP A LOT OF WATER.

16

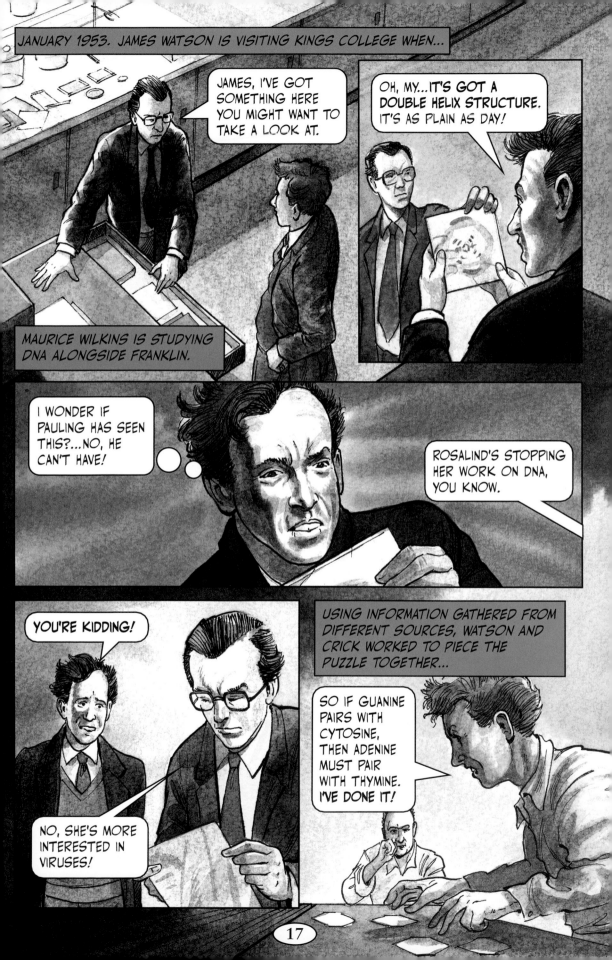

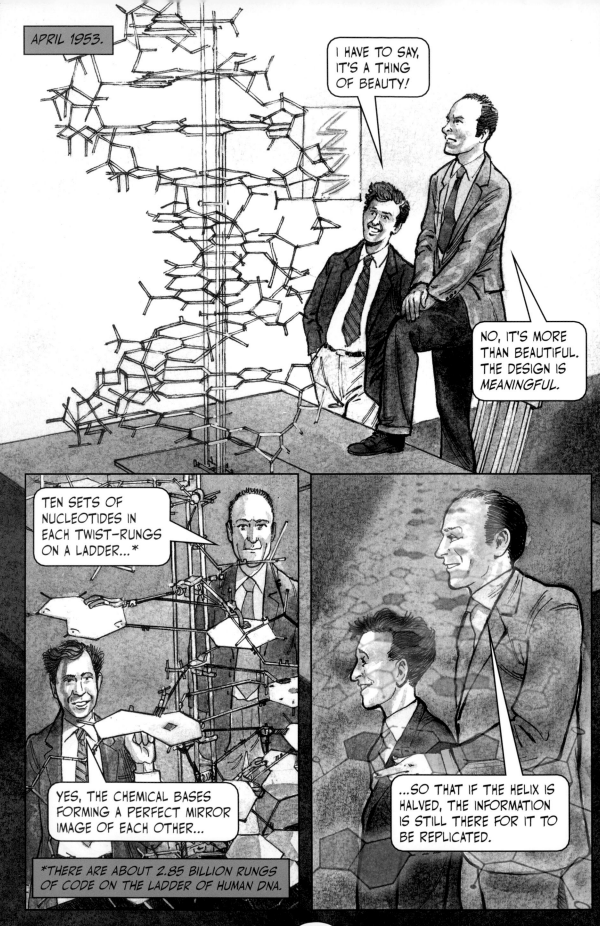

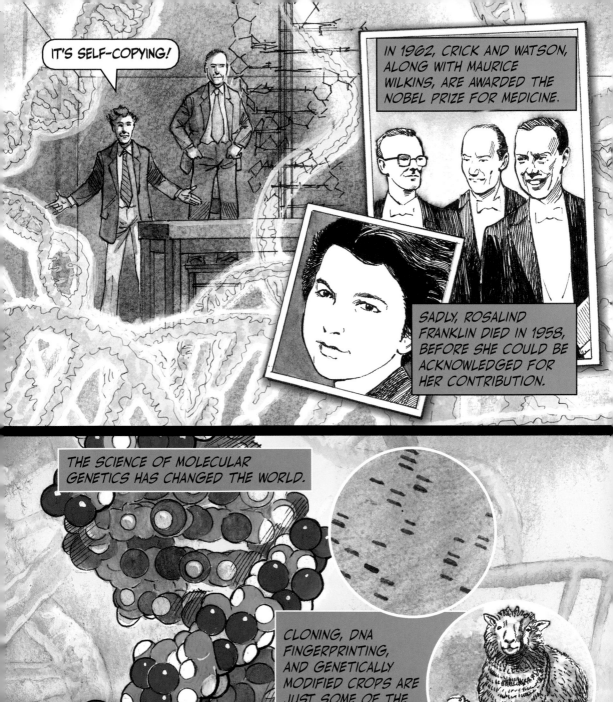

IT'S SELF-COPYING!

IN 1962, CRICK AND WATSON, ALONG WITH MAURICE WILKINS, ARE AWARDED THE NOBEL PRIZE FOR MEDICINE.

SADLY, ROSALIND FRANKLIN DIED IN 1958, BEFORE SHE COULD BE ACKNOWLEDGED FOR HER CONTRIBUTION.

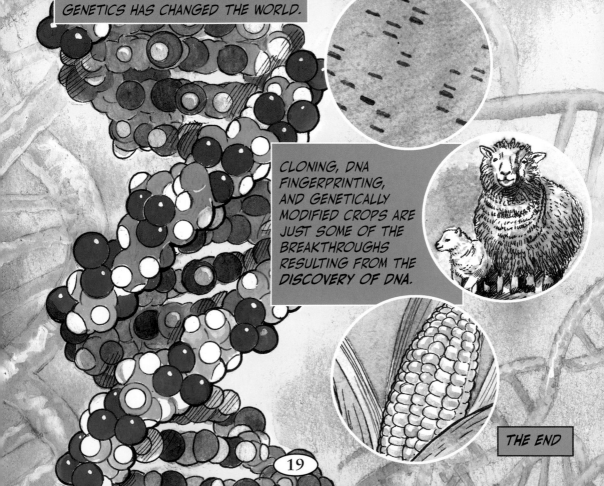

THE SCIENCE OF MOLECULAR GENETICS HAS CHANGED THE WORLD.

CLONING, DNA FINGERPRINTING, AND GENETICALLY MODIFIED CROPS ARE JUST SOME OF THE BREAKTHROUGHS RESULTING FROM THE DISCOVERY OF DNA.

THE END

TH: FIRST H:ART TRANSPLANT

GROOTE SCHUUR HOSPITAL, CAPE TOWN, SOUTH AFRICA, 1966...

THIS NEW HEART-LUNG MACHINE IS A LOT QUIETER THAN THE OLD ONE.

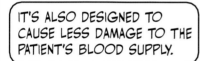

IT'S ALSO DESIGNED TO CAUSE LESS DAMAGE TO THE PATIENT'S BLOOD SUPPLY.

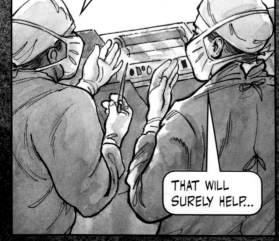

THAT WILL SURELY HELP...

MR. NAKI!

DR. BARNARD, THE NEW HEART IS **READY.**

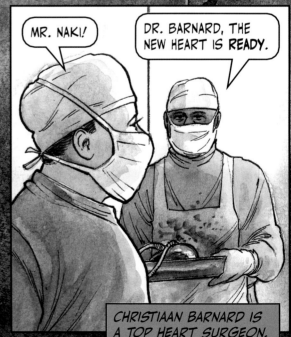

CHRISTIAAN BARNARD IS A TOP HEART SURGEON.

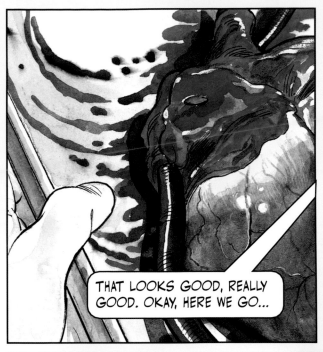

THAT LOOKS GOOD, REALLY GOOD. OKAY, HERE WE GO...

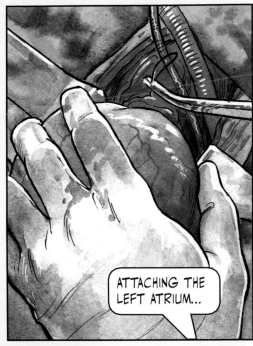

ATTACHING THE LEFT ATRIUM...

TWO HOURS LATER...

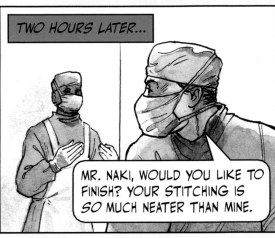

MR. NAKI, WOULD YOU LIKE TO FINISH? YOUR STITCHING IS SO MUCH NEATER THAN MINE.

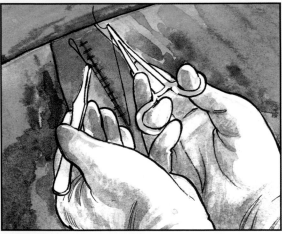

DURING POSTOPERATIVE SCRUB...

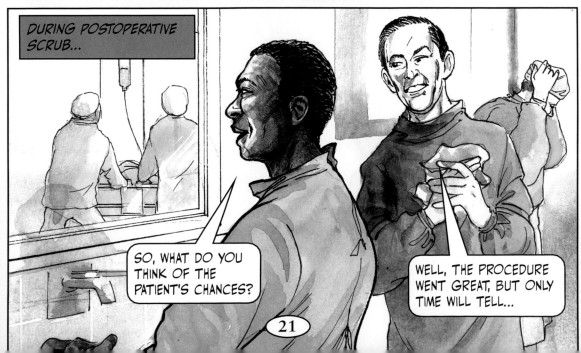

SO, WHAT DO YOU THINK OF THE PATIENT'S CHANCES?

WELL, THE PROCEDURE WENT GREAT, BUT ONLY TIME WILL TELL...

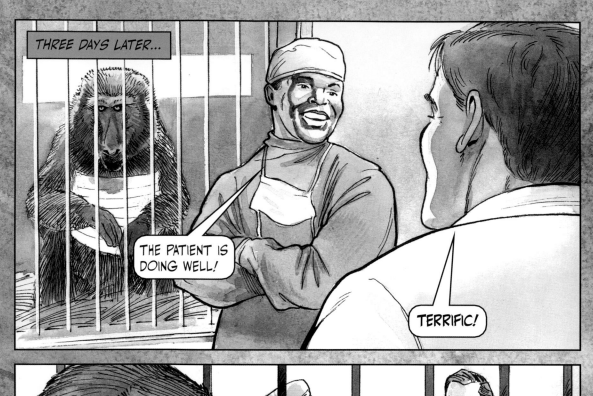

THREE DAYS LATER...

THE PATIENT IS DOING WELL!

TERRIFIC!

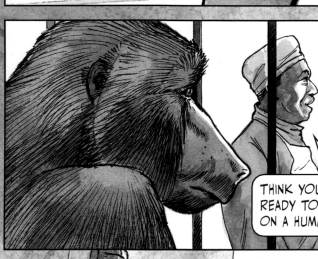

THINK YOU'RE READY TO TRY THIS ON A HUMAN?

YES, I DO. ALL I NEED ARE THE RIGHT PATIENTS TO SHOW UP...

BANG!

CAR ACCIDENT VICTIM— NAME'S DENISE DARVALL.

DECEMBER 3, 1967, EMERGENCY ROOM, GROOTE SCHUUR...

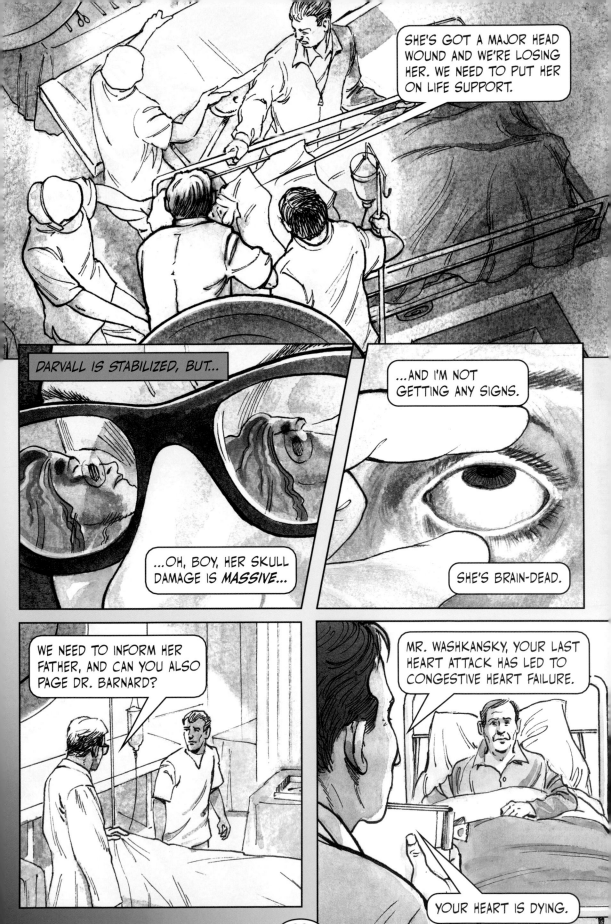

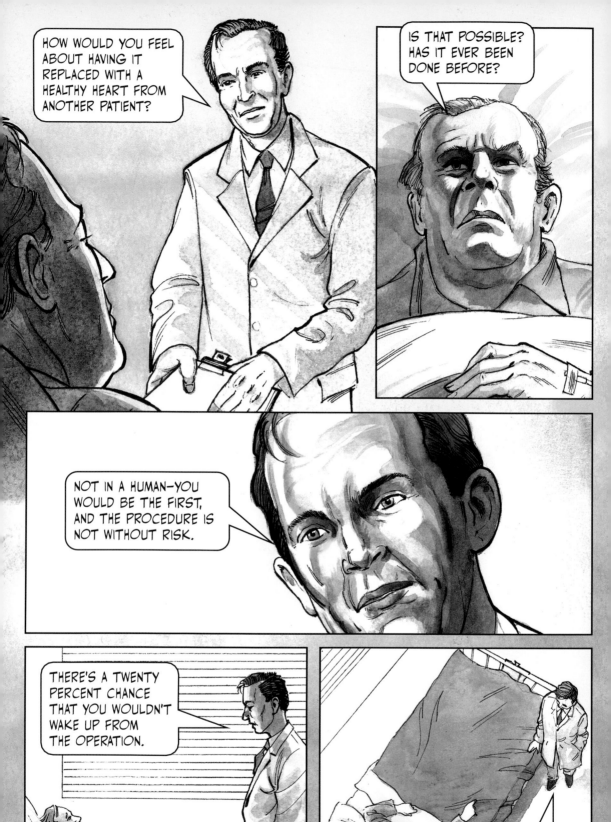

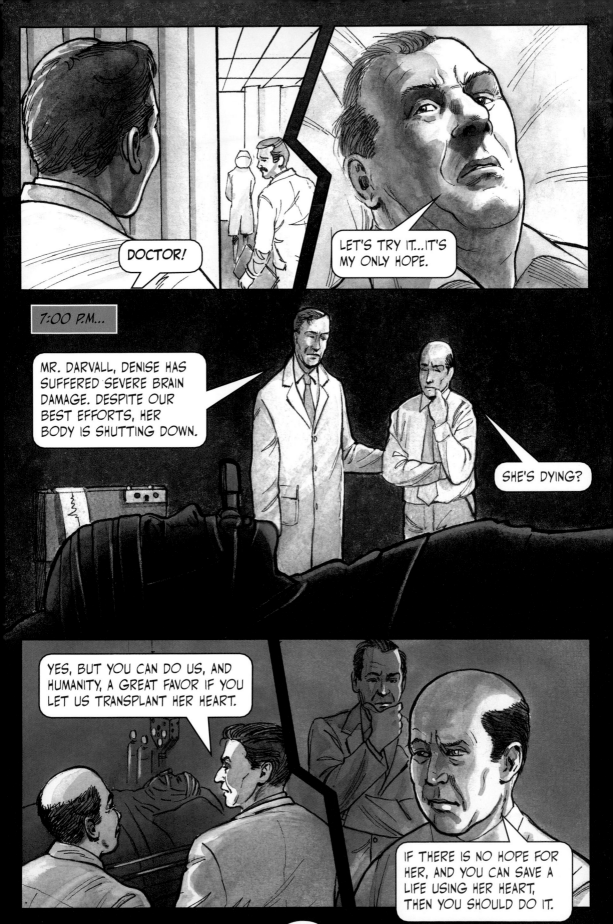

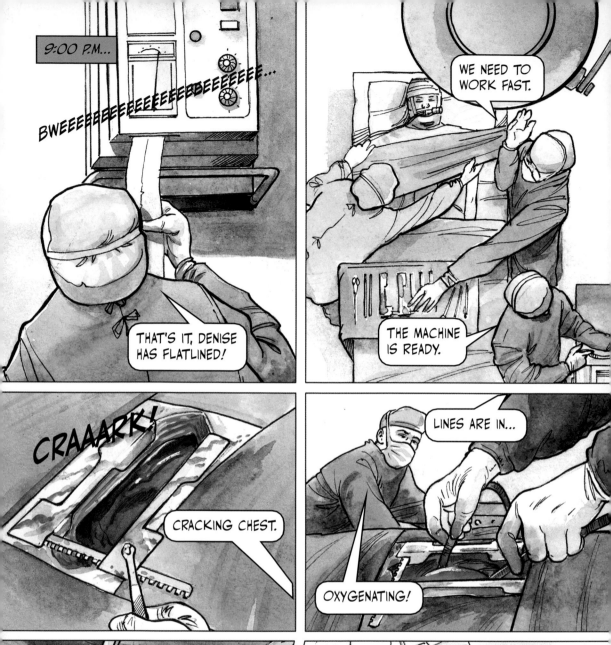

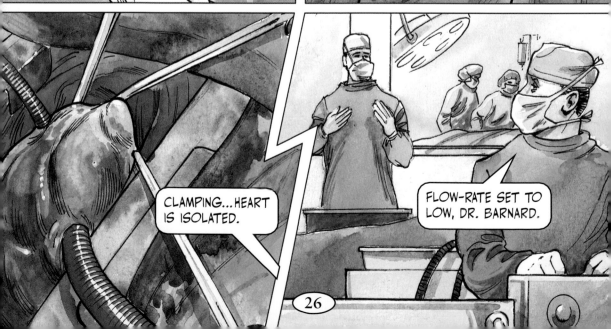

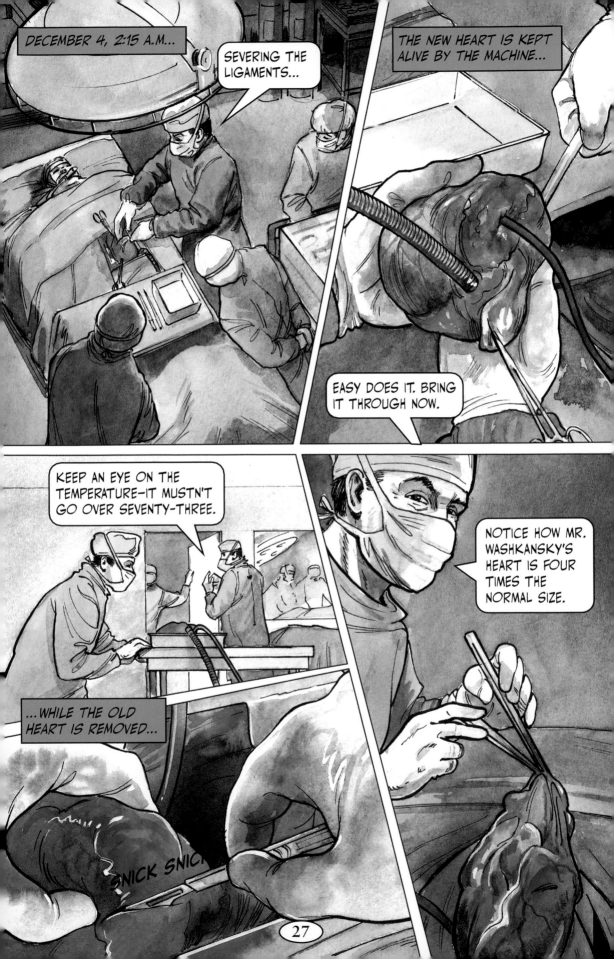

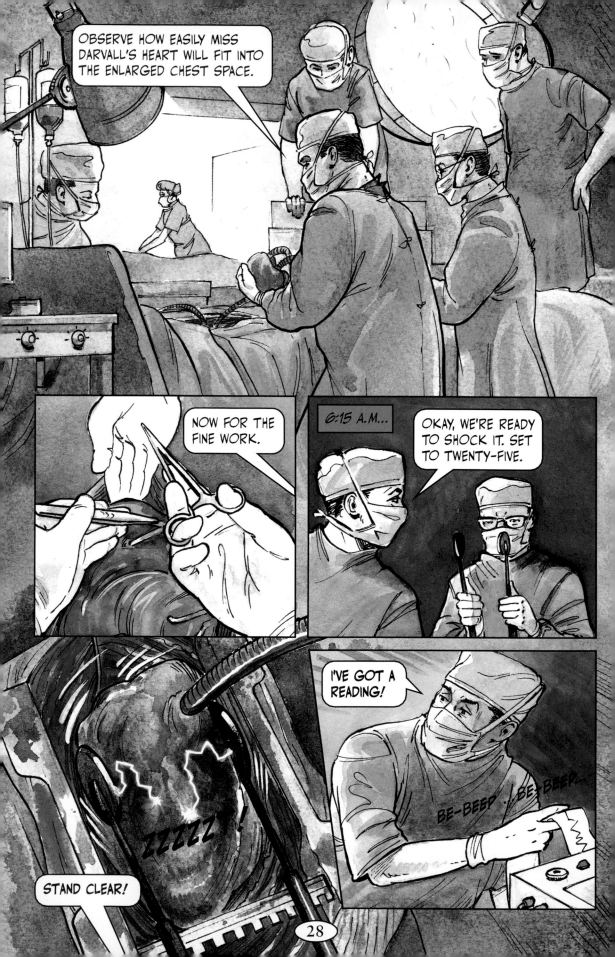

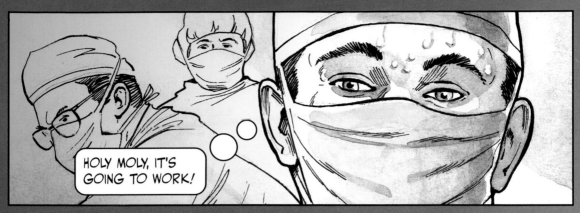

HOLY MOLY, IT'S GOING TO WORK!

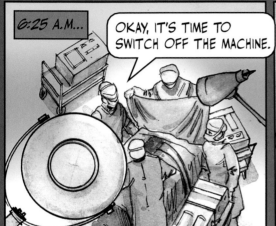

6:25 A.M...

OKAY, IT'S TIME TO SWITCH OFF THE MACHINE.

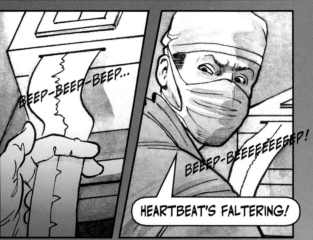

BEEP-BEEP-BEEP...

BEEP-BEEEEEEEEP!

HEARTBEAT'S FALTERING!

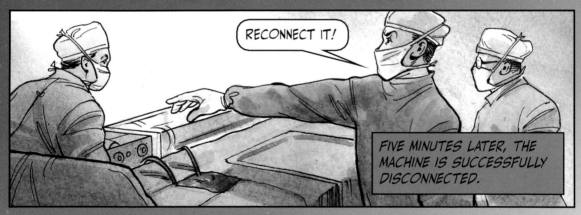

RECONNECT IT!

FIVE MINUTES LATER, THE MACHINE IS SUCCESSFULLY DISCONNECTED.

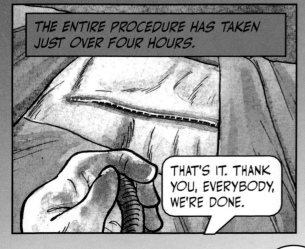

THE ENTIRE PROCEDURE HAS TAKEN JUST OVER FOUR HOURS.

THAT'S IT. THANK YOU, EVERYBODY, WE'RE DONE.

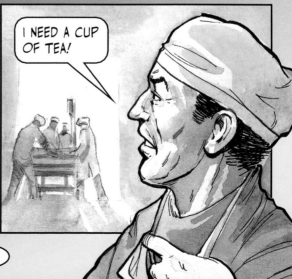

I NEED A CUP OF TEA!

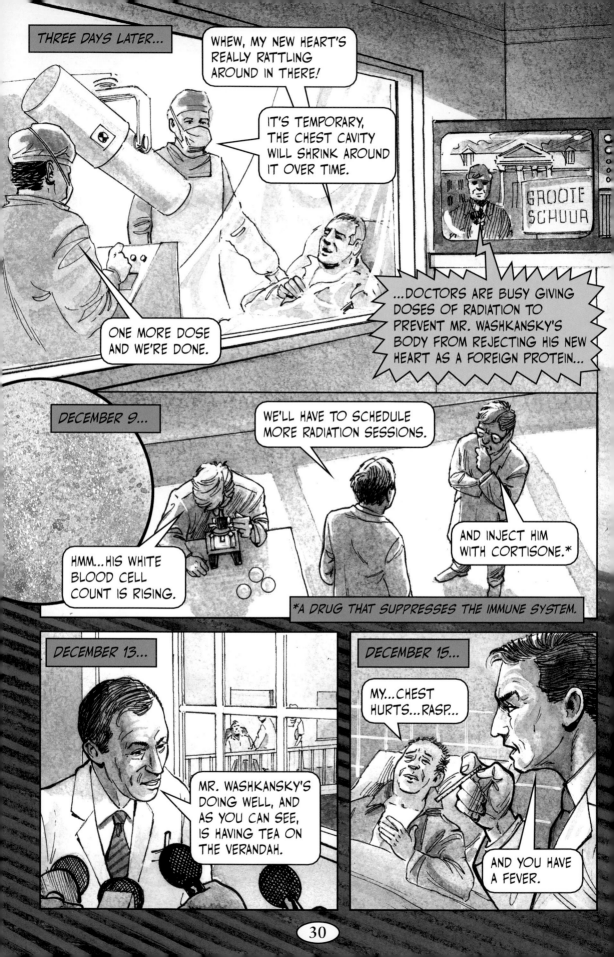

THREE DAYS LATER...

WHEW, MY NEW HEART'S REALLY RATTLING AROUND IN THERE!

IT'S TEMPORARY, THE CHEST CAVITY WILL SHRINK AROUND IT OVER TIME.

ONE MORE DOSE AND WE'RE DONE.

GROOTE SCHUUR

...DOCTORS ARE BUSY GIVING DOSES OF RADIATION TO PREVENT MR. WASHKANSKY'S BODY FROM REJECTING HIS NEW HEART AS A FOREIGN PROTEIN...

DECEMBER 9...

WE'LL HAVE TO SCHEDULE MORE RADIATION SESSIONS.

AND INJECT HIM WITH CORTISONE.*

HMM...HIS WHITE BLOOD CELL COUNT IS RISING.

*A DRUG THAT SUPPRESSES THE IMMUNE SYSTEM.

DECEMBER 13...

MR. WASHKANSKY'S DOING WELL, AND AS YOU CAN SEE, IS HAVING TEA ON THE VERANDAH.

DECEMBER 15...

MY...CHEST HURTS...RASP...

AND YOU HAVE A FEVER.

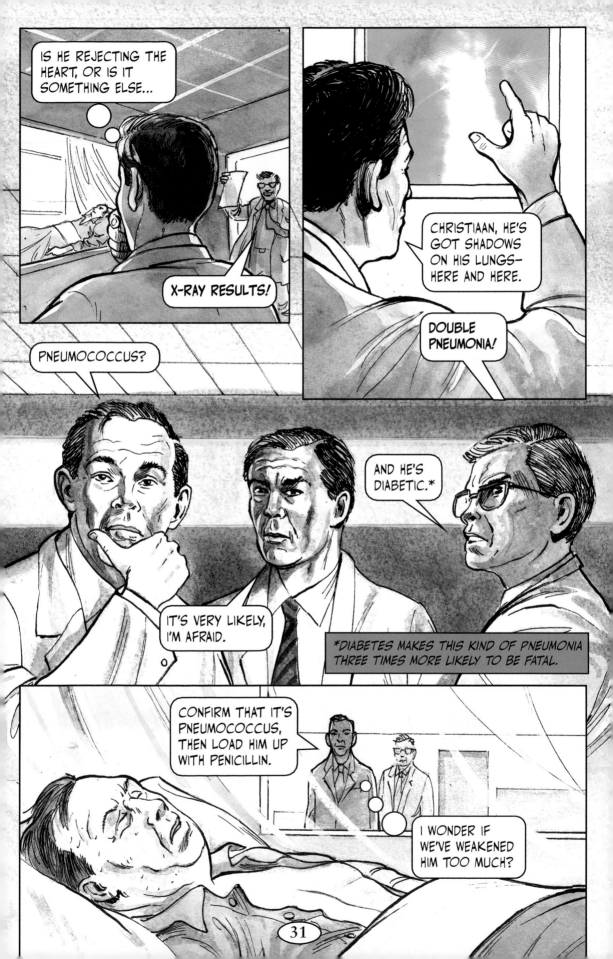

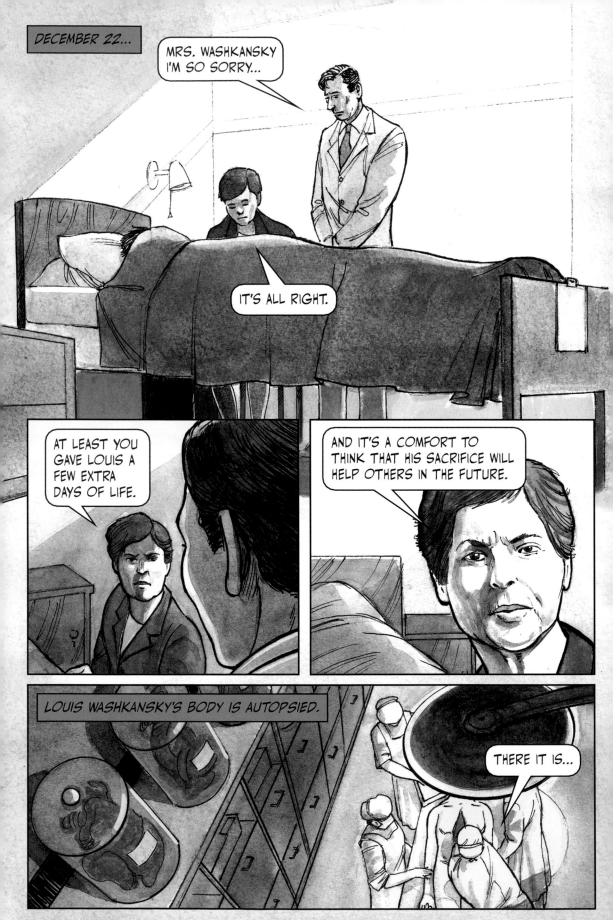

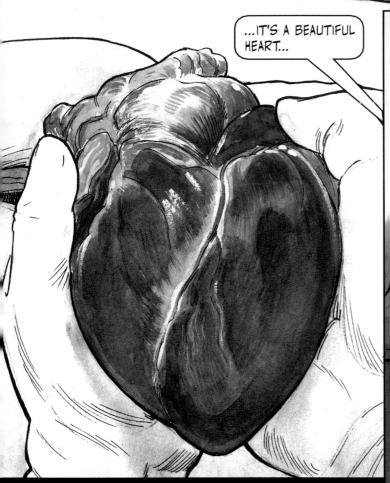

...IT'S A BEAUTIFUL HEART...

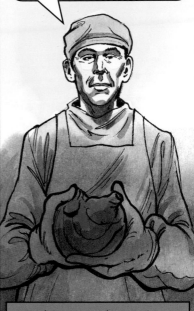

...THAT PUMPED STRONGLY RIGHT TO THE END.

WASHKANSKY HAD DIED BECAUSE OF HIS WEAKENED IMMUNE SYSTEM. HIS ACTUAL TRANSPLANT HAD BEEN A TOTAL SUCCESS.

ALTHOUGH BARNARD'S ACHIEVEMENT PAVED THE WAY FOR MORE HEART TRANSPLANTS, IT WASN'T UNTIL THE DISCOVERY OF NEW ANTI-REJECTION DRUGS THAT TRANSPLANTS BECAME MORE COMMONPLACE...AND RELIABLE.

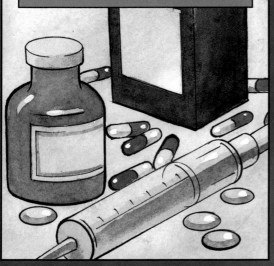

TO DATE, THE WORLD'S LONGEST-LIVING SINGLE HEART TRANSPLANTEE IS AMERICAN TONY HUESMAN.

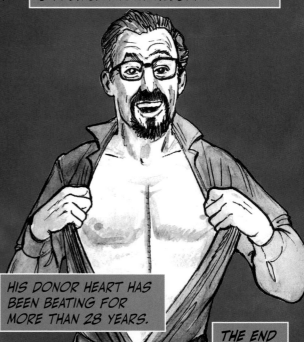

HIS DONOR HEART HAS BEEN BEATING FOR MORE THAN 28 YEARS.

THE END

THE WORLD'S FIRST BIONIC WOMAN

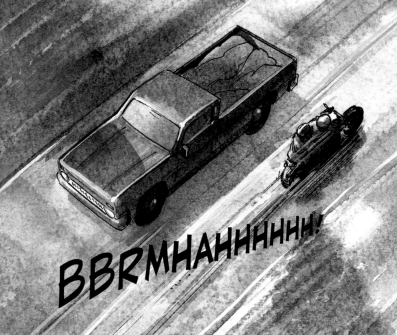

ARKANSAS, 2004. U.S. ARMY VETERAN CLAUDIA MITCHELL IS BEING TAKEN FOR A RIDE IN THE COUNTRY...

BBRMHAHHHHHH!

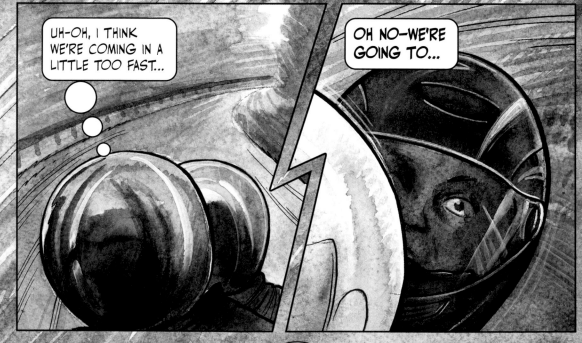

UH-OH, I THINK WE'RE COMING IN A LITTLE TOO FAST...

OH NO—WE'RE GOING TO...

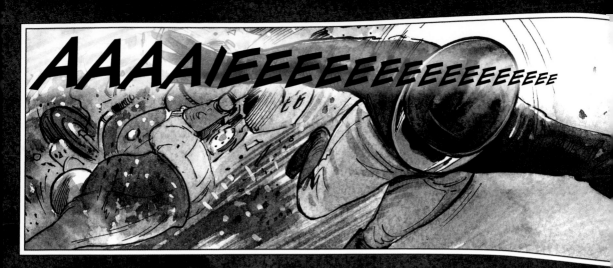

AAAAIEEEEEEEEEEEEEEEEE

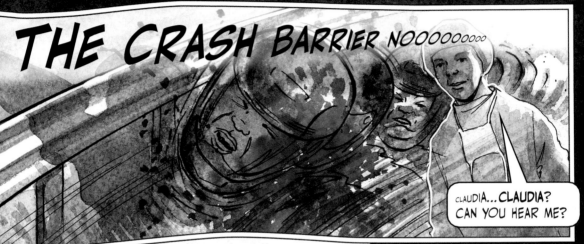

THE CRASH BARRIER NOOOOOOOOO

CLAUDIA...CLAUDIA? CAN YOU HEAR ME?

...UH...I...ER...WHAT HAPPENED?

UH...I FEEL ...KIND OF...

YOU HAD A BAD INJURY, YOU'VE BEEN IN SURGERY. THE DOCTOR WILL TALK TO YOU LATER.

CLAUDIA, YOU'RE IN THE HOSPITAL.

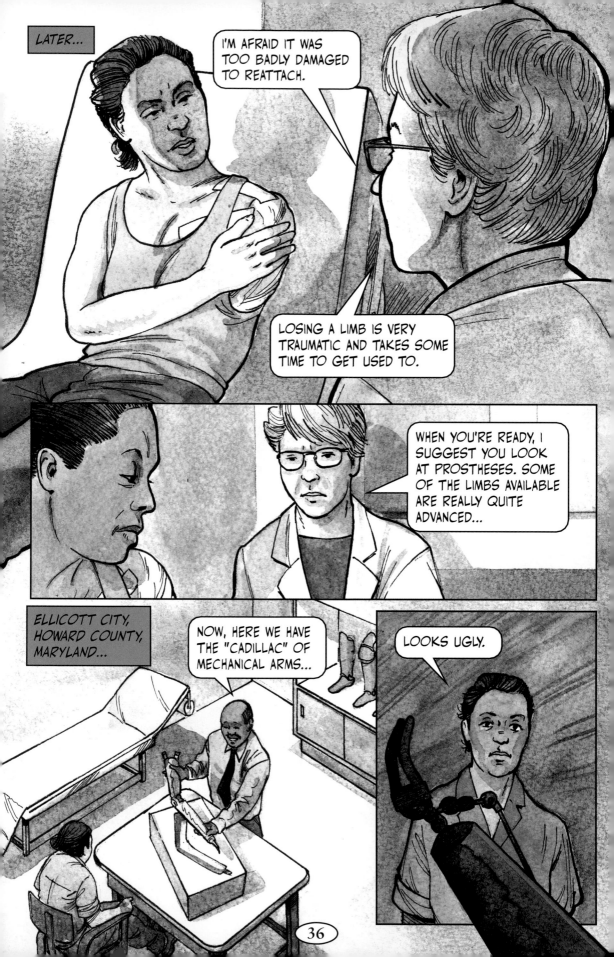

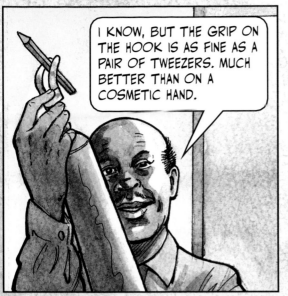

I KNOW, BUT THE GRIP ON THE HOOK IS AS FINE AS A PAIR OF TWEEZERS. MUCH BETTER THAN ON A COSMETIC HAND.

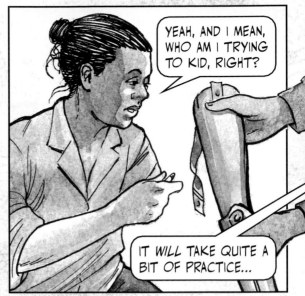

YEAH, AND I MEAN, WHO AM I TRYING TO KID, RIGHT?

IT WILL TAKE QUITE A BIT OF PRACTICE...

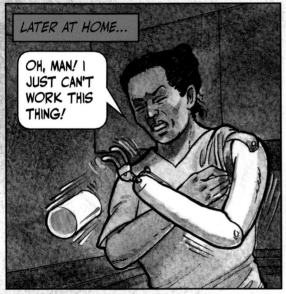

LATER AT HOME...

OH, MAN! I JUST CAN'T WORK THIS THING!

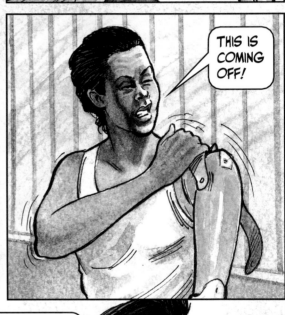

THIS IS COMING OFF!

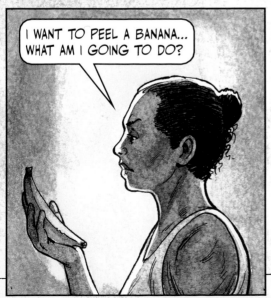

I WANT TO PEEL A BANANA... WHAT AM I GOING TO DO?

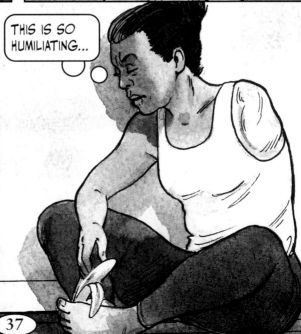

THIS IS SO HUMILIATING...

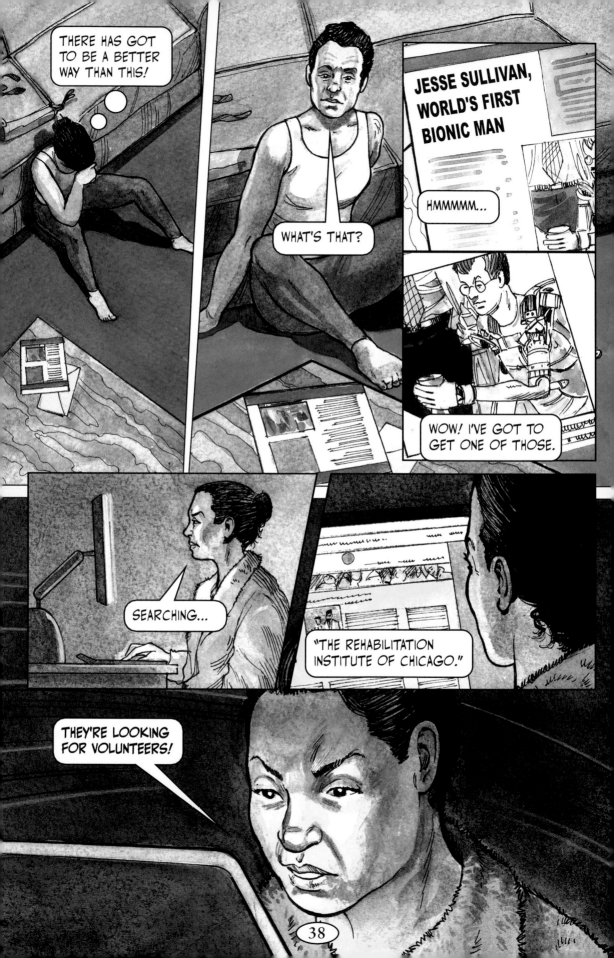

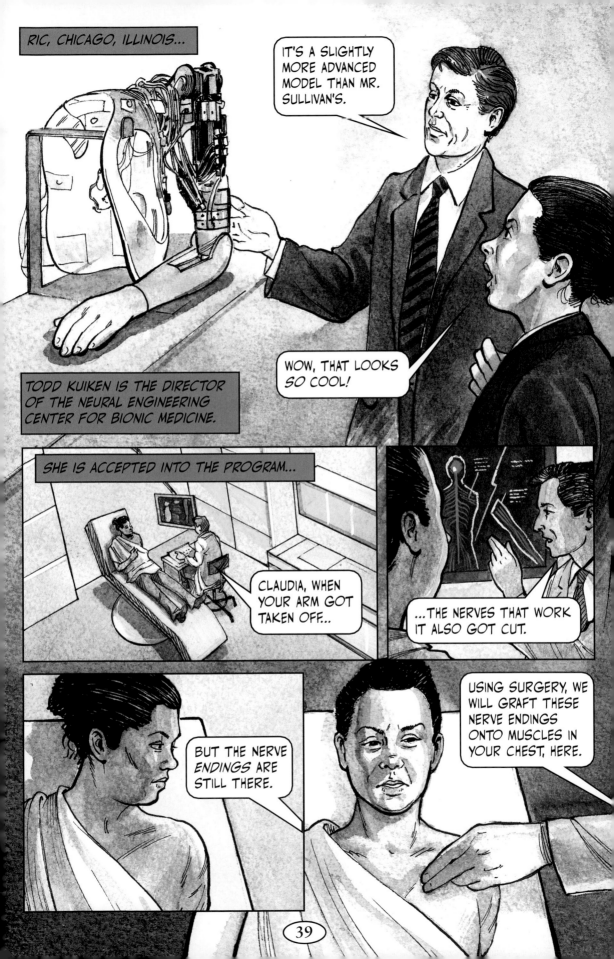

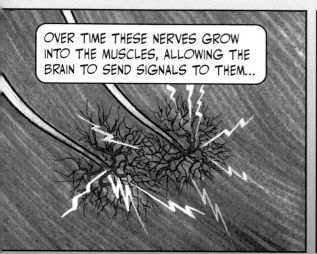

OVER TIME THESE NERVES GROW INTO THE MUSCLES, ALLOWING THE BRAIN TO SEND SIGNALS TO THEM...

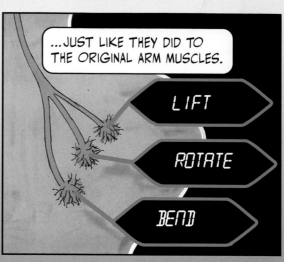

...JUST LIKE THEY DID TO THE ORIGINAL ARM MUSCLES.

LIFT

ROTATE

BEND

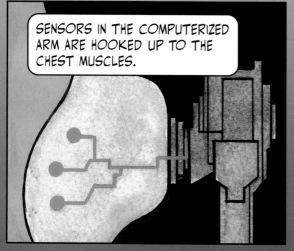

SENSORS IN THE COMPUTERIZED ARM ARE HOOKED UP TO THE CHEST MUSCLES.

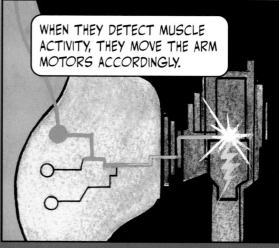

WHEN THEY DETECT MUSCLE ACTIVITY, THEY MOVE THE ARM MOTORS ACCORDINGLY.

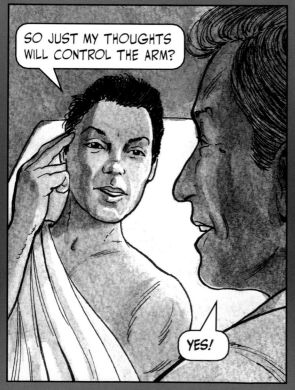

SO JUST MY THOUGHTS WILL CONTROL THE ARM?

YES!

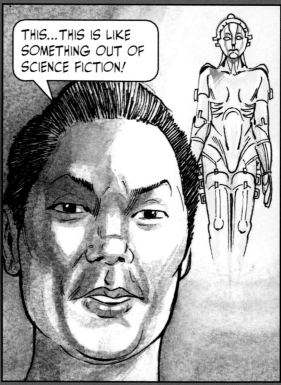

THIS...THIS IS LIKE SOMETHING OUT OF SCIENCE FICTION!

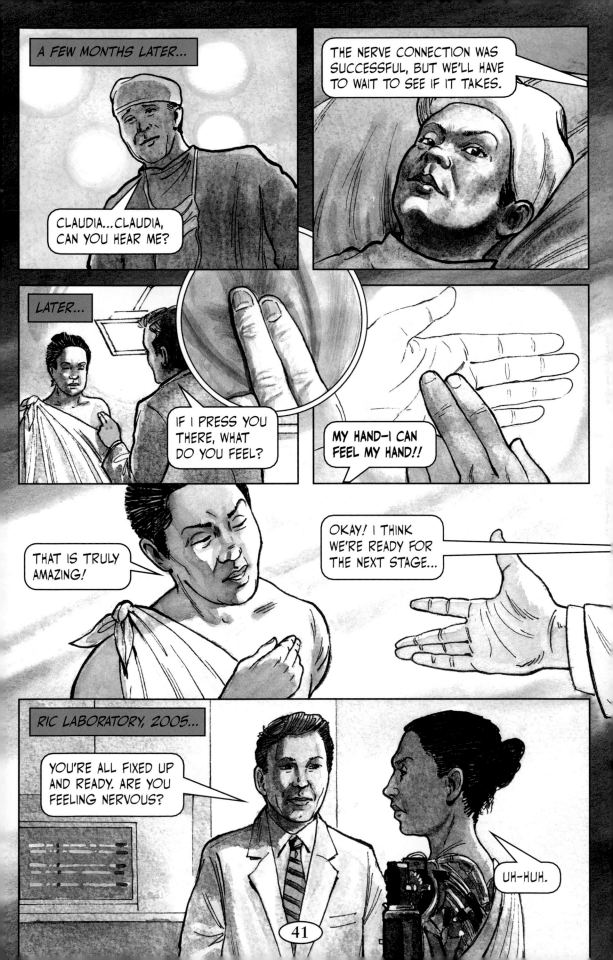

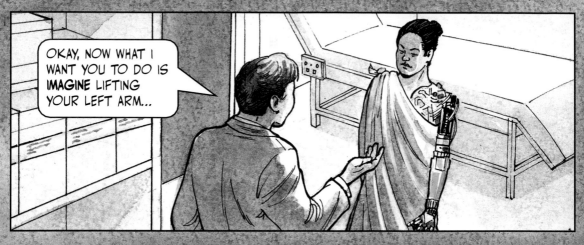

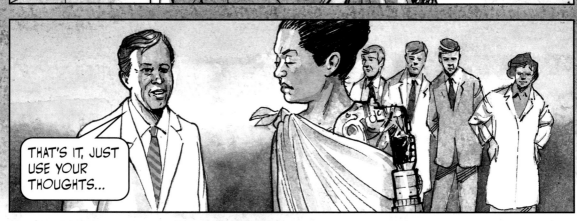

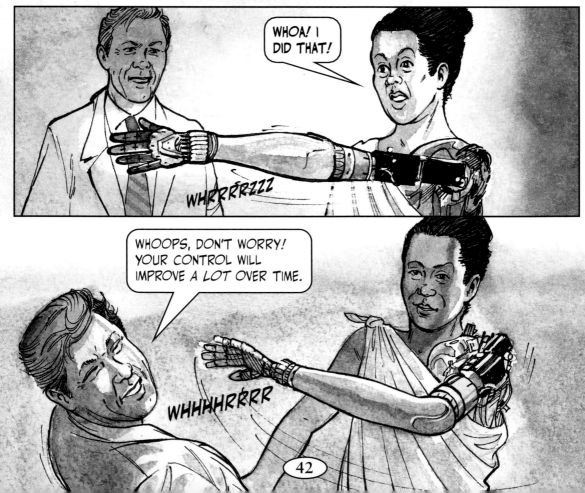

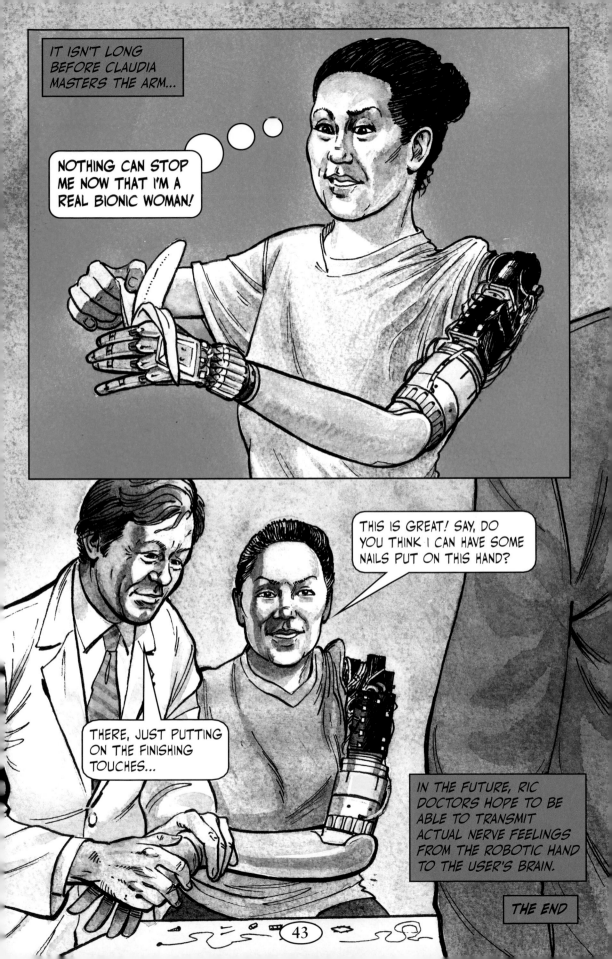

MEDICINE FOR THE 21ST CENTURY

Since the groundbreaking medical developments of the late 20th century, medicine has turned science fiction into fact, from bionic people to cloning.

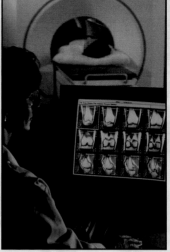

DNA

The story of DNA has continued since its

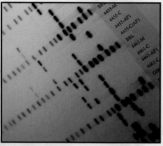

DNA "fingerprint" on film.

discovery. Today, criminals can be caught by forensic scientists using DNA fingerprinting to match prints left at a crime scene with those of the culprit.

Computers play a major role in today's medicine. An MRI scanner linked to a computer uses radio frequency signals to see inside a patient.

DNA has also led to the understanding and prevention of genetic diseases. Drugs have been genetically engineered since the 1980s using animals such as cows, goats, and sheep as the "factories." In the future, scientists think they will "grow" drugs in chicken eggs. Since a chicken can lay 330 eggs a year, cheap drugs could be available to all.

CLONING

In 1996, the first mammal, a sheep named Dolly, was cloned from a single cell. Although many people disagree with the science of cloning, it has been proposed as a method of preserving endangered species.

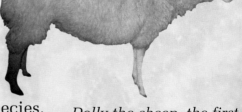

Dolly the sheep, the first cloned mammal, died in 2003.

PROSTHETICS

Except for the brain and nervous system, almost every part of our bodies can be replaced, from blood and veins to newly grown skin, and electronic prosthetics (see right).

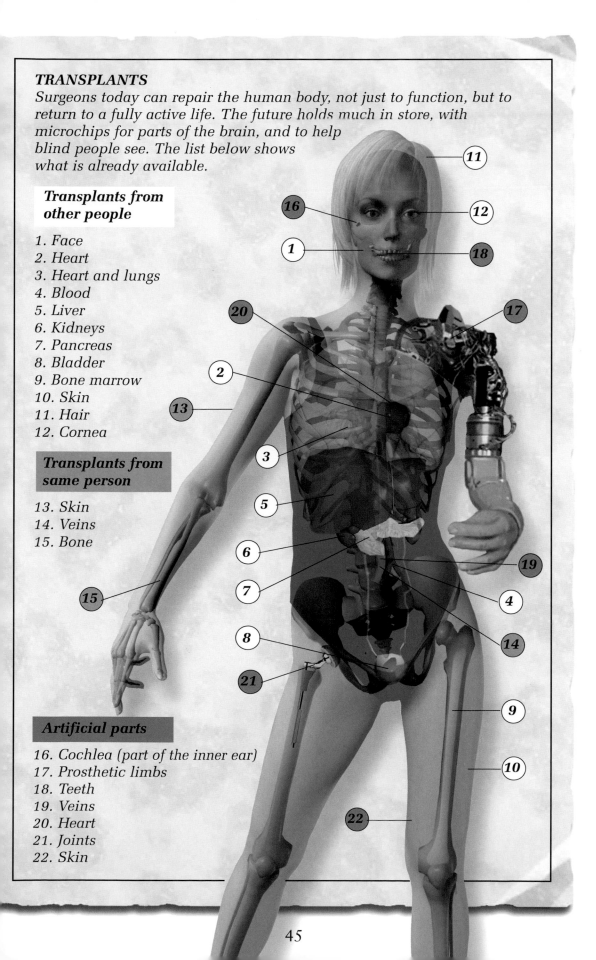

TRANSPLANTS

Surgeons today can repair the human body, not just to function, but to return to a fully active life. The future holds much in store, with microchips for parts of the brain, and to help blind people see. The list below shows what is already available.

Transplants from other people

1. Face
2. Heart
3. Heart and lungs
4. Blood
5. Liver
6. Kidneys
7. Pancreas
8. Bladder
9. Bone marrow
10. Skin
11. Hair
12. Cornea

Transplants from same person

13. Skin
14. Veins
15. Bone

Artificial parts

16. Cochlea (part of the inner ear)
17. Prosthetic limbs
18. Teeth
19. Veins
20. Heart
21. Joints
22. Skin

GLOSSARY

amputation Cutting off a limb using surgery.

anatomy The science of studying the structure of humans and animals, often through cutting them open.

astrology Observing stars and planets, and how they affect people.

autopsy Medical investigation of a body, to find out the cause of death.

bacteriologist A person who studies bacteria—simple, living things that multiply and can cause disease.

cell The smallest unit of a living thing, which has a cytoplasm and a nucleus wrapped in a skin.

cytoplasm The material inside a cell other than the nucleus.

diabetic A medical disorder that affects the production of energy within human (or animal) cells.

elementary analysis Detailed examination of the structure of something.

evolution The way living things are thought to have developed over millions of years.

faltering Losing strength.

gene Part of a chromosome that passes on hereditary information.

genetic Relating to genes or heredity.

graft Transplant surgically.

helix A three-dimensional shape like a spiral staircase.

heredity The passing on of characteristics from parent to offspring.

immune system The body's ability to protect itself against disease.

immunization The process of programming (inoculating) the body to protect itself from certain diseases.

isolated Separated from.

ligament Structure that supports an organ and holds it in place.

molecule Smallest part of a chemical.

nucleotides Basic structural unit (the rungs in the ladder) of DNA.

nucleus Important part of a cell, which holds the genetic material.

oxygenating Enriching with oxygen.

pneumococcus Bacteria associated with pneumonia.

pneumonia Inflammation of a lung, caused by bacteria or a virus. Inflammation of both lungs is called double pneumonia.

protein A complicated family of molecules, important to our bodies.

pus A thick, yellowish liquid produced in infected body parts.

strains Different types of the same organism.

theories A set of ideas to explain something.

viruses Body invaders that multiply inside cells, causing disease.

white blood cells Blood cells that fight foreign matter and disease.

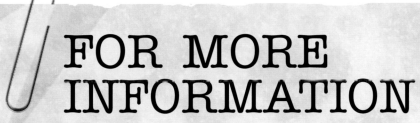

FOR MORE INFORMATION

ORGANIZATIONS

Dolan DNA Learning Center
334 Main Street,
Cold Spring Harbor, NY 11724
(515) 367-5170
E-mail: dnalc@cshl.edu
Web site: http://dnalc.org

National Museum of Health and Medicine
6900 Georgia Avenue, NW
Washington, D.C. 20306
(202) 782-2200
E-mail: nmhminfo@afip.osd.mil
Web site: http://nmhm.washingtondc.museum

FURTHER READING

Cobb, Allan B. *The Bionic Human.* New York: Rosen, 2003.

de la Bedoyere, Camilla. *The Discovery of DNA.* Milwaukee: Gareth Stevens Inc, 2006.

Marx, Christy. *Watson and Crick and DNA.* New York: Rosen, 2005.

Travers, Bridget and Fran Locher Freiman. *Medical Discoveries: Medical Breakthroughs and the People Who Developed Them.* Chicago: UXL, 1996.

Woods, Michael and Mary Woods. *The History of Medicine (Major Inventions Through History).* Minneapolis: Twenty-First Century Books, 2006.

INDEX

A

amputation, 6, 46
anatomy, 4, 5, 46
artificial limbs, 6
Astbury, W. T., 15
Avery, Oswald, 12

B

Bakken, Earl, 7
Barnard, Christiaan, 7, 20–33
bionic, 34, 39, 43, 44
brain, 40, 43, 44, 45

C

cells, 9, 10, 46
chromosomal code, 12
cloning, 19, 44
Crick, Francis, 7, 16, 17, 19

D

Darvall, Denise, 22–26
DNA, 7–19
fingerprinting, 19, 44
Dolly, 44
Donald, Ian, 7

E

evolution, 8, 46

F

Fleming, Alexander, 7
Flemming, Walther, 11, 12
forensic science, 44

Franklin, Rosalind, 16, 17, 19

G

Gray's Anatomy, 4, 5

H

heart transplant, 20-33
helix, 18, 46
double helix structure, 17
triple helix structure, 15
Hounsfield, Godfrey, 7
Huesman, Tony, 33

J

Jenner, Edward, 6

K

Kuiken, Todd, 39

L

Lister, Joseph, 7

M

Miescher, Friedrich, 9–11
Mitchell, Claudia, 34–43
molecule, 10, 11, 15, 16, 46
Morgan, Thomas Hunt, 12

N

Naki, Mr., 20, 21
Nobel Prize, 19
nucleus, 10, 11, 46

O

Origin of the Species, 8

P

Paré, Ambroise, 6
Pasteur, Louis, 6
Pauling, Linus, 15–17
pneumonia, 13, 31, 46
Polo, Marco, 6
prostheses, 36, 44, 45

R

Roentgen, Wilhelm, 7

S

Sullivan, Jesse, 38

V

viruses, 17, 46

W

Washkansky, Louis, 23, 26–33
Watson, James, 16, 17, 19
white blood cell count, 30, 46
Wilkins, Maurice 19

X

X-rays, 7, 16, 31

Web Sites

Due to the changing nature of Internet links, the Rosen Publishing Group, Inc., has developed an online list of Web sites related to the subject of this book. This site is updated regularly. Please use this link to access the list:

http://www.rosenlinks.com/gd/med/

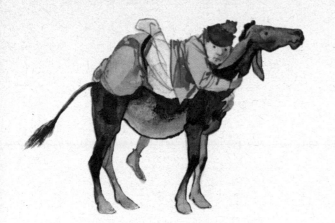

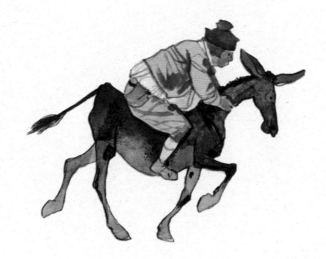

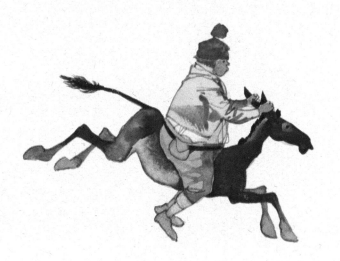

A Treasury of the

WORLD'S GREATEST
FAIRY TALES

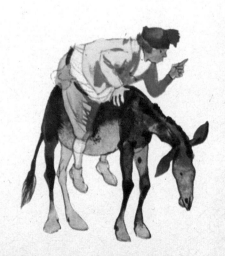

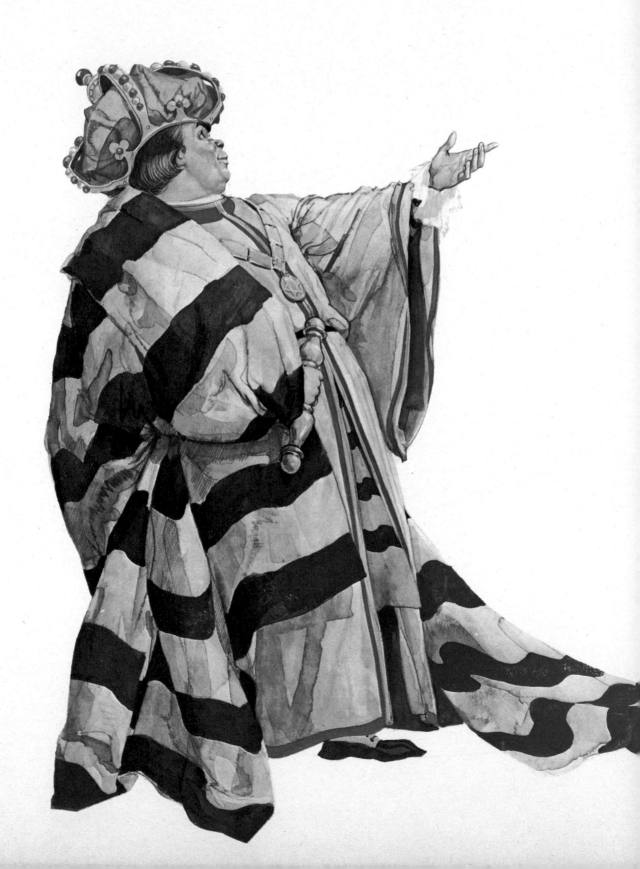

A Treasury of the

WORLD'S GREATEST FAIRY TALES

THE DANBURY PRESS

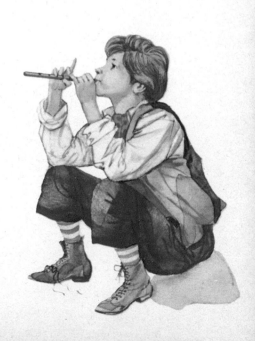

Story adaptations by
HELEN HYMAN

Published by The Danbury Press, a division of Grolier Enterprises, Inc.
Publisher—Robert B. Clarke
Marketing Director—Robert G. Bartner
Creative Director—Gilbert Evans

Library of Congress Catalog Card Number: 72-86579

Text © 1972 by Fratelli Fabbri Editori, Milan

Illustrations © 1966, 1969 by Fratelli Fabbri Editori, Milan

Once upon a time...

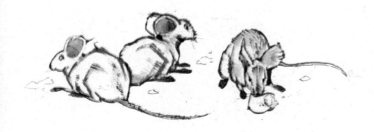

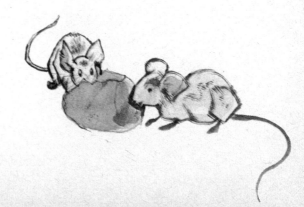

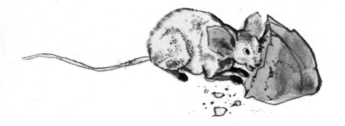

CONTENTS

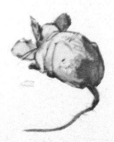

A Treasury of the

WORLD'S GREATEST
FAIRY TALES

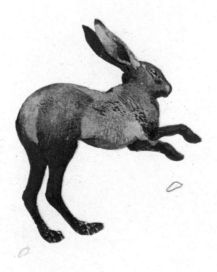

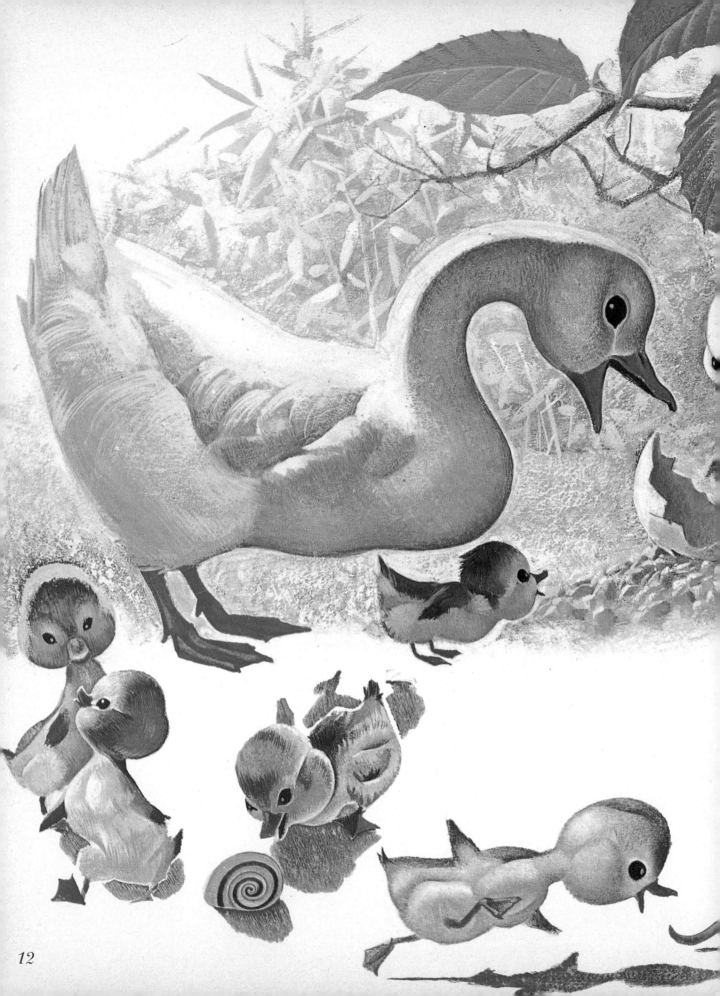

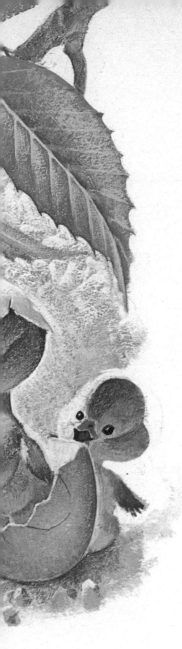

THE UGLY DUCKLING

Once upon a time, in the tall grasses of a green canal, a mother duck sat patiently hatching her eggs. At last she heard the first egg crack, then the second, and soon six fluffy yellow ducklings were hatched into the world. Only one large egg was left unhatched in the nest. The mother watched it anxiously and was relieved when it too began to crack open. But her relief changed to dismay when out hopped the ugliest duckling she had ever seen.

Instead of being small and round and soft and yellow like the other ducklings, he was large and awkward and gray. He seemed to grow uglier every day. But he was kind and friendly to everyone, even though his brothers and sisters were ashamed of him and all the ducks in the canal laughed at him.

"That's no duckling," they cackled meanly. "He's probably a worthless young turkeycock."

Only his mother loved him and defended him.

"He's really not so ugly when you look at him closely. He's quite pretty," she kept on insisting. Carefully she taught him everything she taught her other children and refused to leave him behind when she took them for their first swimming lesson.

"Quack!" she said proudly. "See how beautifully he swims, better than all the others. No one can say now that he's not a duckling."

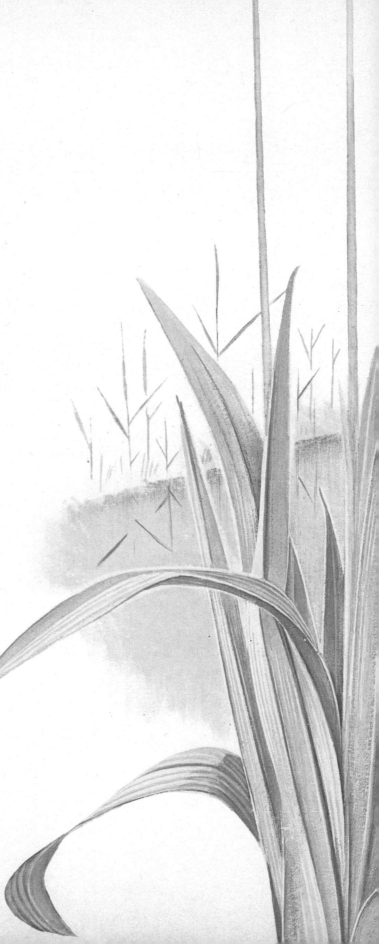

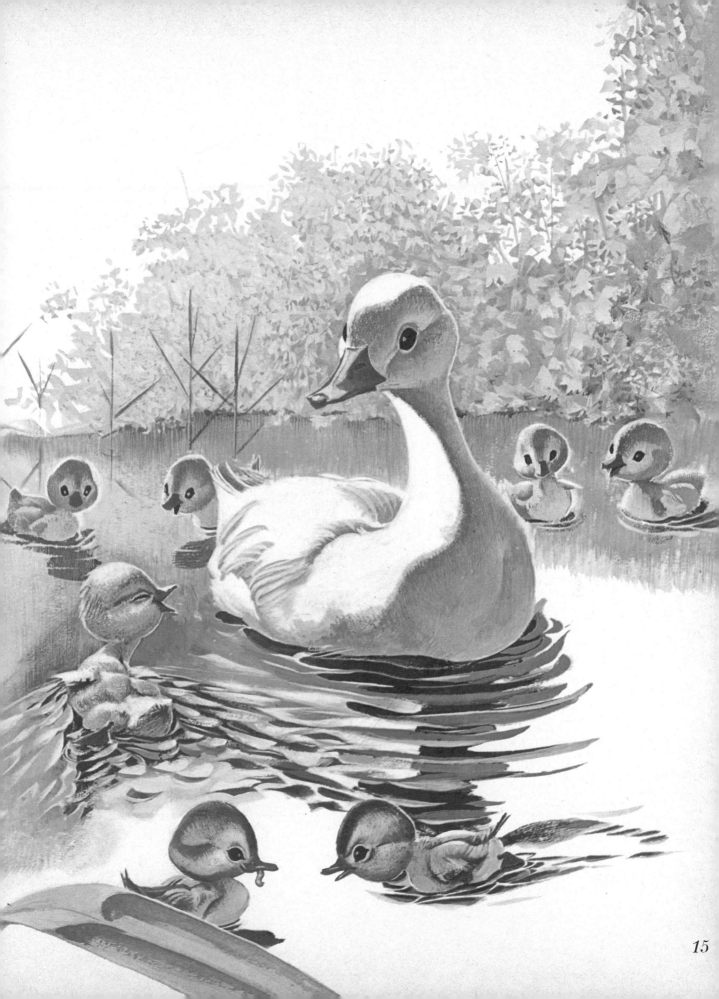

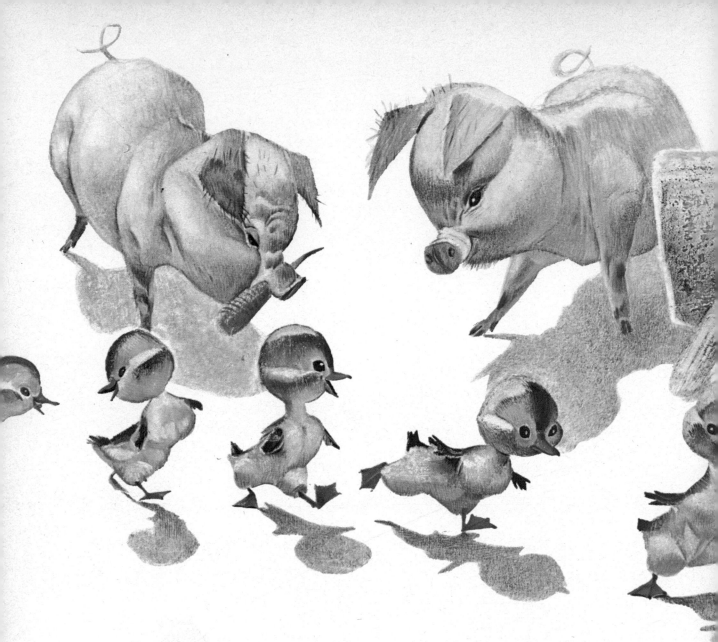

But the other ducks were not at all impressed, and when his mother lined up her ducklings and took them all to visit the barnyard, his brothers and sisters were so ashamed that they did not want him along. And it was even worse in the barnyard, where all the new animals he met scorned and ridiculed him. Even the pigs snorted at him, and the geese honked at him viciously.

"Leave him alone," cried his mother. "He's not doing any harm."

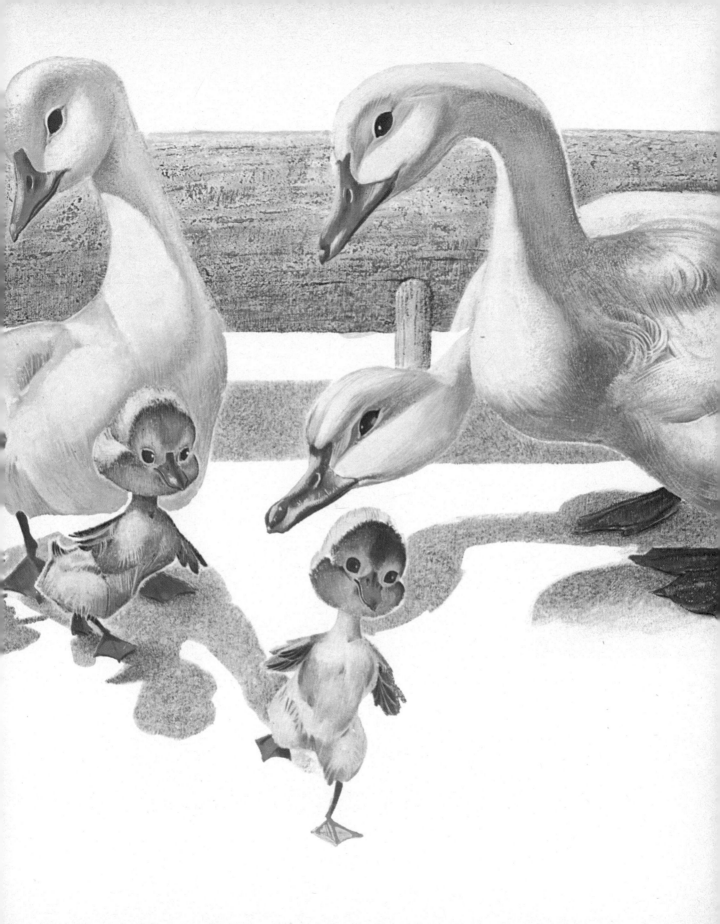

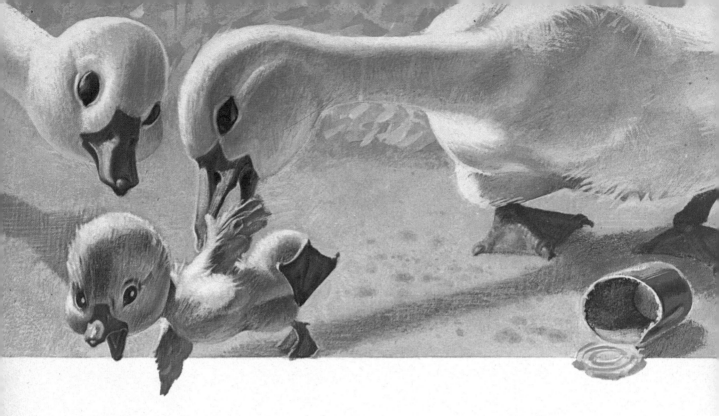

"He's too ugly to look at, and we shall tease him all we like!" they answered cruelly, as they kept right on honking and snorting.

"He's not handsome, I'll admit," replied his mother, stroking him gently and scratching his neck, "but he's good and kind, and he's still young. I'm sure he'll outgrow this stage soon and end up just like the others—and even stronger."

The little duckling did not believe her words and knew that she was heartbroken because he was so different and so ugly. She became sadder and sadder as time went on and the teasing became worse and worse. The ducks bit him, the hens pecked at him, the geese chased him, and even the girl who fed the poultry kicked him. He was the laughing stock of the whole barnyard.

No matter where he turned he met meanness and cruelty. He tried to hide, but wherever he went someone found him and teased him some more. Finally, he could stand all the cackling and squawking no longer, so he jumped over the barnyard fence and ran away. He kept on running even though he really had no idea where he was going. Things were not much better outside the barnyard either, because even the wild creatures ran away from him.

"I guess I'm so ugly, everyone's afraid of me!" he quacked miserably to himself.

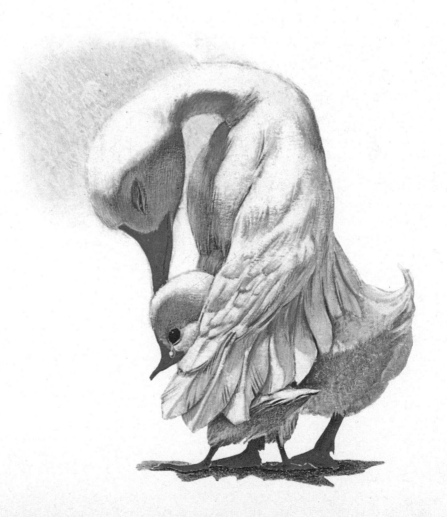

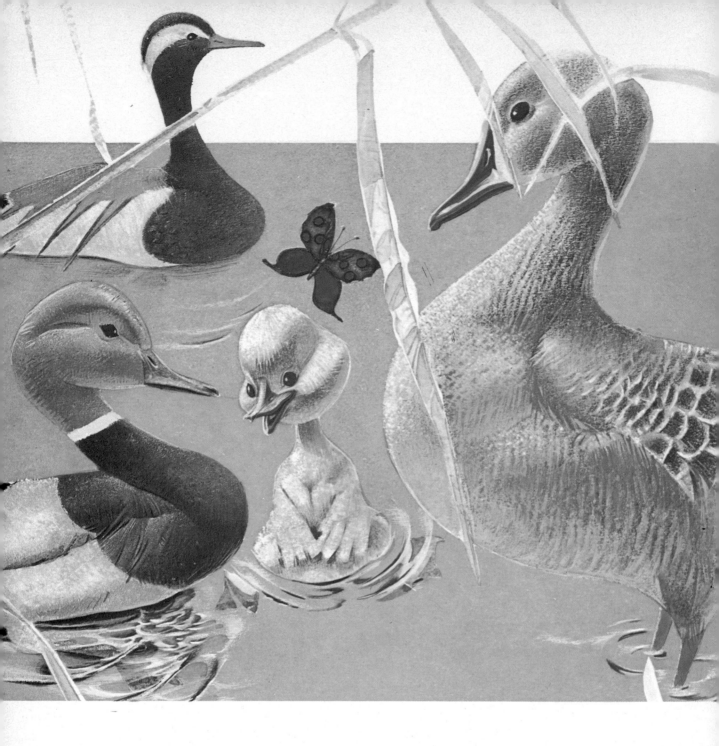

He found some wild ducks and geese for company for
a while, but one day these friendly birds were shot by
hunters and carried off by some fierce-looking hunting
dogs. But the dogs ignored the scared little duckling,
hiding in the tall grass nearby.

"I guess I'm even too ugly for them to take," he sighed
thankfully.

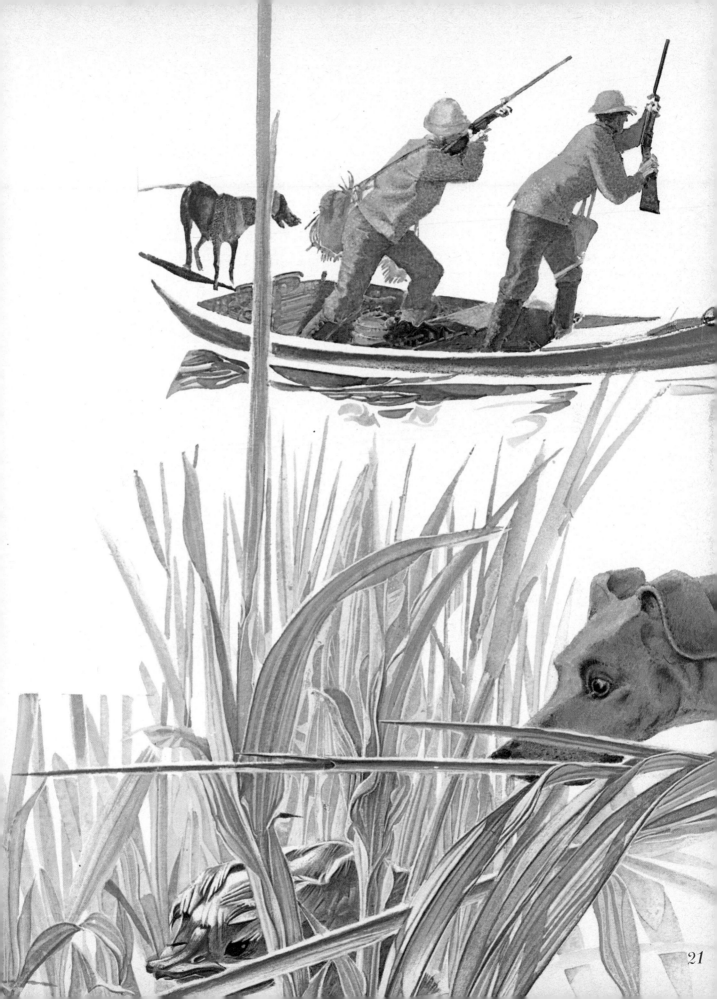

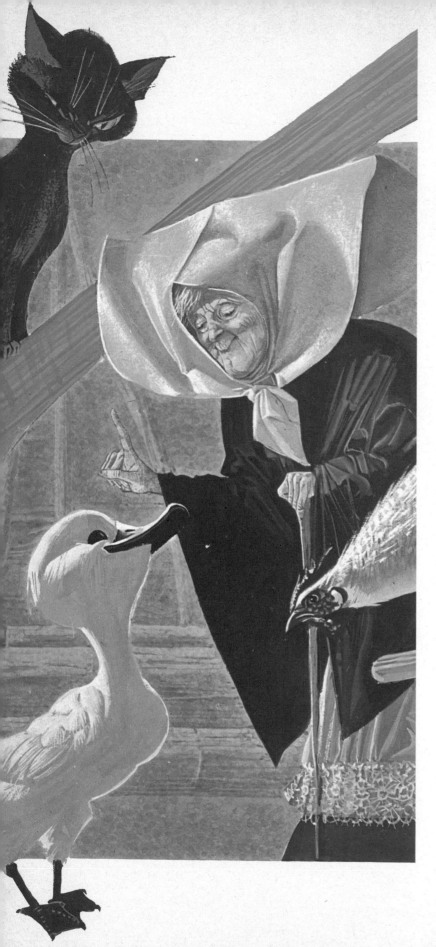

The poor duckling feared that the dogs and hunters might come back, so he ran away from the pond and kept on running till he came to a little hut in the woods, where a very old lady lived with her hen and her cat. She loved them both dearly, because the hen laid tasty eggs for her and the cat purred constantly to cheer her. The old lady's eyesight was so poor that she thought the duckling was a full-grown duck because he was so oversized.

"How lucky I am!" she cried. "I have a beautiful hen to lay beautiful hens' eggs for me, and now I have a fine duck to lay some fine duck eggs."

She brought the duckling into her house and treated him kindly, but the cat felt himself to be master of the house and the hen thought she was its mistress, and both were jealous of their new guest.

"Can you really lay eggs?" asked the hen suspiciously.

"No," answered the duckling honestly.

"Then of what earthly use are you to anyone?" snapped the hen, who proudly laid her daily egg just to show off.

"Can you purr?" asked the cat.

"I can quack," replied the duckling. "But I can't purr."

"Then of what earthly use are you to anyone?" sneered the cat, purring loudly just to show off.

Then both of them began to torment the poor duckling, so that once again he had to run away.

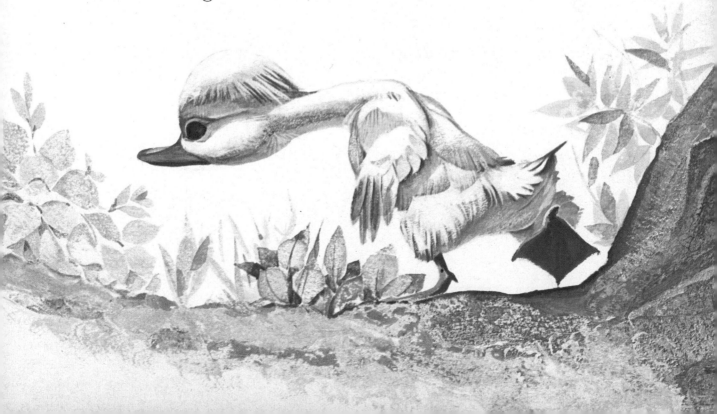

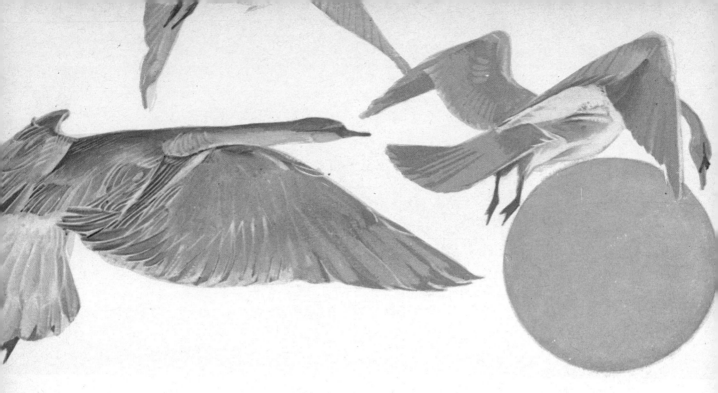

"It's good to be out of that house and in the wide world again," the duckling said to himself, though he was so lonely he did not believe a word he was saying.

But he soon found a nice pond to swim in and amused himself splashing and diving and chasing insects and catching minnows. After a time, however, the water grew colder and the wind stronger; the leaves began to turn yellow and then brown, and autumn arrived. Just before winter came, the duckling heard a strange sound in the sky. He looked into the sunset and saw a flock of graceful swans flying over him. He had never seen any creatures so beautiful and stared in wonder at their snow-white plumage, their splendid wings, and their long slender necks.

The duckling did not know that these birds were swans, but he knew he loved them more than he had ever loved anything in his life before. He did not envy them, either, because it would have been beyond his wildest dreams to wish such beauty for himself. He just watched them worshipfully as they flew off to warmer lands across the sea. All through the long, cold winter he remembered their beauty with pleasure.

And the winter was long and so very cold! The duckling had to keep swimming round in circles, or the water would have frozen him in tight. But still, as the ice on the pond grew thicker, it became harder and harder for him to swim at all.

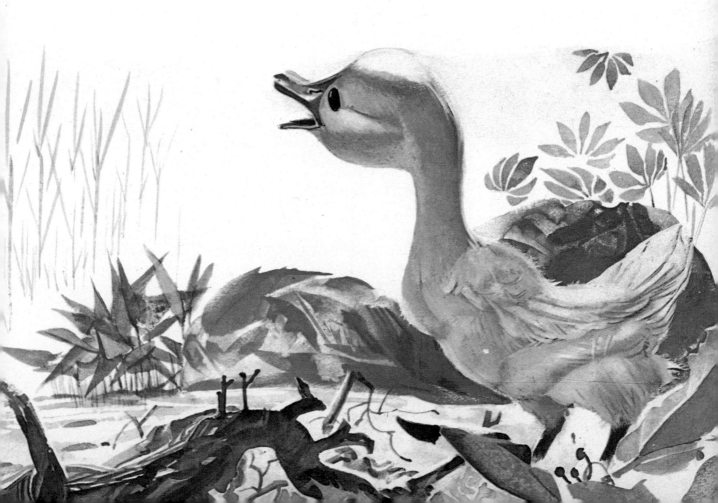

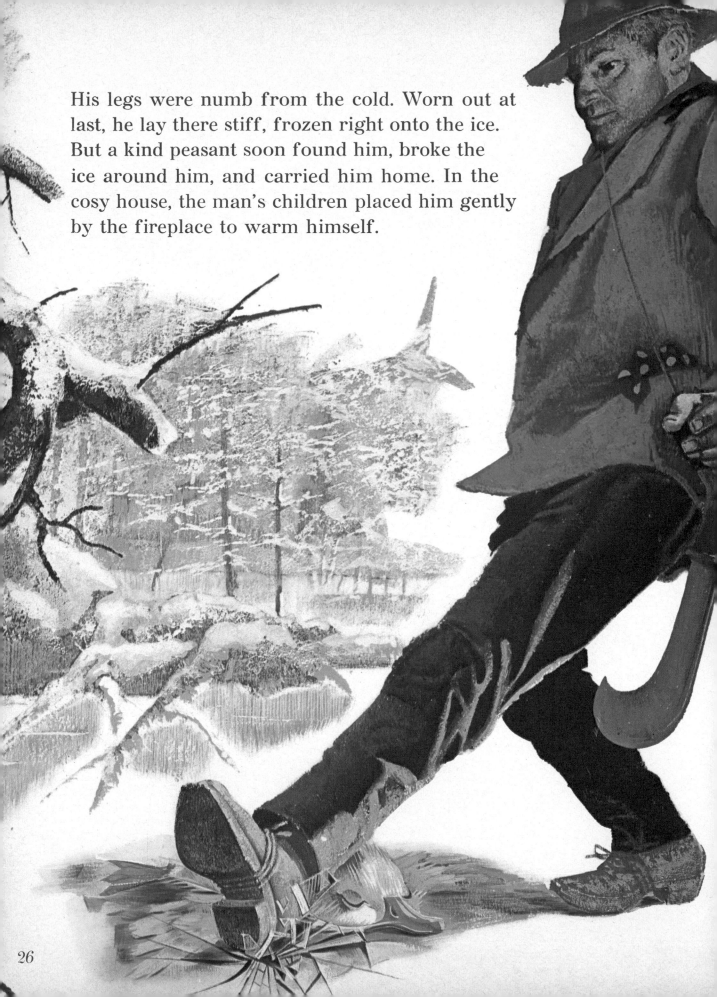

His legs were numb from the cold. Worn out at last, he lay there stiff, frozen right onto the ice. But a kind peasant soon found him, broke the ice around him, and carried him home. In the cosy house, the man's children placed him gently by the fireplace to warm himself.

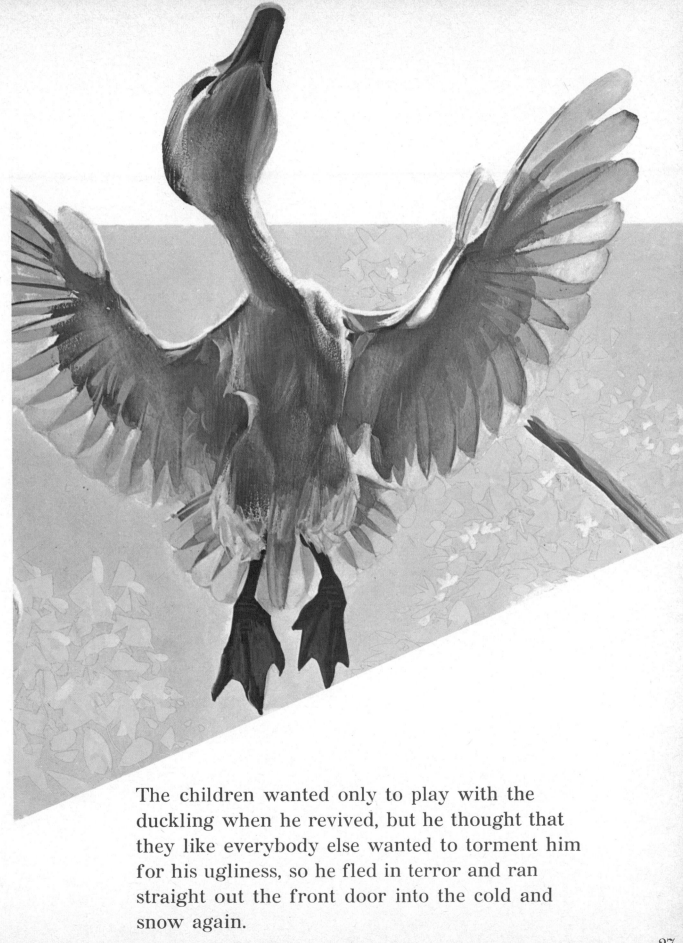

The children wanted only to play with the duckling when he revived, but he thought that they like everybody else wanted to torment him for his ugliness, so he fled in terror and ran straight out the front door into the cold and snow again.

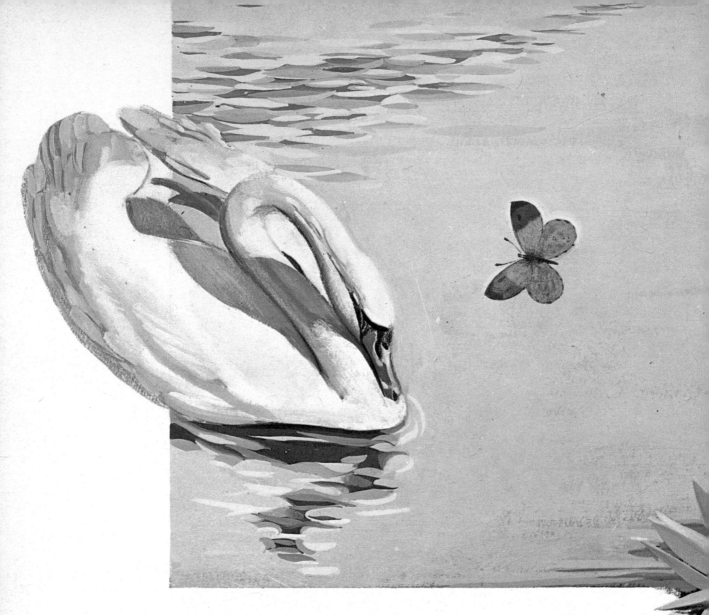

Somehow the duckling managed to live through the rest of the hard winter, and when spring came he felt bigger and stronger. Then, one day as he was swimming happily, coming toward him he saw three of the glorious birds he so worshiped.

"I'll go over to those beautiful creatures," he thought, "and they will surely kill me because I am so ugly. But I would rather be killed by such kingly birds than live on only to be bitten by ducks, pecked at by hens, and chased by everyone else."

So, bowing his head humbly, he swam toward the graceful swans.

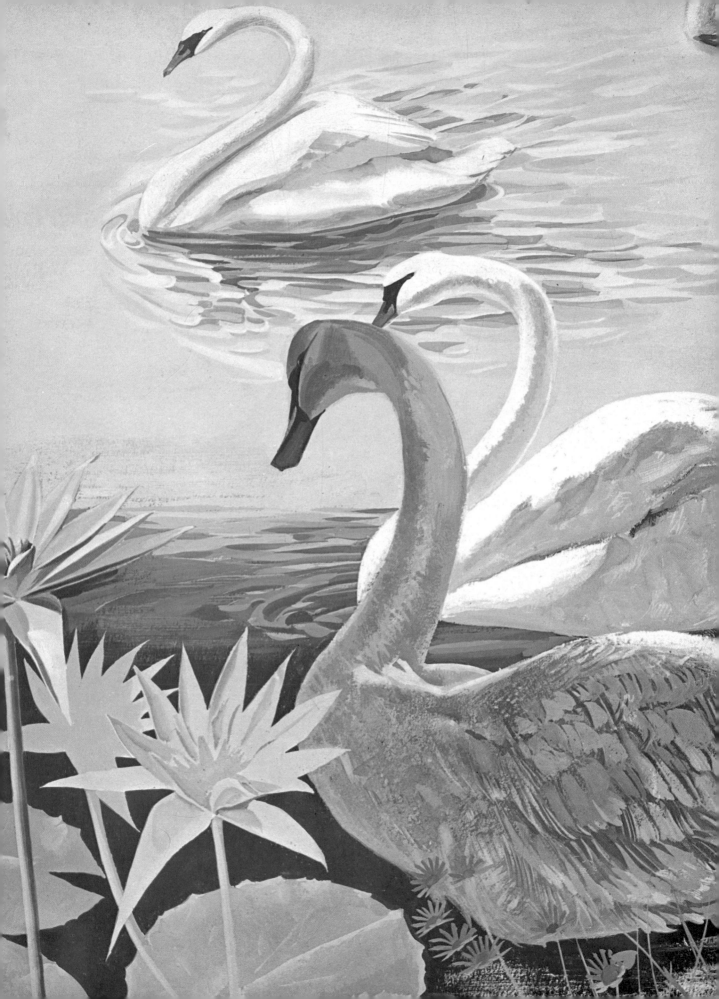

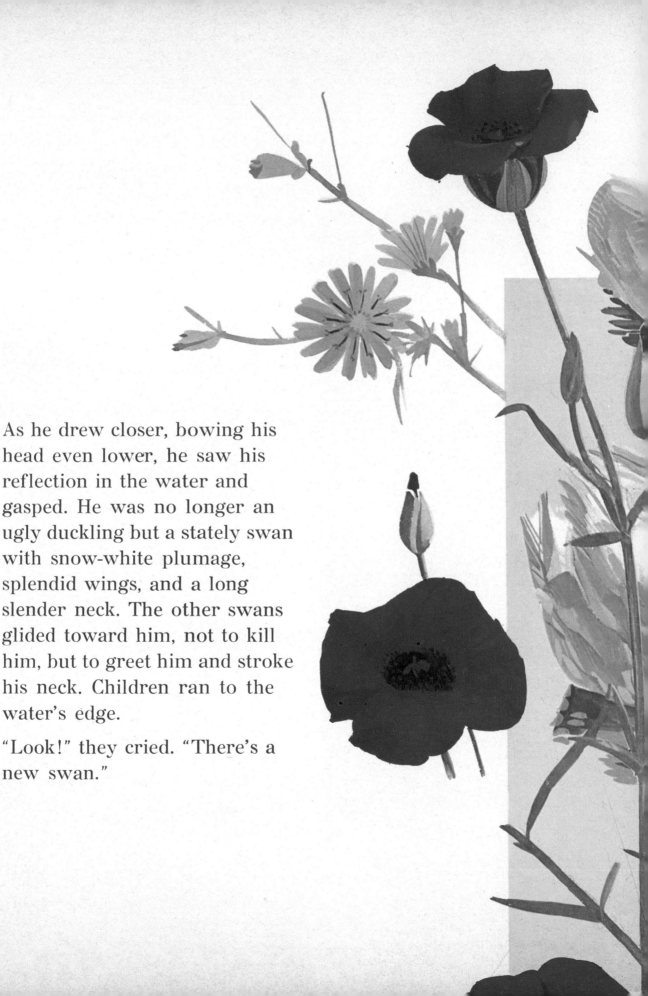

As he drew closer, bowing his head even lower, he saw his reflection in the water and gasped. He was no longer an ugly duckling but a stately swan with snow-white plumage, splendid wings, and a long slender neck. The other swans glided toward him, not to kill him, but to greet him and stroke his neck. Children ran to the water's edge.

"Look!" they cried. "There's a new swan."

"Yes," said their parents. "And the new one is the most beautiful of all."

As everyone gathered round to admire him, the new swan hid his head modestly and thought, "I never dreamed I could ever know such happiness when I was the despised ugly duckling."

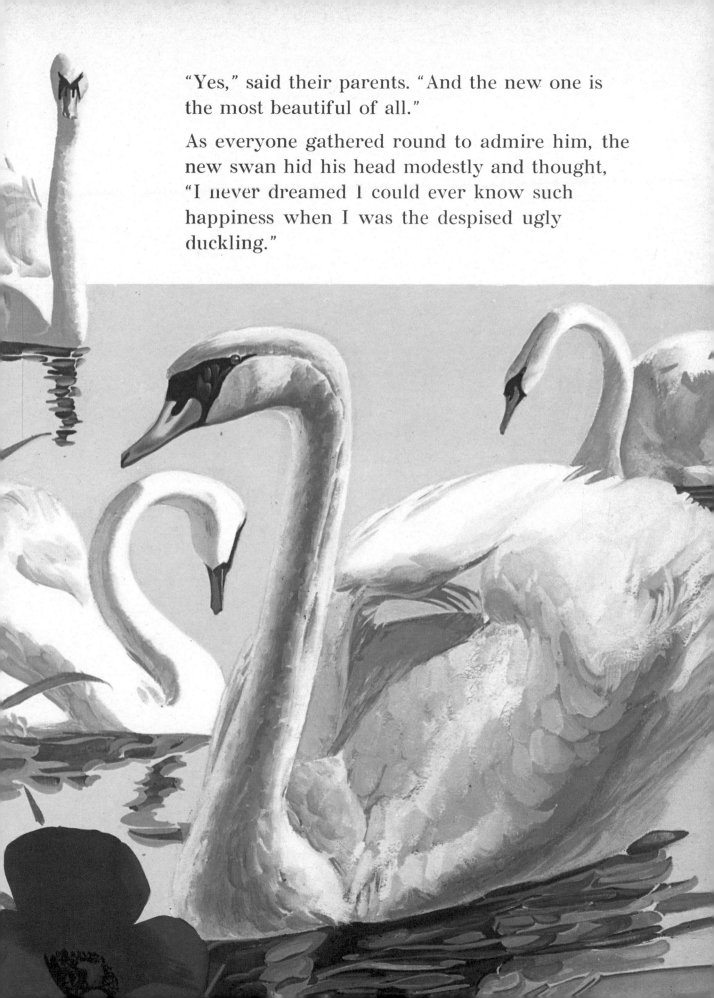

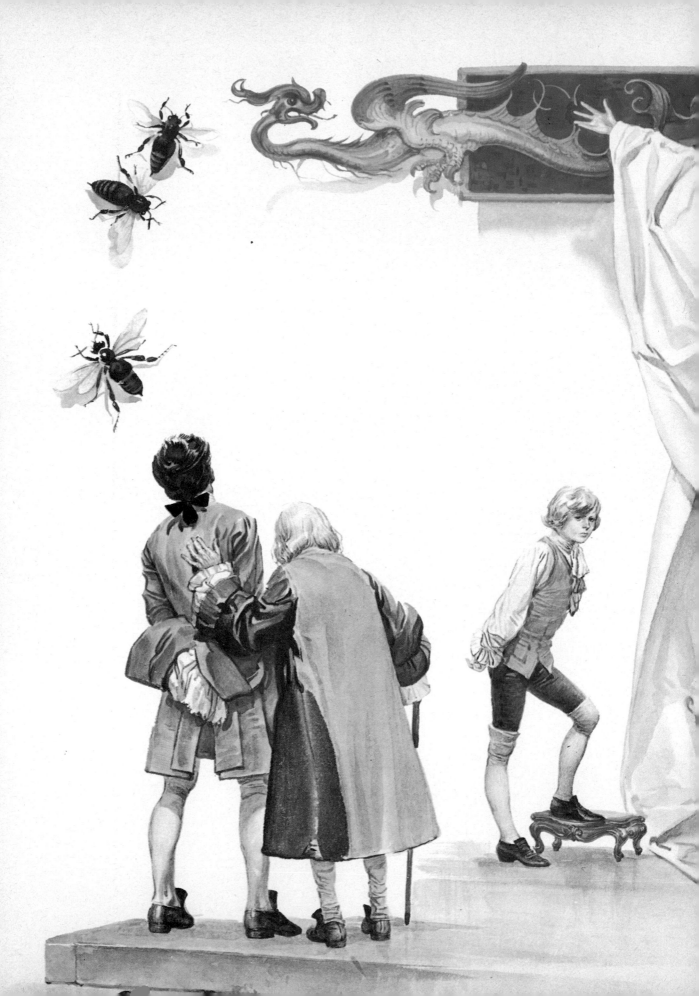

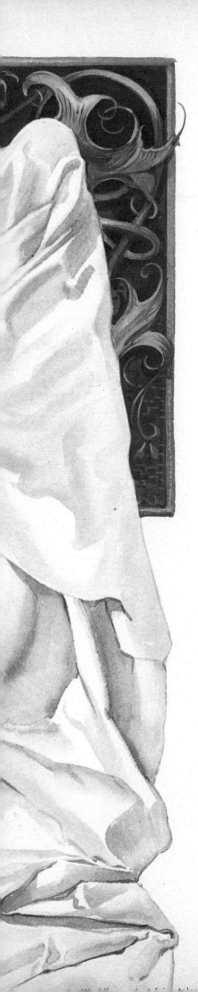

THE ENCHANTED PRINCESS

Once upon a time, there was a very fine cabinetmaker who lived with his wife and two sons. The elder son Hans was good and generous; but Henry, the younger one, was mean and selfish. But, as so often happens, the foolish father loved the mean son best.

The old cabinetmaker was known far and wide for the beauty and perfection of his work. People came from everywhere to buy his handsome chairs and sturdy chests, so that he made a good living and was able to keep his family in comfort.

But one year great misfortune came to their land. The crops were ruined by floods, and the cattle were killed off by disease. The cabinetmaker soon found his purse empty, and also that many people owed him money. This was a most unusual situation, because in the past his customers had always paid quickly. But since he had no money left, he had to try to collect what was owed him, and so he went from house to house.

"Alas, good sir," wailed one debtor, "my cows all died and I am ruined!"

"Would that I could pay you," sighed another. "But my harvest rotted and I am penniless."

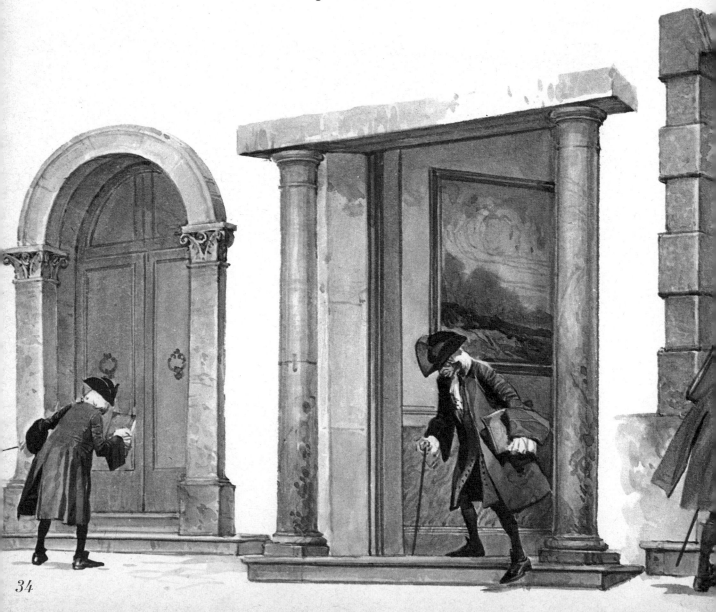

"Give me till springtime, I beg you," pleaded a third.

At every house the poor man heard the same tale of woe and, much discouraged, started for home as poor as before. On his way he stopped at the inn for a glass of ale, and while there he heard a traveler tell a strange tale.

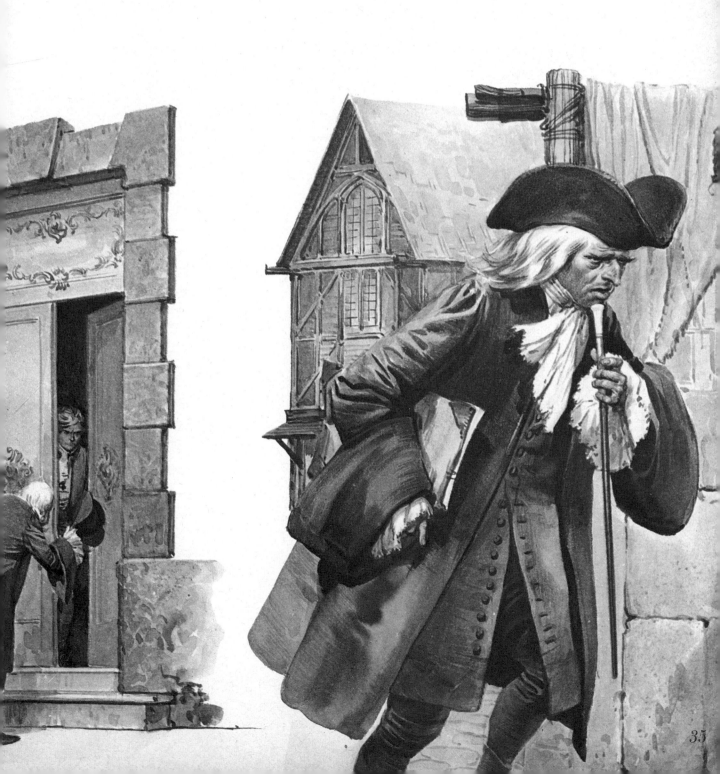

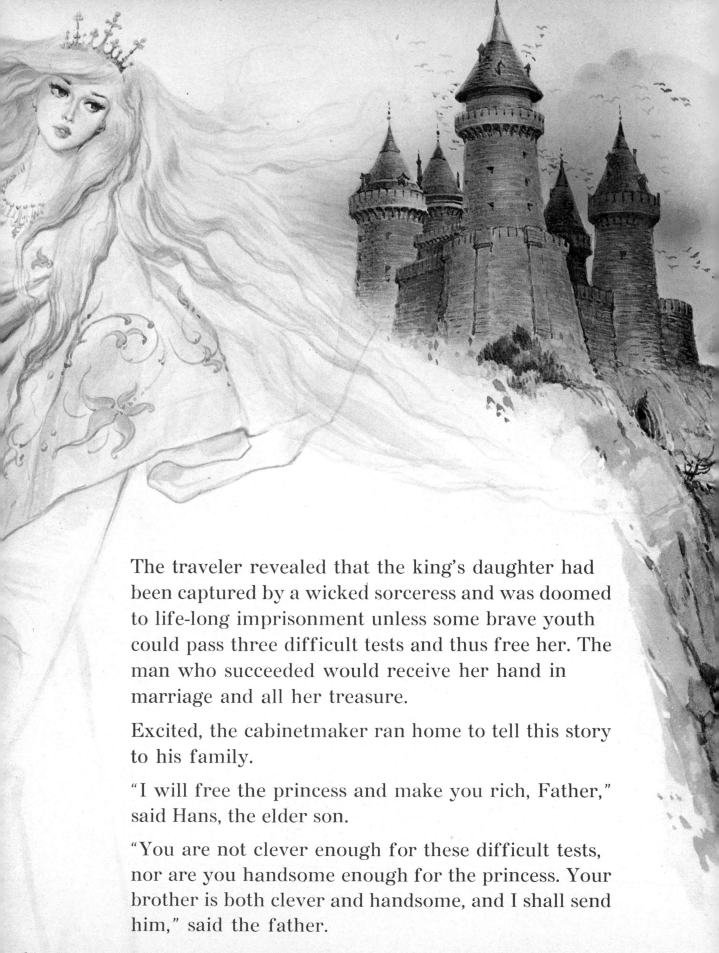

The traveler revealed that the king's daughter had been captured by a wicked sorceress and was doomed to life-long imprisonment unless some brave youth could pass three difficult tests and thus free her. The man who succeeded would receive her hand in marriage and all her treasure.

Excited, the cabinetmaker ran home to tell this story to his family.

"I will free the princess and make you rich, Father," said Hans, the elder son.

"You are not clever enough for these difficult tests, nor are you handsome enough for the princess. Your brother is both clever and handsome, and I shall send him," said the father.

The next day he bid farewell to his favorite son, confident that Henry would succeed. Henry, who was just as confident, promised to send back a golden coach drawn by six white horses to bring his parents to the castle after he had finished his task. Then he rode off, feeling like a king already and treating all whom he met in his way with haughtiness and cruelty. He threw stones at the birds who flew over him and chased rabbits back into their burrows. When he saw an anthill and the ants busy at work, he brutally rode over it and crushed them.

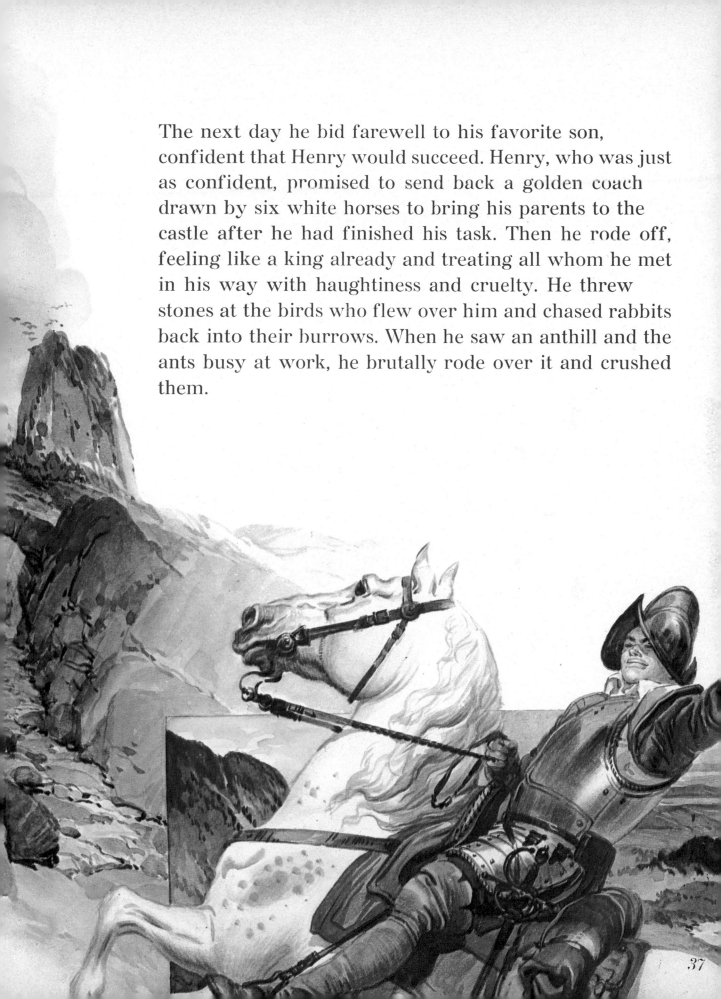

Farther on, he passed a pond where twelve wild ducks swam freely. Cunningly he lured them to the bank and shot them. Later he found a busy beehive and killed every bee just for his own amusement.

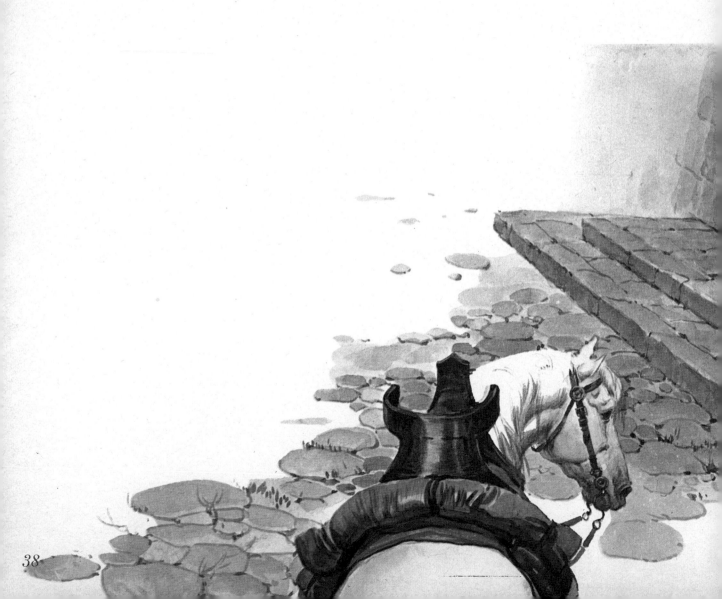

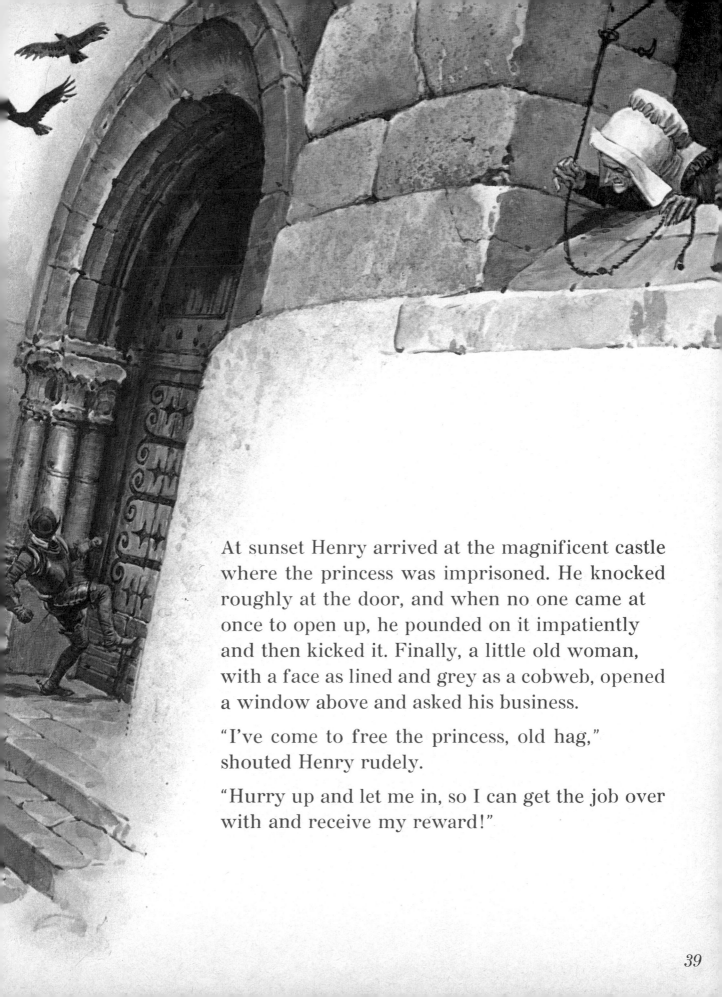

At sunset Henry arrived at the magnificent castle where the princess was imprisoned. He knocked roughly at the door, and when no one came at once to open up, he pounded on it impatiently and then kicked it. Finally, a little old woman, with a face as lined and grey as a cobweb, opened a window above and asked his business.

"I've come to free the princess, old hag," shouted Henry rudely.

"Hurry up and let me in, so I can get the job over with and receive my reward!"

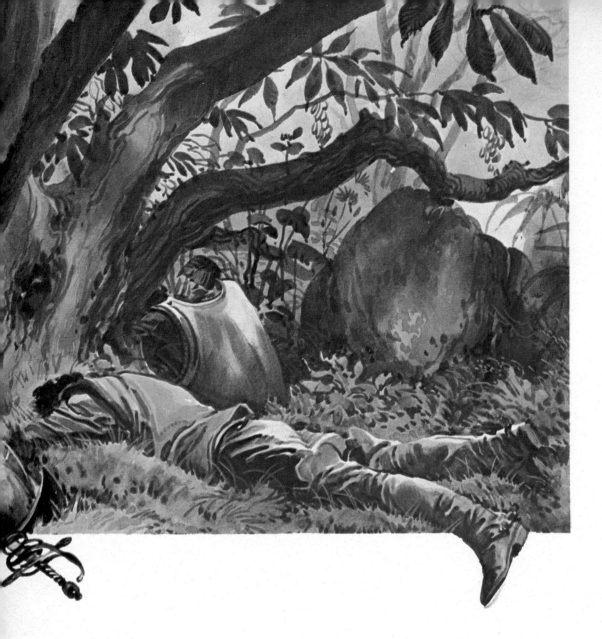

"Now, now, my son, don't rush things," said the old woman. "Tomorrow is another day. Return here at sunrise, and don't be late."

She then slammed the window shut, and Henry could do nothing but wait impatiently till morning. When sunrise came, the old woman was ready for him with a basketful of tiny seeds which she scattered far and wide over a nearby meadow.

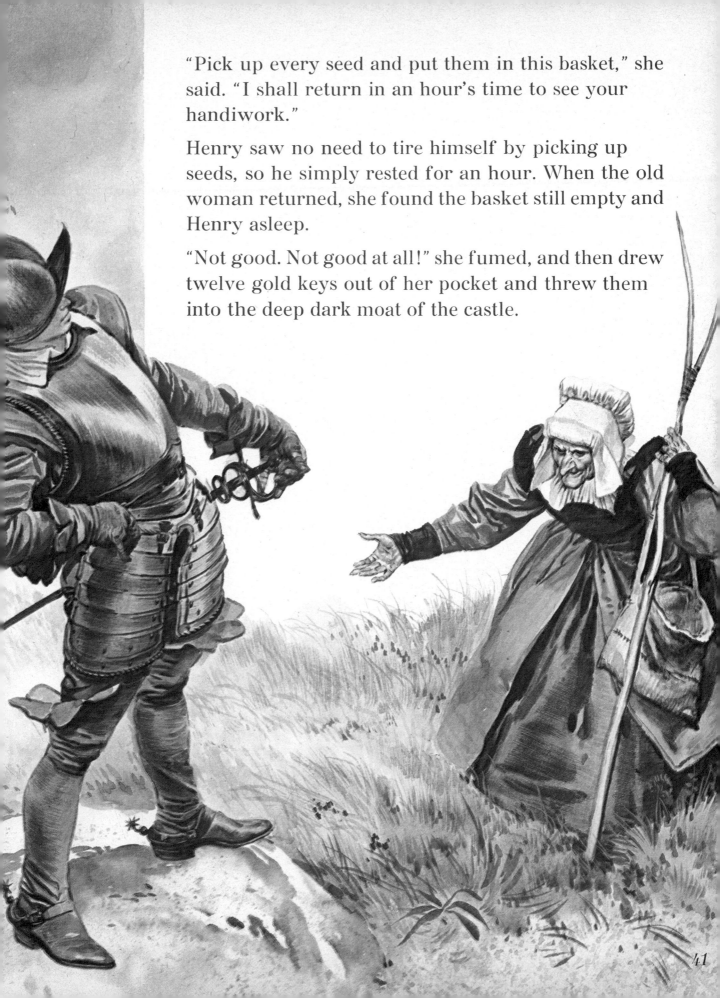

"Pick up every seed and put them in this basket," she said. "I shall return in an hour's time to see your handiwork."

Henry saw no need to tire himself by picking up seeds, so he simply rested for an hour. When the old woman returned, she found the basket still empty and Henry asleep.

"Not good. Not good at all!" she fumed, and then drew twelve gold keys out of her pocket and threw them into the deep dark moat of the castle.

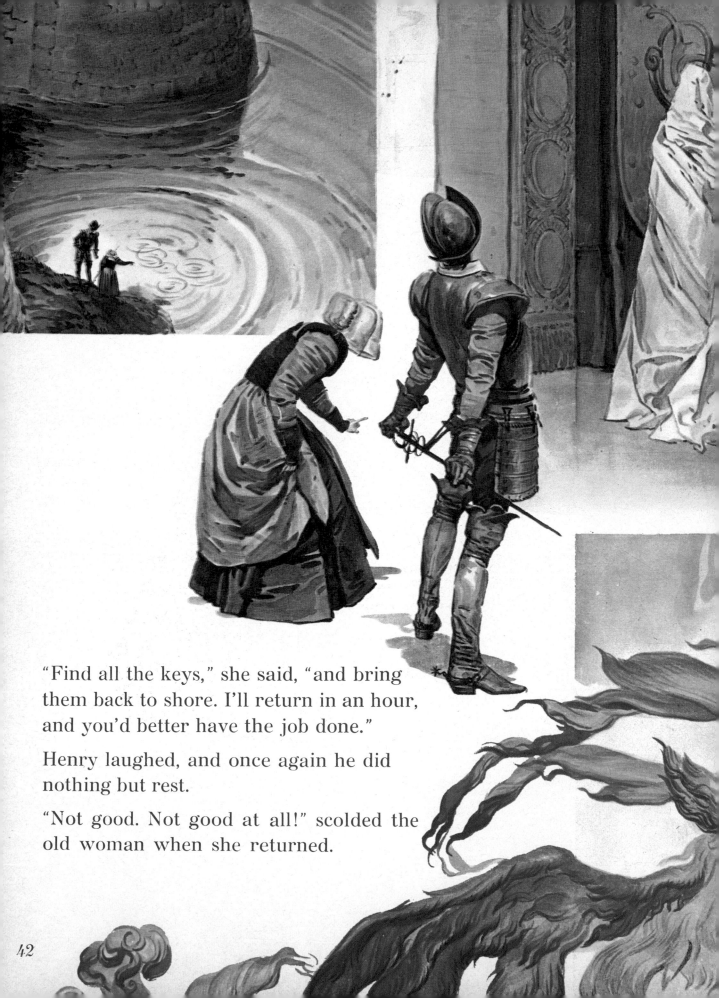

"Find all the keys," she said, "and bring them back to shore. I'll return in an hour, and you'd better have the job done."

Henry laughed, and once again he did nothing but rest.

"Not good. Not good at all!" scolded the old woman when she returned.

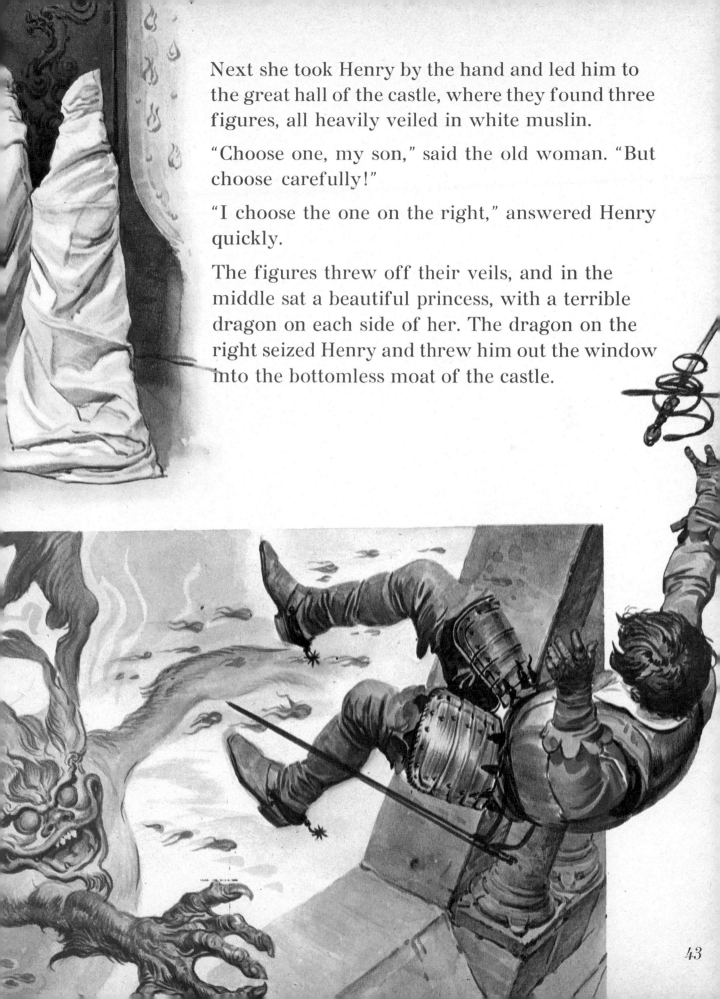

Next she took Henry by the hand and led him to the great hall of the castle, where they found three figures, all heavily veiled in white muslin.

"Choose one, my son," said the old woman. "But choose carefully!"

"I choose the one on the right," answered Henry quickly.

The figures threw off their veils, and in the middle sat a beautiful princess, with a terrible dragon on each side of her. The dragon on the right seized Henry and threw him out the window into the bottomless moat of the castle.

43

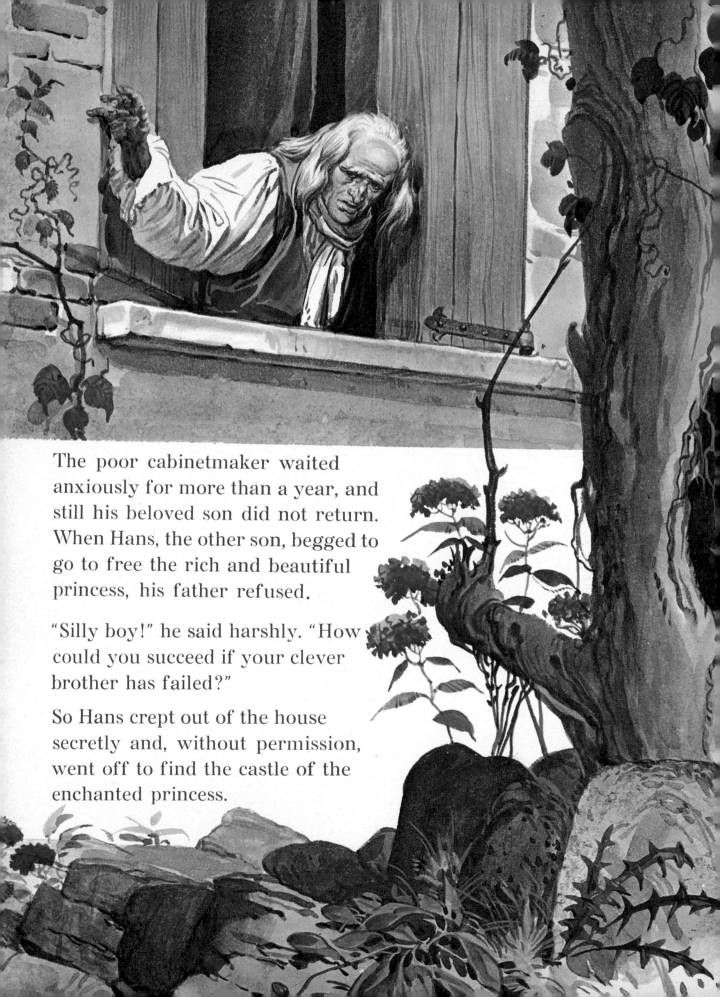

The poor cabinetmaker waited anxiously for more than a year, and still his beloved son did not return. When Hans, the other son, begged to go to free the rich and beautiful princess, his father refused.

"Silly boy!" he said harshly. "How could you succeed if your clever brother has failed?"

So Hans crept out of the house secretly and, without permission, went off to find the castle of the enchanted princess.

The journey took longer for Hans than for his brother, because good and gentle Hans stopped to make friends with all the wild creatures he met along the way. He did not throw stones at the birds, and so they sang him to sleep with their sweetest songs.

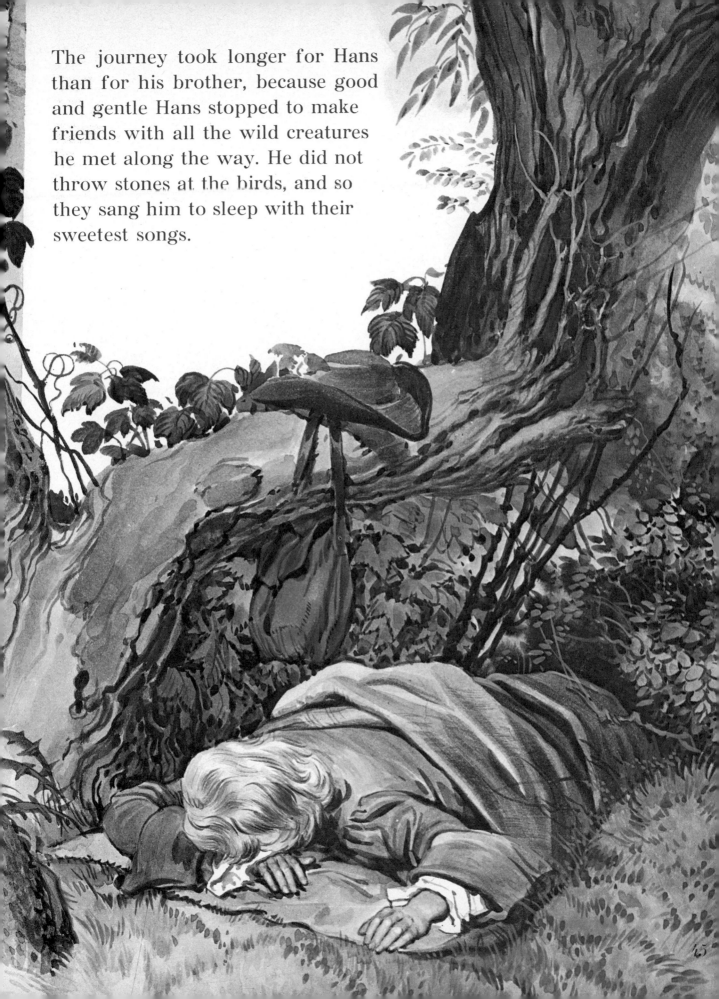

Hans was never too busy, or too tired, or too intent on his journey to be kind and thoughtful to all he met. When he came to the ants busily rebuilding their anthill, he did not disturb them and even stayed to help. Ducks were swimming on the pond, and he called them to the bank, not to kill them but to feed them crumbs.

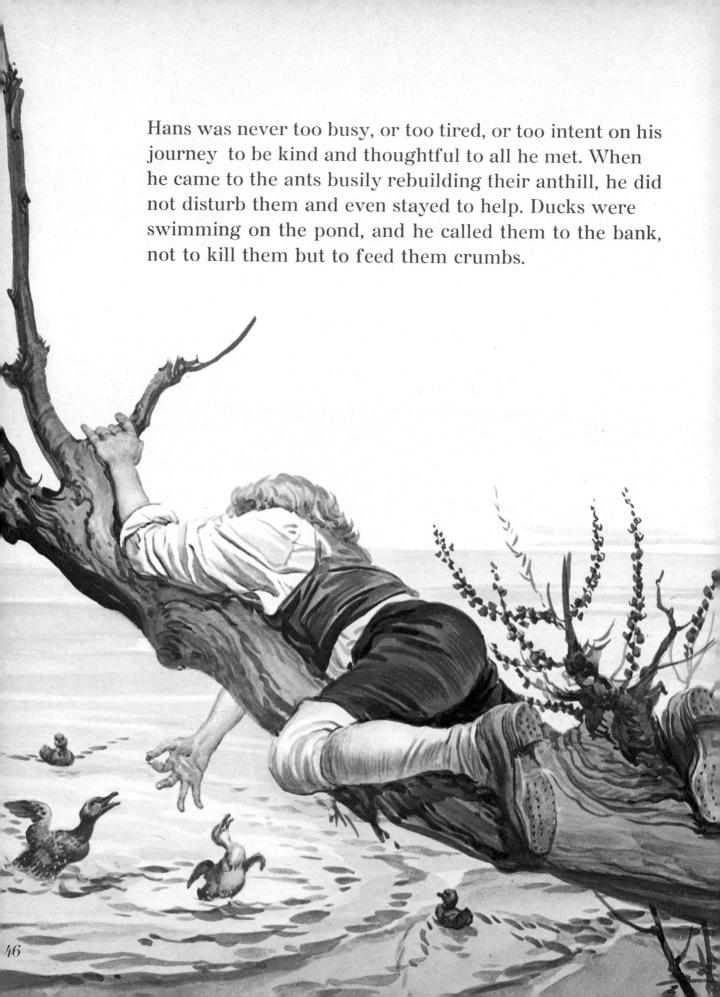

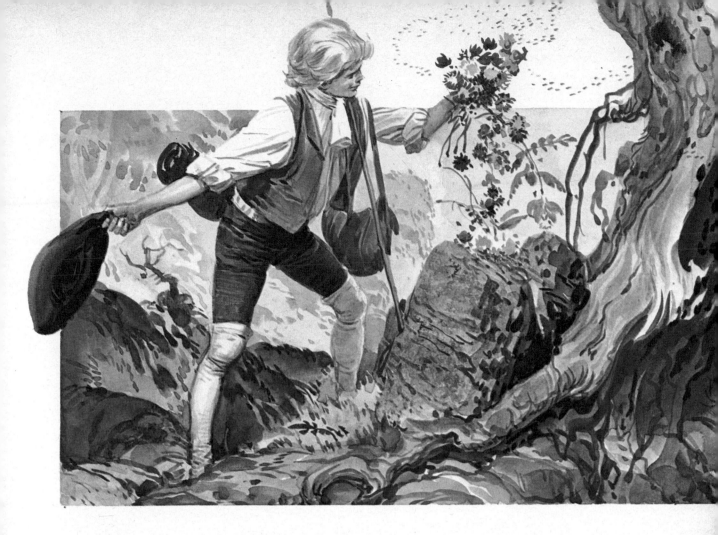

Beautiful wildflowers grew by the path as he approached
the beehive. He picked some for the bees to help them
with their honeymaking. When he came to the castle, he
knocked softly on the door. The old woman immediately
opened her window and asked him what he wanted.

"If I may be so bold, gentle mistress," Hans said politely,
"I would like to try to free the beautiful princess."

"You may try," the crone answered. "But if you fail to pass
the three tests, it will cost you your life."

"I already know the dangers," he replied. "But it is my
fondest wish to succeed. Please, tell me what I must do."

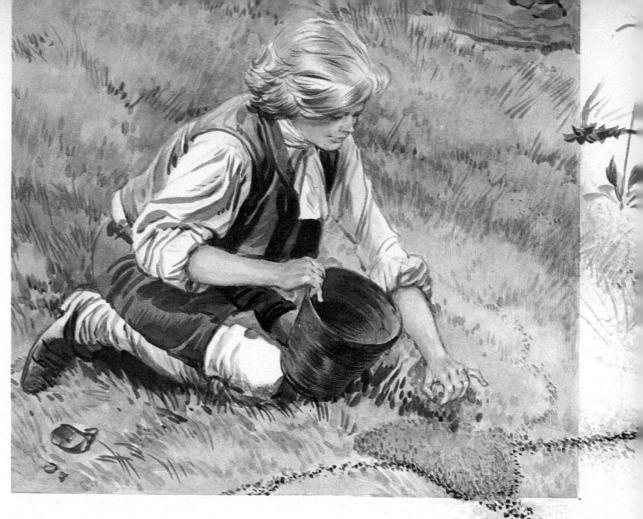

Once again the old woman scattered the basket of seeds and told Hans she would be back in an hour to inspect his work. Hans worked without stopping, but the basket was not even half full when the hour was nearly over. Suddenly, a swarm of ants crawled over the field, and each one carried a single seed to the basket. When the old woman came back, the basket was full.

"That's good," she said approvingly. Then, once more she threw twelve gold keys into the deepest part of the moat.

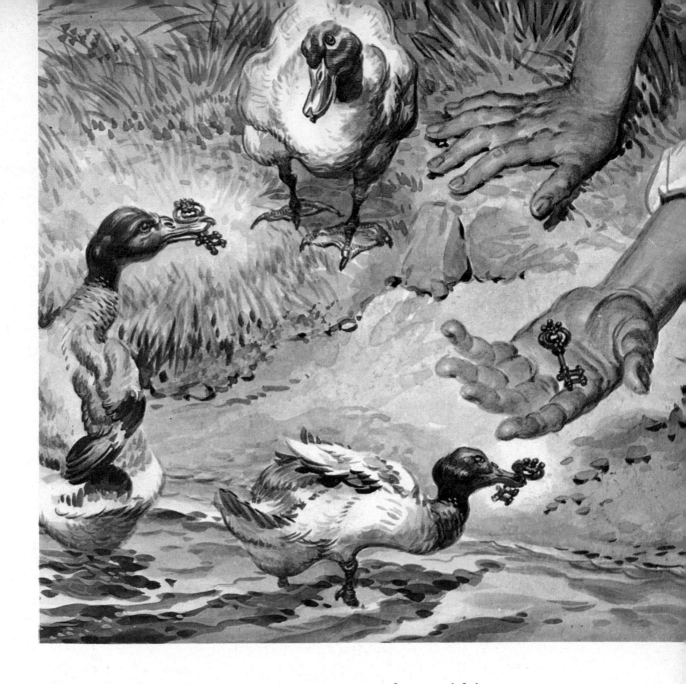

After ordering Hans to recover every key within the
hour, she went away again. Again Hans was in despair at
his task; time after time he dove in but could not find
a single key. Then, suddenly, twelve wild ducks flew by
and dove deep into the water. When they came up
again, each was carrying one gold key.

"That's good, too," murmured the old woman when she
saw the keys. Next she led Hans into the castle.

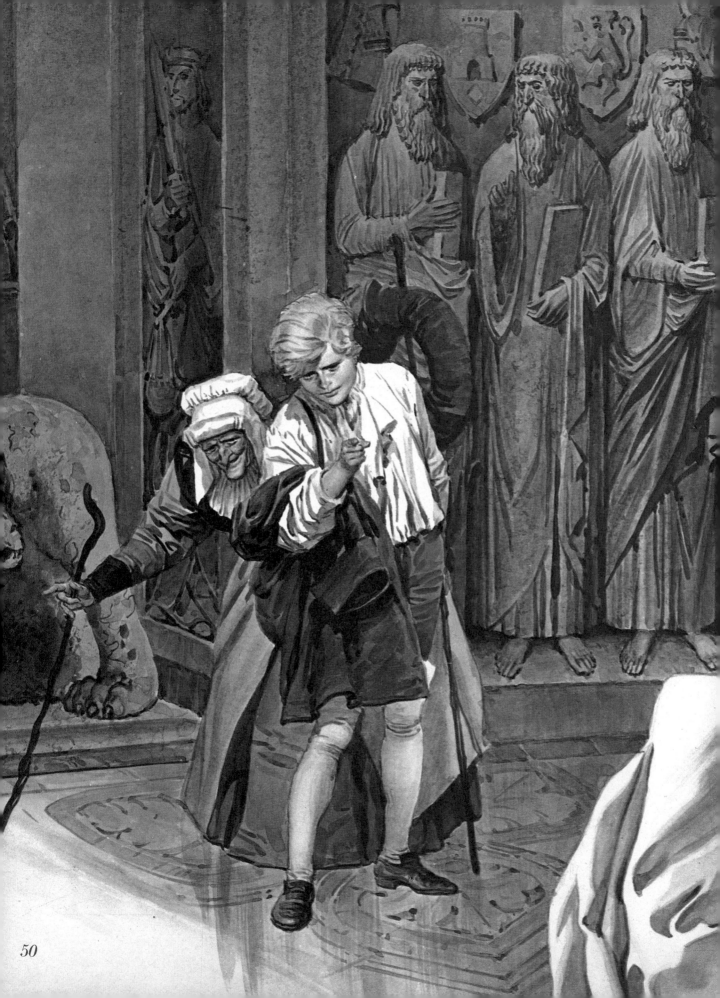

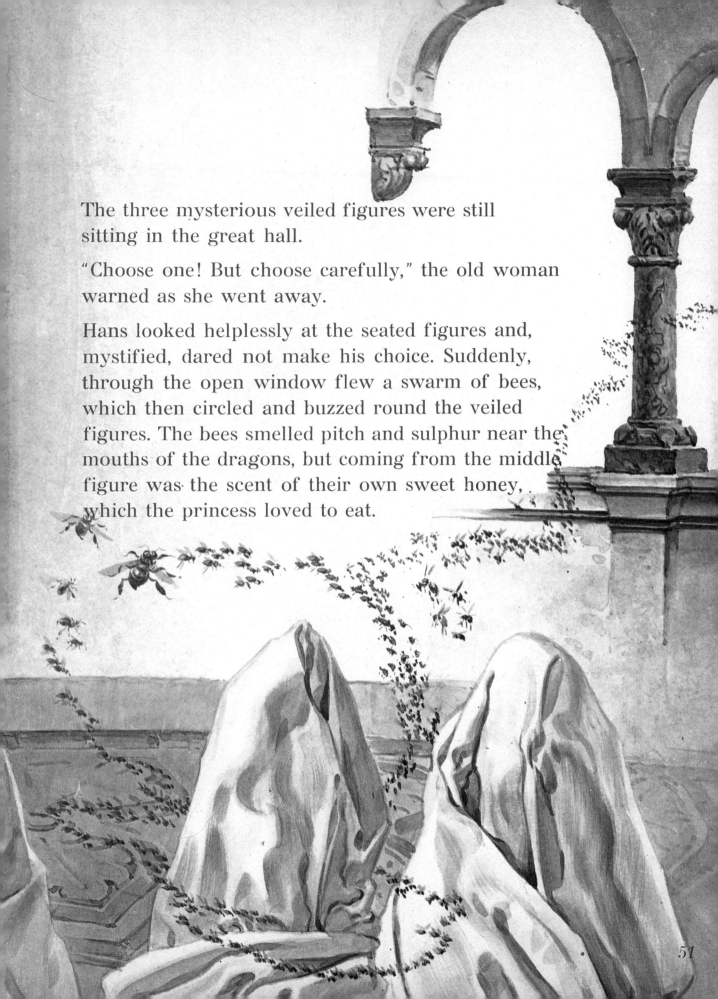

The three mysterious veiled figures were still sitting in the great hall.

"Choose one! But choose carefully," the old woman warned as she went away.

Hans looked helplessly at the seated figures and, mystified, dared not make his choice. Suddenly, through the open window flew a swarm of bees, which then circled and buzzed round the veiled figures. The bees smelled pitch and sulphur near the mouths of the dragons, but coming from the middle figure was the scent of their own sweet honey, which the princess loved to eat.

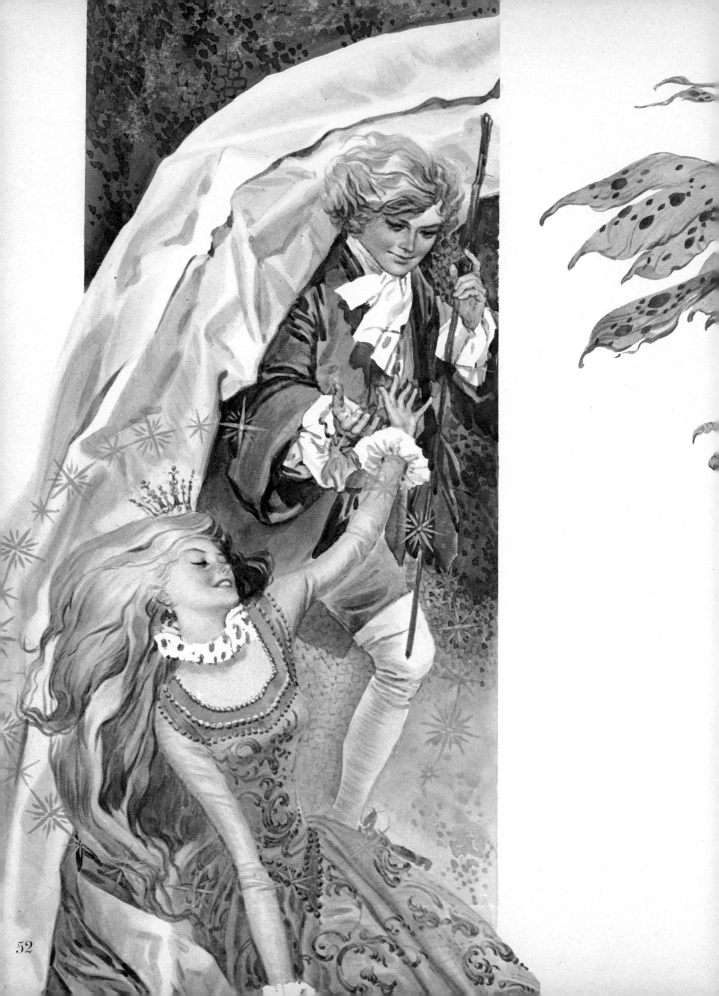

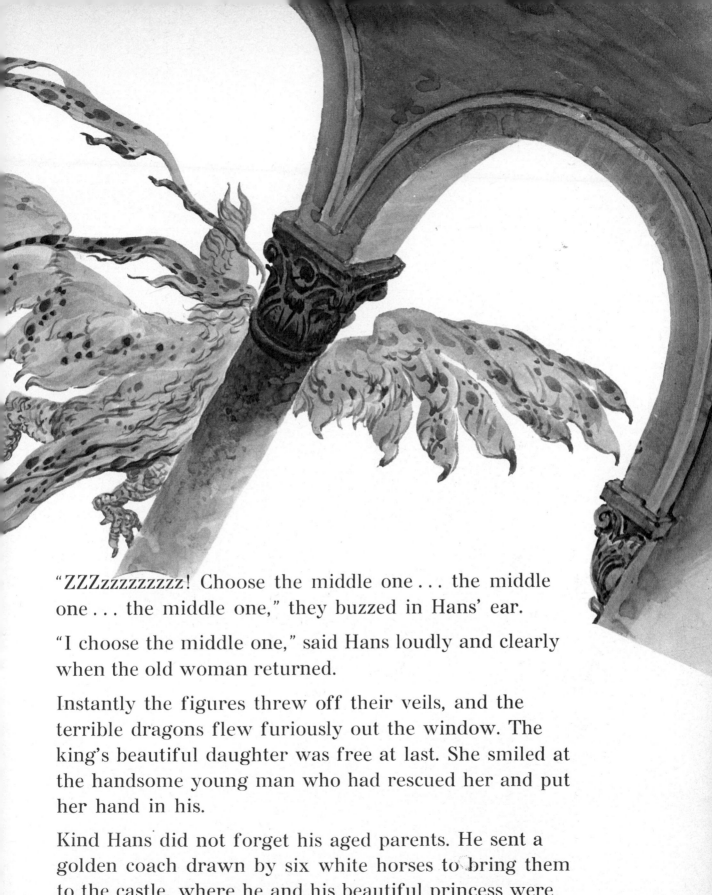

"ZZZzzzzzzzzz! Choose the middle one . . . the middle one . . . the middle one," they buzzed in Hans' ear.

"I choose the middle one," said Hans loudly and clearly when the old woman returned.

Instantly the figures threw off their veils, and the terrible dragons flew furiously out the window. The king's beautiful daughter was free at last. She smiled at the handsome young man who had rescued her and put her hand in his.

Kind Hans did not forget his aged parents. He sent a golden coach drawn by six white horses to bring them to the castle, where he and his beautiful princess were married in splendor. All of them lived happily and without fear of evil dragons ever after.

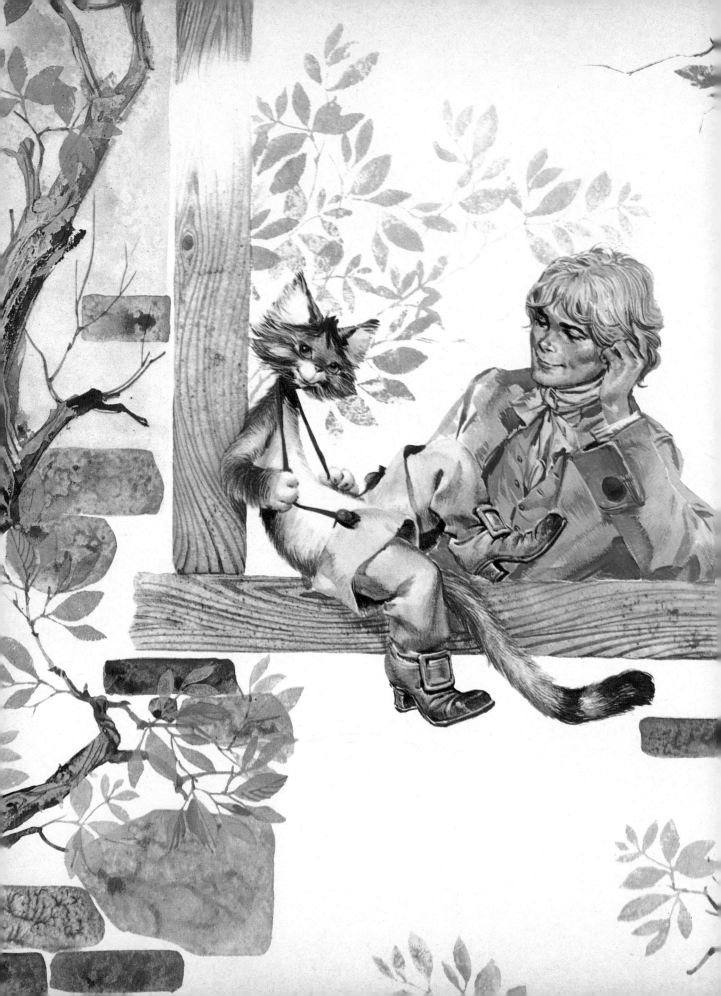

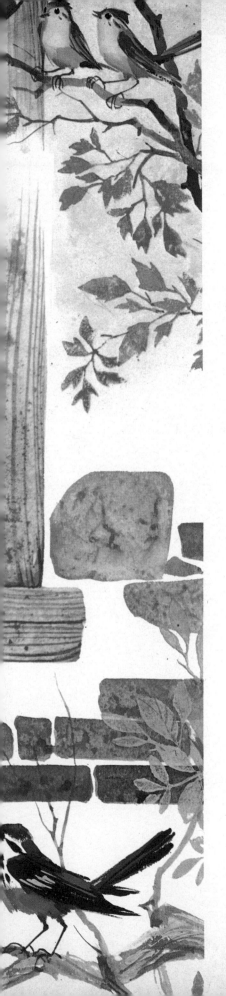

PUSS-IN-BOOTS

Once upon a time there was a miller who was so poor that when he died he had only three things to leave to his three sons. To the eldest son the miller left his mill. To the second son he left his hard-working donkey. But all he had to leave to his handsome youngest son was his cat.

"What good is a cat to me?" the youngest son sighed unhappily. "How will I ever make my fortune in the world?"

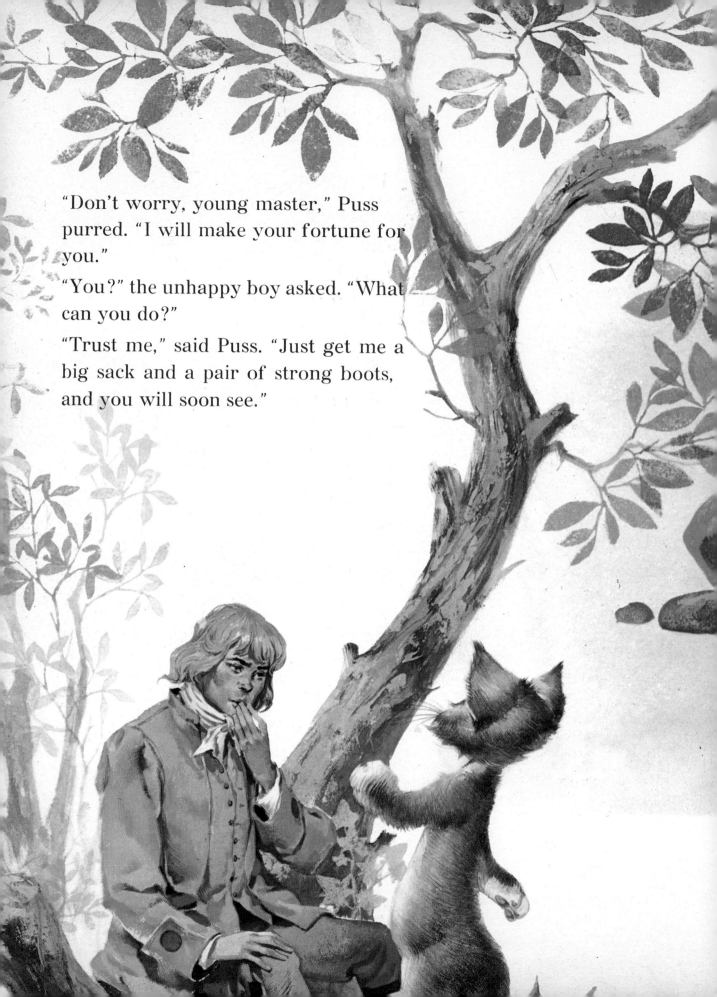

"Don't worry, young master," Puss purred. "I will make your fortune for you."

"You?" the unhappy boy asked. "What can you do?"

"Trust me," said Puss. "Just get me a big sack and a pair of strong boots, and you will soon see."

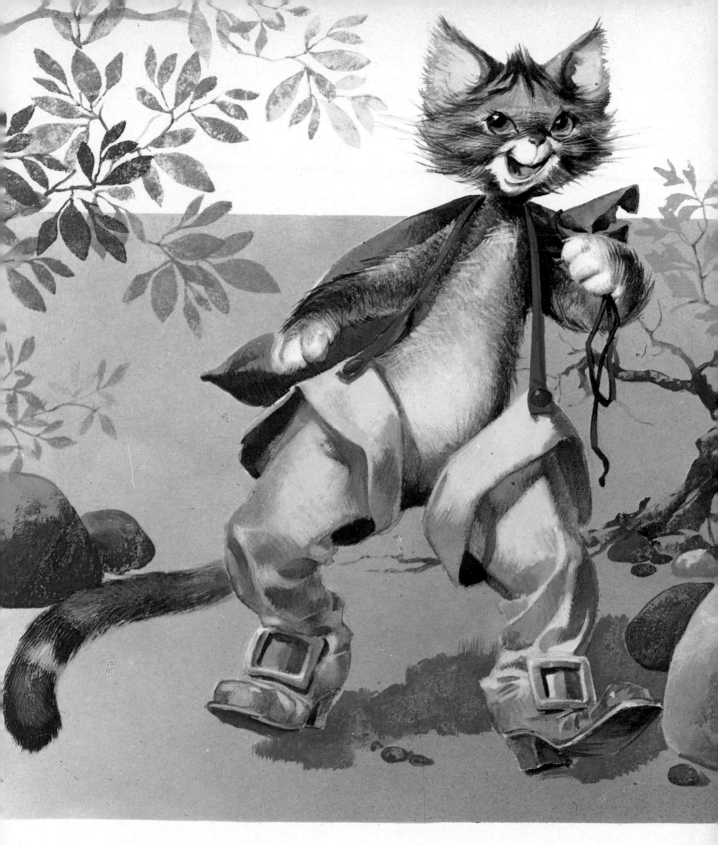

Still doubtful, the young man found a pair of boots and a
sack for his cat. In a few minutes Puss-In-Boots set out
through the forest to make his master's fortune.

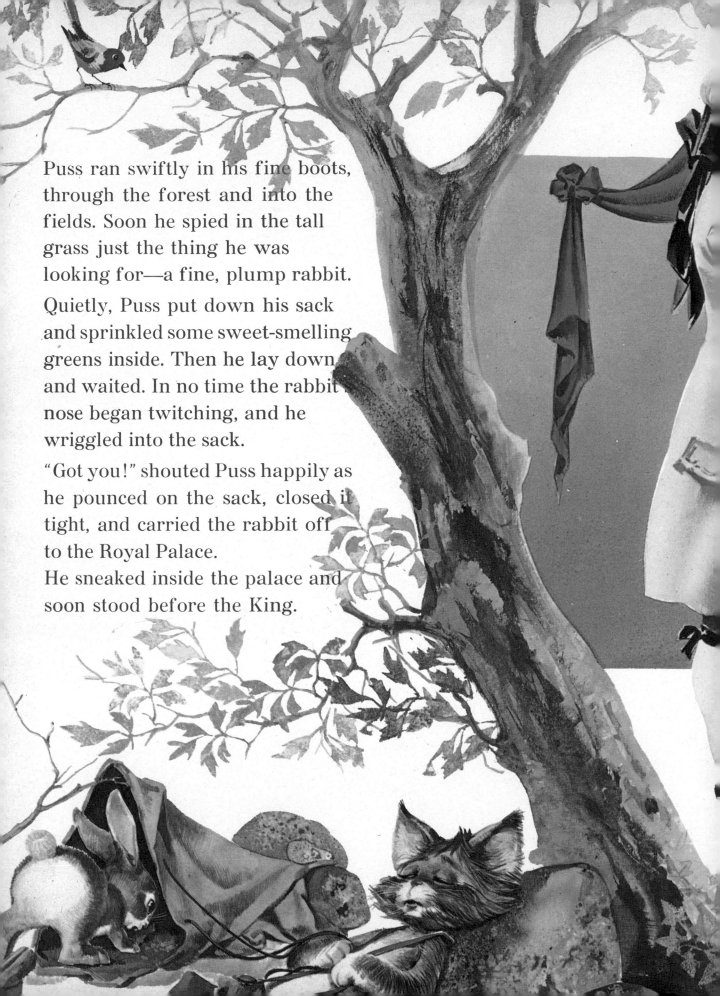

Puss ran swiftly in his fine boots,
through the forest and into the
fields. Soon he spied in the tall
grass just the thing he was
looking for—a fine, plump rabbit.

Quietly, Puss put down his sack
and sprinkled some sweet-smelling
greens inside. Then he lay down
and waited. In no time the rabbit
nose began twitching, and he
wriggled into the sack.

"Got you!" shouted Puss happily as
he pounced on the sack, closed it
tight, and carried the rabbit off
to the Royal Palace.
He sneaked inside the palace and
soon stood before the King.

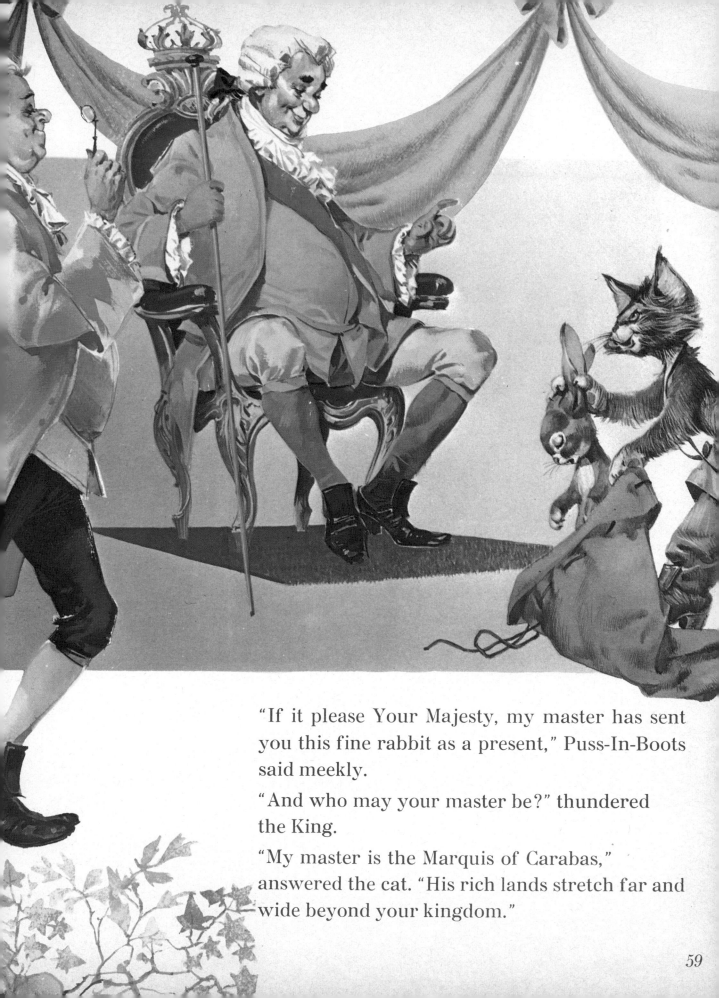

"If it please Your Majesty, my master has sent you this fine rabbit as a present," Puss-In-Boots said meekly.

"And who may your master be?" thundered the King.

"My master is the Marquis of Carabas," answered the cat. "His rich lands stretch far and wide beyond your kingdom."

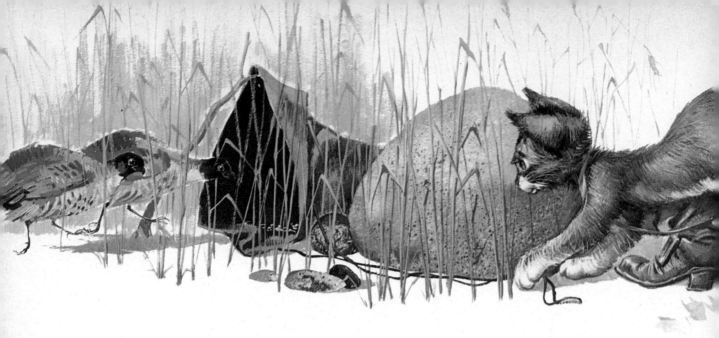

His Majesty was delighted, because kings enjoy presents just as much as ordinary people do. Every day after that, Puss stopped in to visit the King and share a goblet of royal cocoa. Every day he brought a different present—a pair of colorful pheasants, a dozen peacock eggs, or a fine speckled trout. And as he presented each to the King, he would announce loudly:

"I bring you this gift from my master, the Marquis of Carabas."

One morning Puss learned that the King and his beautiful daughter were setting out on a trip to visit neighboring kingdoms.

As soon as he heard the news, Puss rushed back to the mill to find his master.

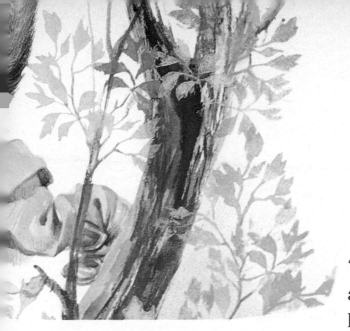

"Come quickly, master," he called and made the young man follow him to the riverbank.

"Now," said Puss, "take off your clothes and jump in the river."

"But why?" asked his master. "It's too cold to go swimming."

"Trust me," answered Puss.

So the young man threw off his shirt and jumped in. The frogs watched in astonishment as he shivvered in the cold water. Puss quickly hid his master's ragged shirt under a rock and then sat looking down the road.

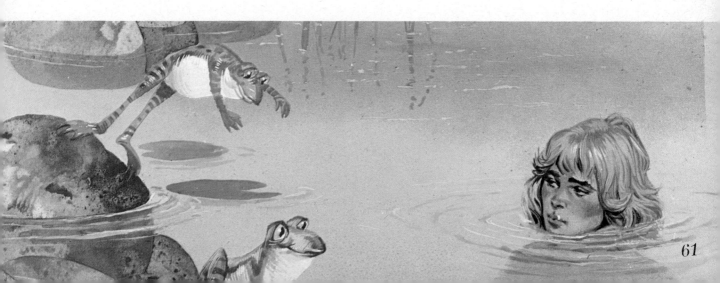

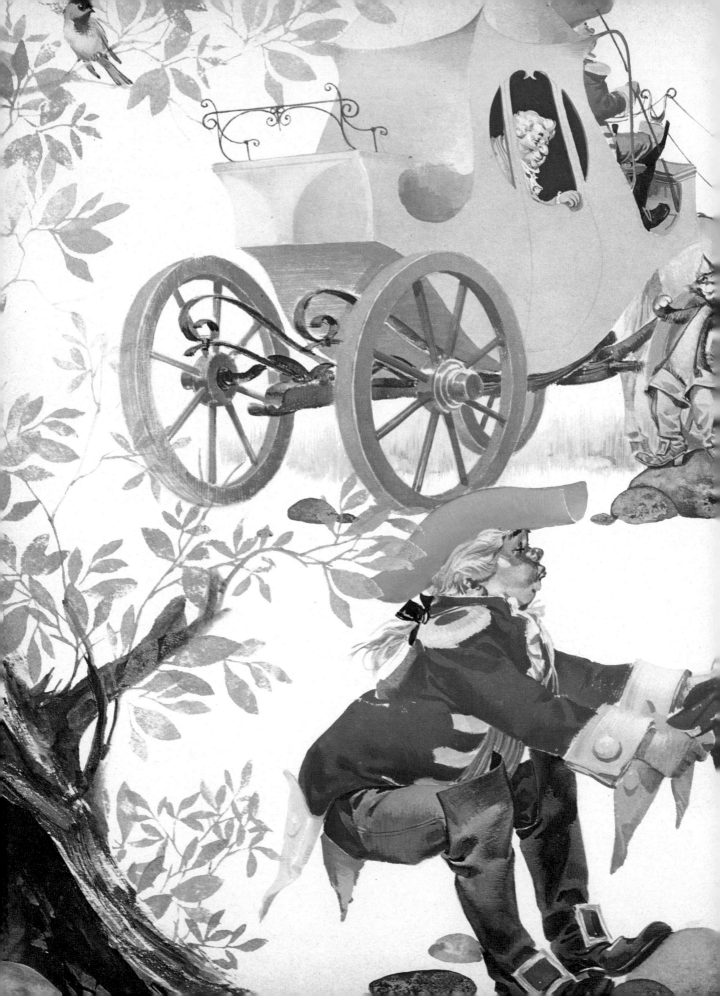

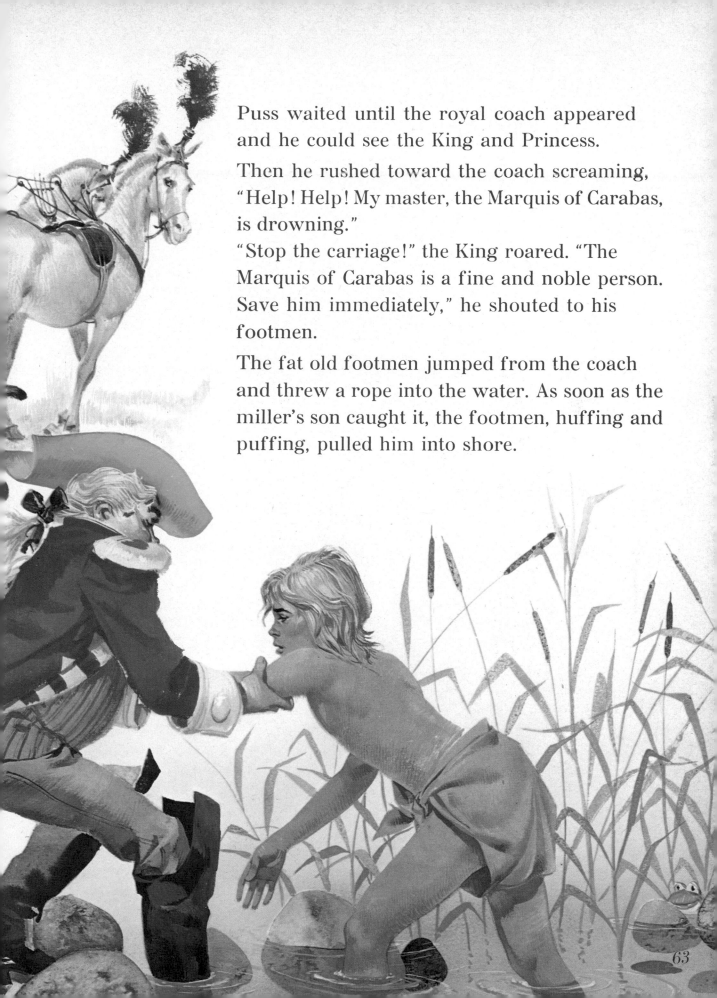

Puss waited until the royal coach appeared and he could see the King and Princess.

Then he rushed toward the coach screaming, "Help! Help! My master, the Marquis of Carabas, is drowning."

"Stop the carriage!" the King roared. "The Marquis of Carabas is a fine and noble person. Save him immediately," he shouted to his footmen.

The fat old footmen jumped from the coach and threw a rope into the water. As soon as the miller's son caught it, the footmen, huffing and puffing, pulled him into shore.

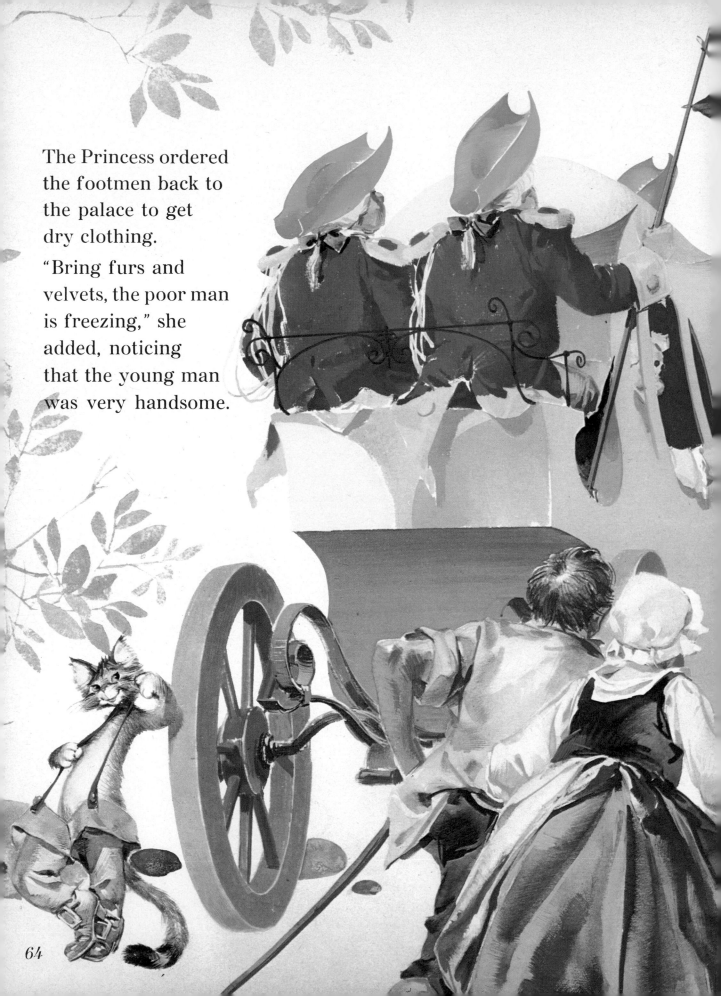

The Princess ordered the footmen back to the palace to get dry clothing.

"Bring furs and velvets, the poor man is freezing," she added, noticing that the young man was very handsome.

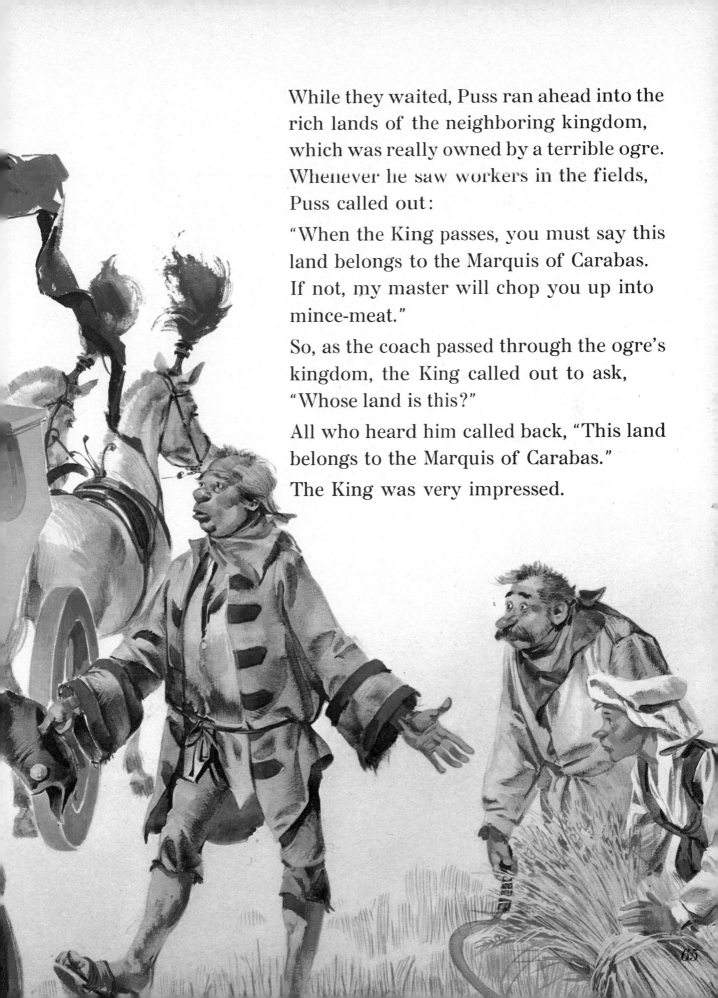

While they waited, Puss ran ahead into the rich lands of the neighboring kingdom, which was really owned by a terrible ogre. Whenever he saw workers in the fields, Puss called out:

"When the King passes, you must say this land belongs to the Marquis of Carabas. If not, my master will chop you up into mince-meat."

So, as the coach passed through the ogre's kingdom, the King called out to ask, "Whose land is this?"

All who heard him called back, "This land belongs to the Marquis of Carabas."

The King was very impressed.

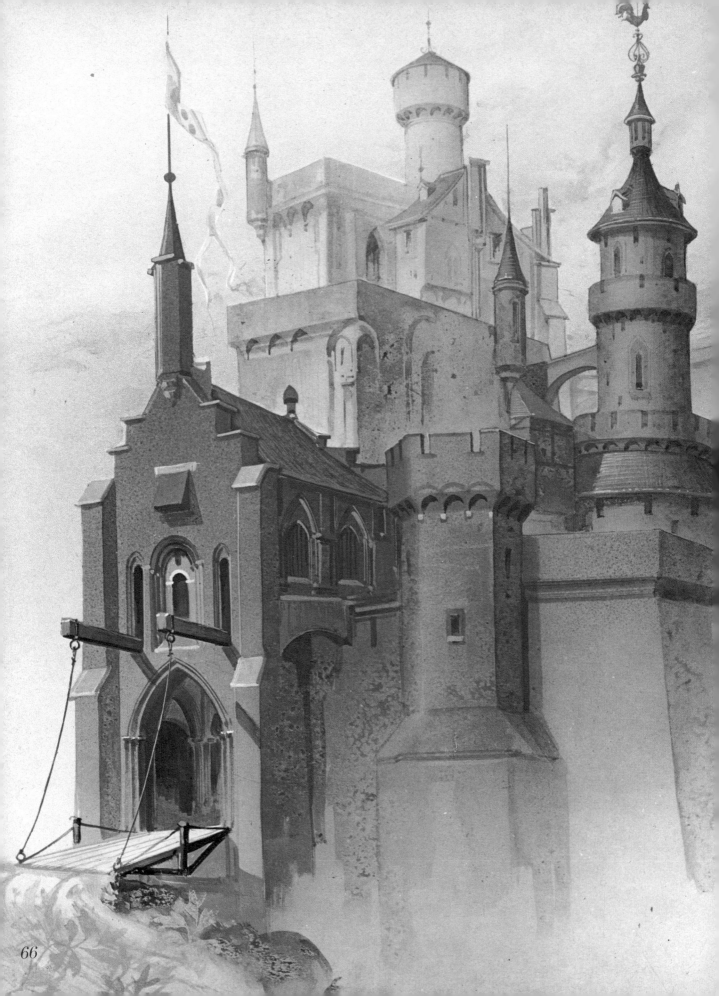

Meanwhile Puss rushed ahead to the castle of the rich ogre. He smiled sweetly when he stood before the terrible fellow, for he had a shrewd plan.

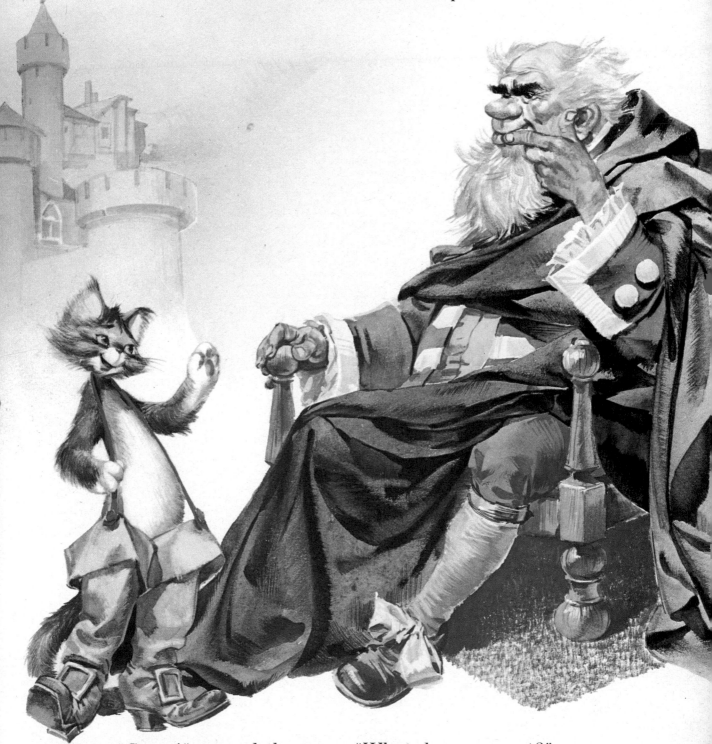

"Grrrr!" roared the ogre. "What do you want?"

"I've heard you can change yourself into a lion. Can you really?" Puss asked slyly.

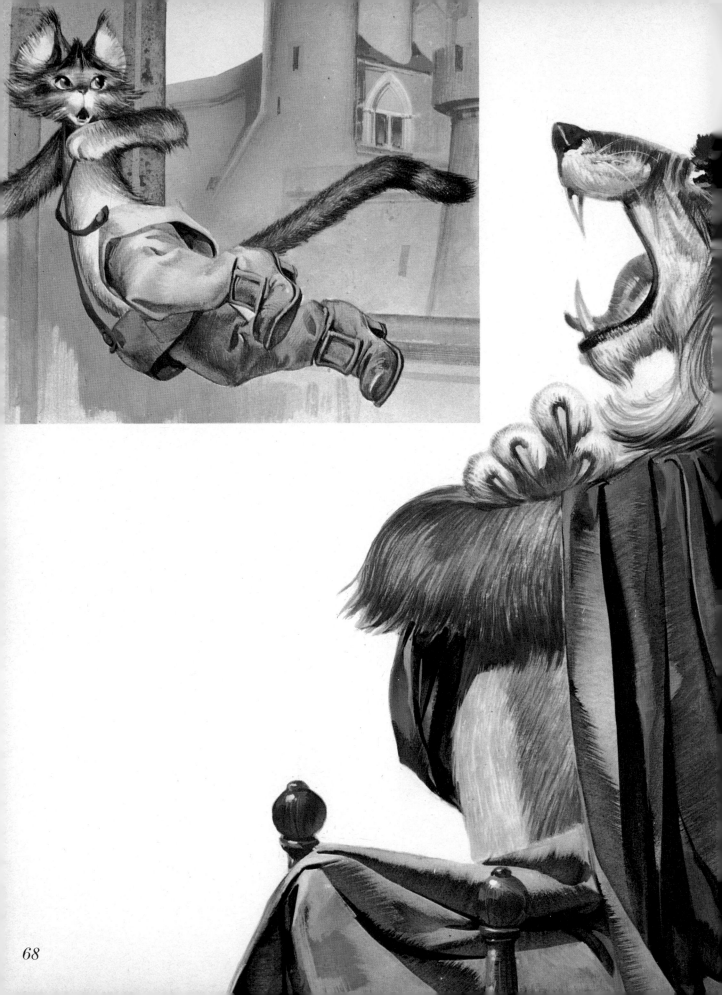

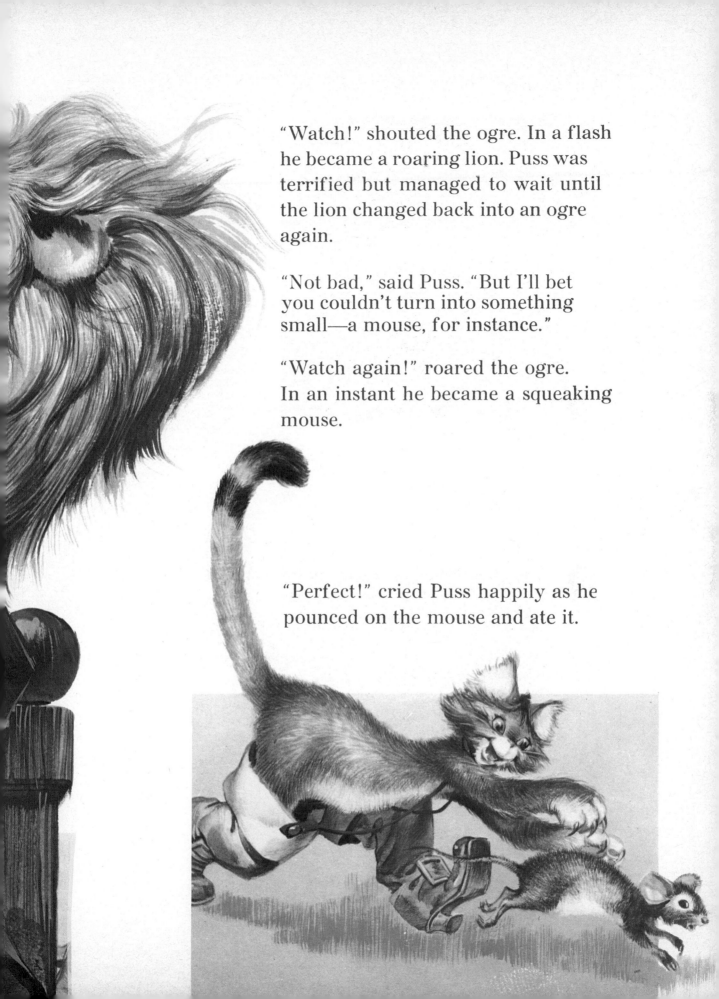

"Watch!" shouted the ogre. In a flash he became a roaring lion. Puss was terrified but managed to wait until the lion changed back into an ogre again.

"Not bad," said Puss. "But I'll bet you couldn't turn into something small—a mouse, for instance."

"Watch again!" roared the ogre. In an instant he became a squeaking mouse.

"Perfect!" cried Puss happily as he pounced on the mouse and ate it.

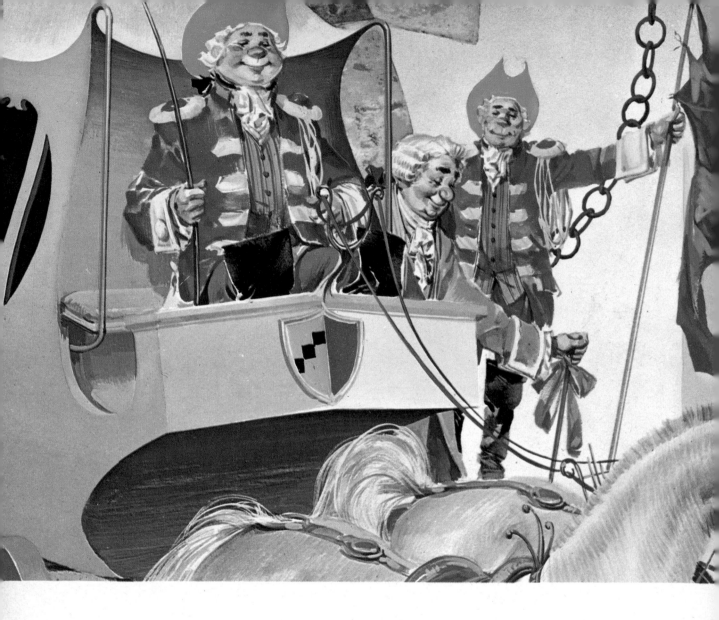

At that moment the royal coach was approaching the castle. During the ride, the King had decided that the Marquis of Carabas was a very rich man, and the golden-haired Princess had discovered that she was in love with the handsome lad, and he with her.

When Puss heard the coach, he rushed to the castle gate.

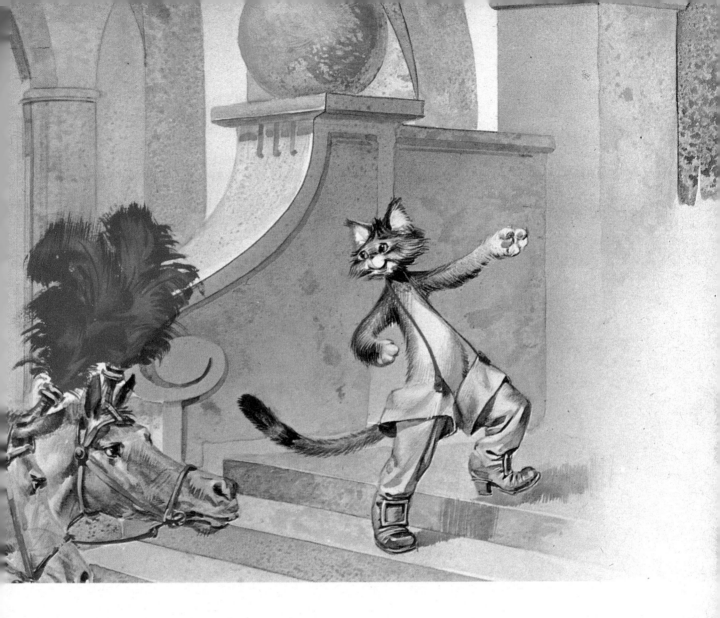

"Welcome, Your Majesties," he said breathlessly.

Then he turned to the miller's son and winked at him.

"Welcome home, my master, Marquis of Carabas," he said proudly. "Your banquet is waiting."

So with Puss leading the way, the royal party entered the ogre's castle, which now belonged to the miller's son.

As the royal guests enjoyed themselves at the splendid banquet which had been prepared for the ogre and his friends, the King announced joyfully:

"My daughter, the Princess, and the Marquis of Carabas will be married in two days!"

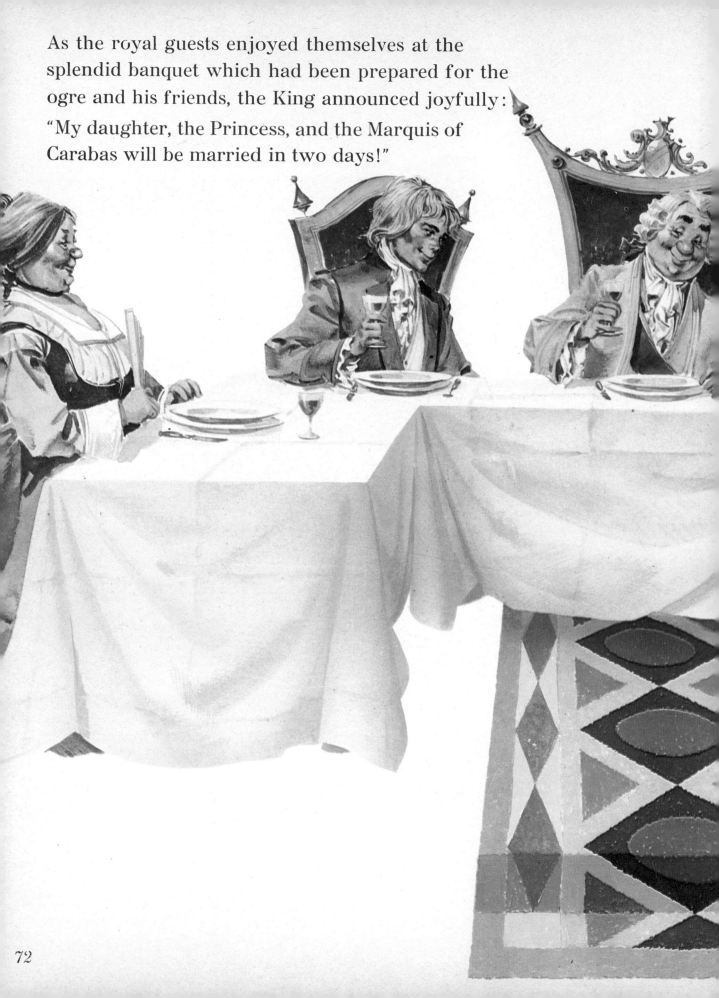

After the wedding the beautiful princess and the miller's son, now the rich Marquis of Carabas, sailed away on their honeymoon. Of course, they took along their faithful friend, Puss-In-Boots. And all three lived happily ever after.

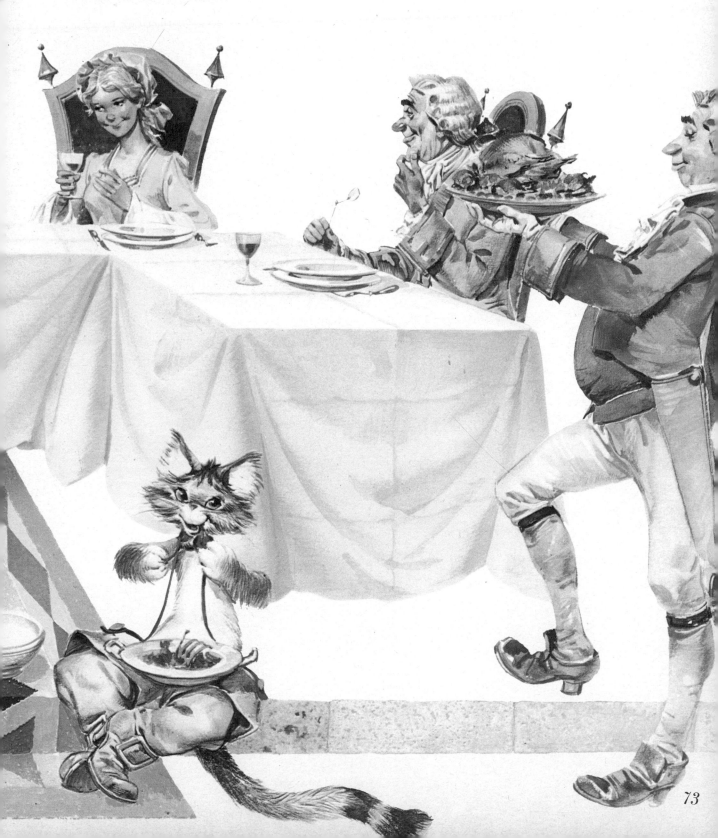

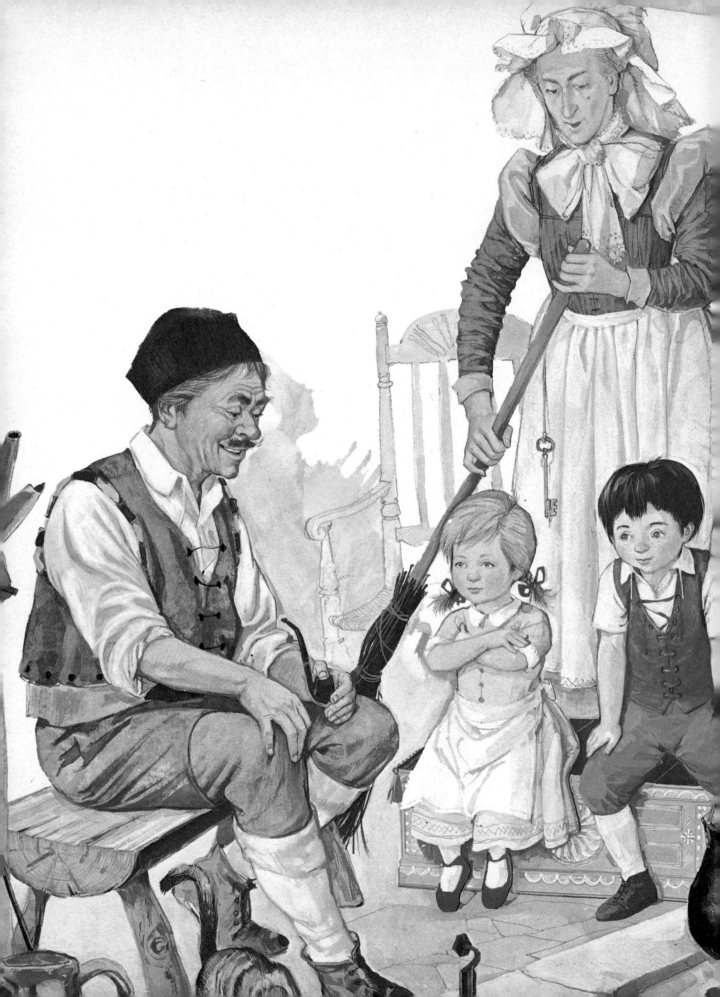

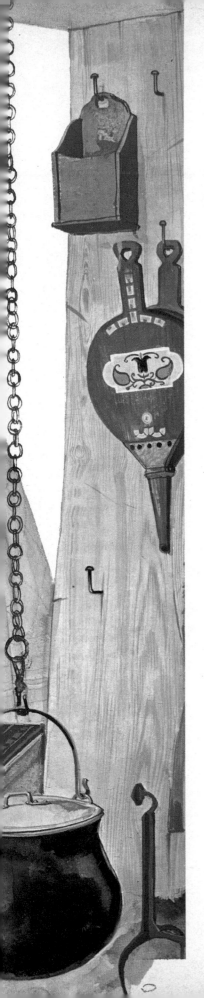

HANSEL AND GRETEL

Once upon a time a poor woodcutter lived on the edge of a dark forest with his little son and daughter, Hansel and Gretel, and a new wife. His first wife had died many years before, and his second was unfortunately a cruel and hardhearted woman who cared nothing for her stepchildren. The poor man tried hard to support his family, but somehow all his efforts failed. The children loved their father and tried not to complain when they were cold and hungry, but the stepmother endlessly blamed her husband for all their misfortunes.

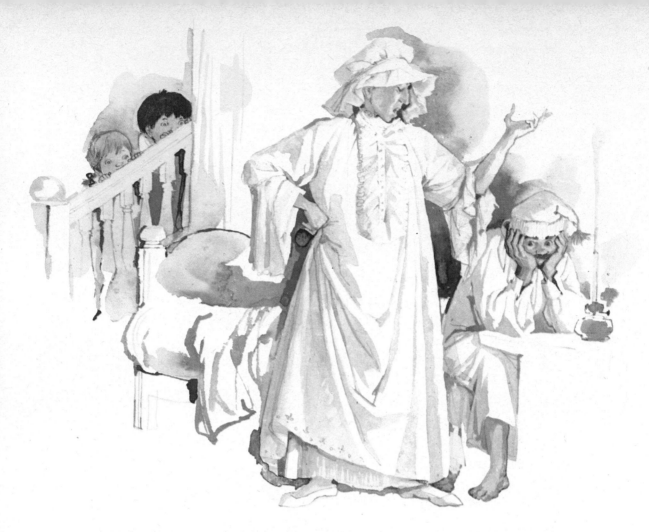

One night when Hansel and Gretel had gone to bed
hungrier than ever, their father, thinking them asleep,
admitted to his wife that the family was penniless and
would soon die of starvation.

"There's only one thing to do, husband," she said harshly,
not knowing the children heard every word. "We must
take those children of yours deep into the forest and
leave them there. Then we shall only have ourselves to feed."
The woodcutter was horrified at her cruelty, but she
nagged him without ceasing, so that finally the poor man
had to give in.

Gretel sobbed in her bed, but Hansel comforted her and
promised to care for her always. As soon as his parents
were asleep, Hansel tiptoed into the garden and filled his
pockets with glistening white pebbles, and then he crept
back into bed again.

The next morning they ate only dry bread for breakfast,
and then all of them set out for the forest to gather
kindling wood. Hansel walked behind his parents,
carefully dropping the little white pebbles, one by one,
to mark a path to find his way home again.

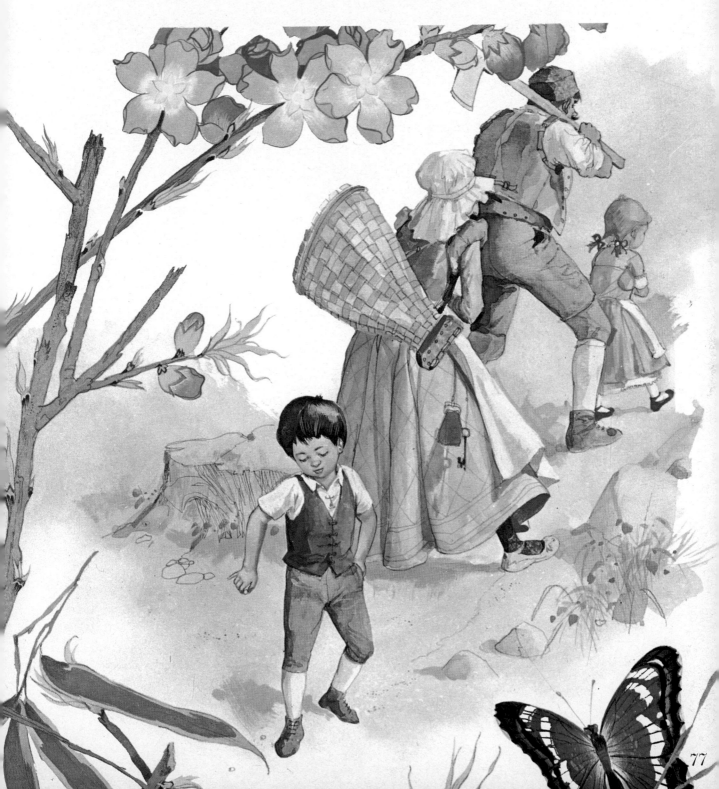

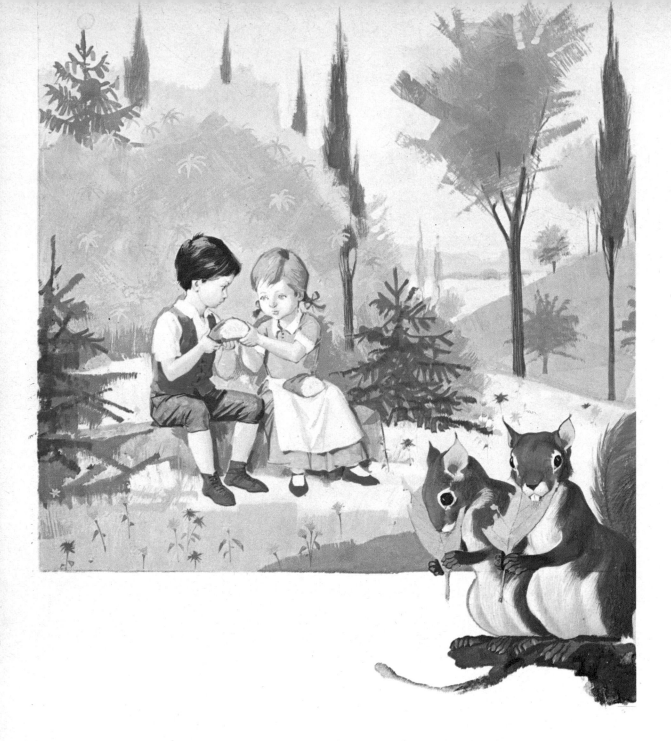

Deep in the forest their father made a little fire of brush
for the children and told them to rest by it to keep warm
while he and their stepmother went to find bigger logs.
The warmth of the fire made the children very drowsy,
and soon they fell asleep. When they woke, it was nearly
dark and only a pale moon shone through the treetops.
Gretel began to cry, but Hansel soothed her gently.

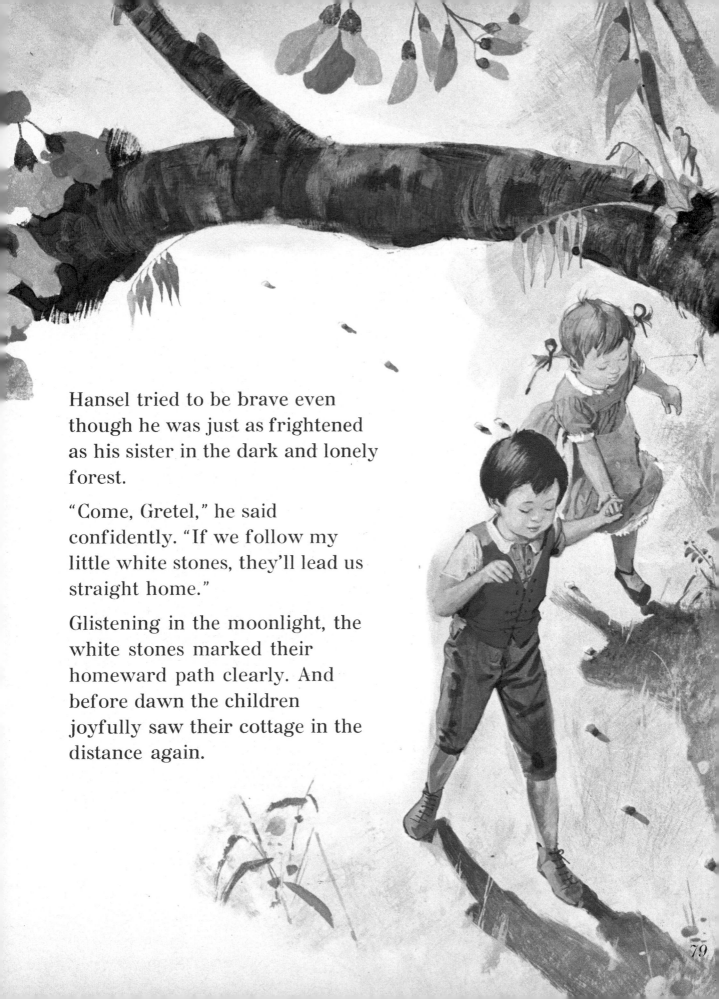

Hansel tried to be brave even though he was just as frightened as his sister in the dark and lonely forest.

"Come, Gretel," he said confidently. "If we follow my little white stones, they'll lead us straight home."

Glistening in the moonlight, the white stones marked their homeward path clearly. And before dawn the children joyfully saw their cottage in the distance again.

Their father rejoiced and embraced them and shared his morning crust. But their stepmother only scolded them for their lateness, and afterward nagged her husband to go into the forest again the next day with the children to lose them. Once again she forced him to agree.

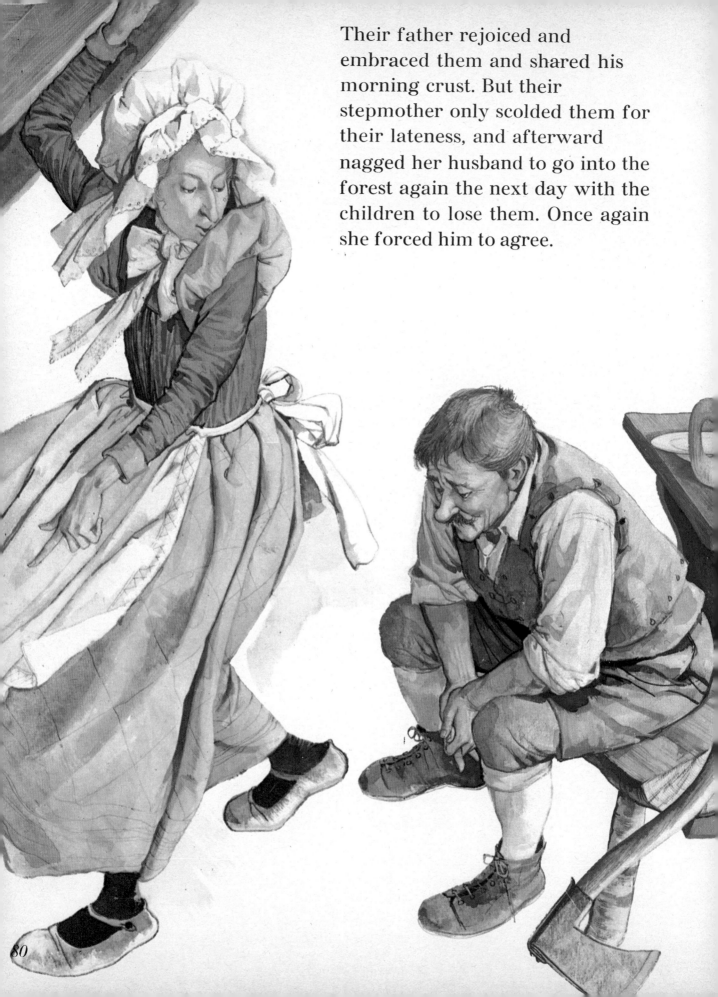

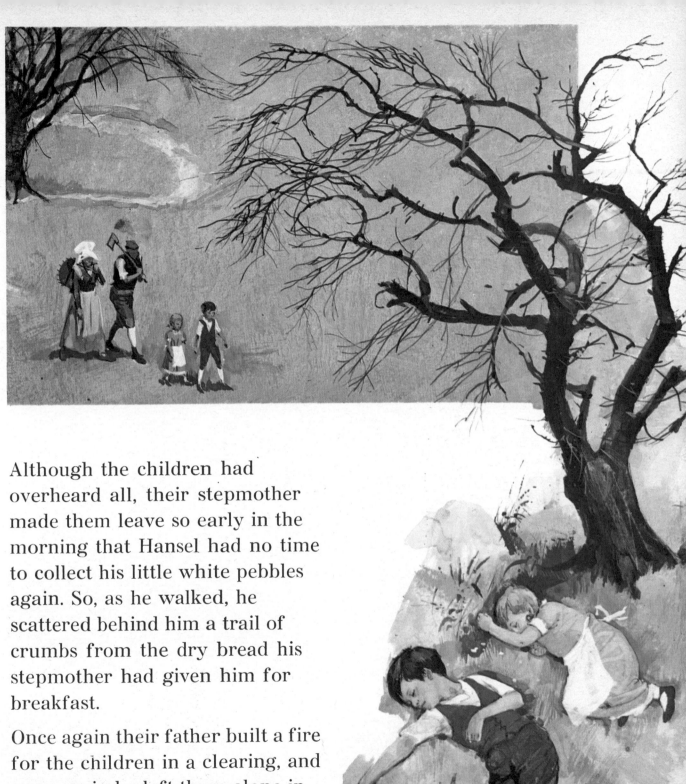

Although the children had overheard all, their stepmother made them leave so early in the morning that Hansel had no time to collect his little white pebbles again. So, as he walked, he scattered behind him a trail of crumbs from the dry bread his stepmother had given him for breakfast.

Once again their father built a fire for the children in a clearing, and once again he left them alone in the forest, where they were soon fast asleep.

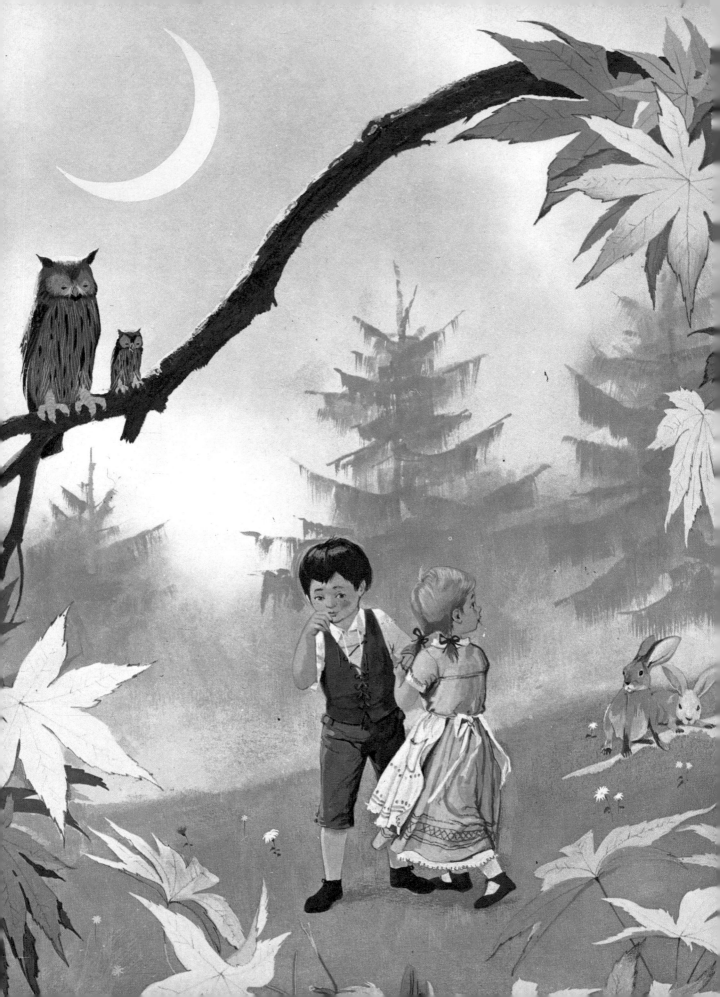

When they woke, night had already fallen and pale moonlight peeked through the trees. But this time it did not light the path of crumbs Hansel had made in the morning, because the path had vanished. The birds had feasted on his trail of breadcrumbs, and not a morsel was left. First they tried one path and then another, but each one led them deeper and deeper into the forest. Soon Hansel knew they were hopelessly lost and tried as best he could to comfort his little sister—even though he badly needed comforting himself.

"Don't worry, Gretel," he said bravely. "We'll find our way home easily in the morning, when it's light."

"But I'm very hungry," sobbed his sister.

"So am I," Hansel replied. "But I'm sure we'll find some nuts or sweet berries in the morning."

"I'm tired, too. I want to sleep in my own bed," Gretel went on, crying harder.

"So do I," Hansel answered. "But this moss is just as soft, so lie down here with me and we'll be safe and warm."

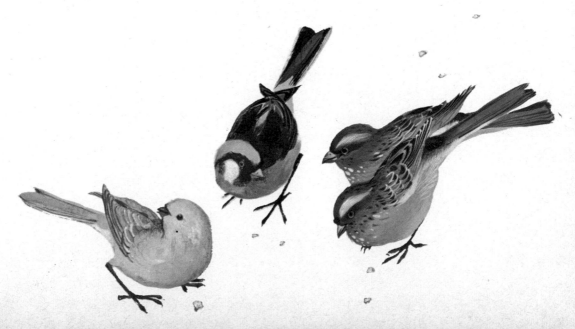

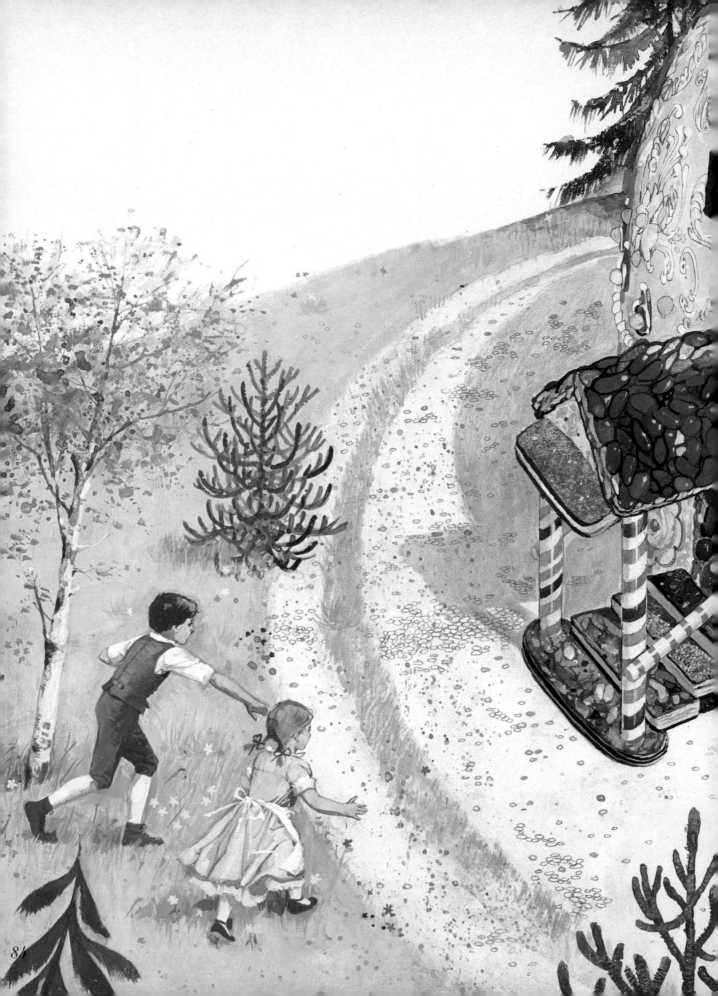

84

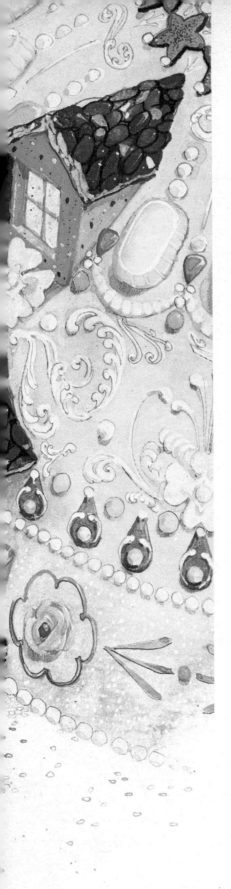

The children slept peacefully on their mossy bed, but the next morning they found they were just as lost in the daylight as in the dark and were hungrier than ever. They immediately set out to find berries, and since the little forest birds always know where the best berries grow, the children followed them and soon were able to eat their fill of sweet, juicy fruit.

As they were eating, Hansel and Gretel noticed that one little white bird was not picking berries like the others, but sat on a branch and seemed to sing out especially for them. When the song was over, the bird flew away—but he soared through the air so slowly that the children were able to follow him. Finally he led them to a clearing in the woods, where they found the most wonderful house they had ever seen. The roof was made of sugared gingerbread, the walls of marvelous little cakes frosted together, the windowpanes were crystal sugar, and the doorway was made of jelly beans and had candycane pillars. With cries of delight, the children broke off little pieces of the sweets and were munching them happily when the door opened and a little old lady appeared to see who was nibbling away at her house.

"Poor hungry darlings," she cried. "Come inside, and I'll give you some real nourishing food."

She led the children into her cosy little sugar-cake cottage and prepared a delicious breakfast of pancakes smothered in butter and syrup, with apples and nuts for dessert and as much milk as they could drink. Then she tucked them into clean, warm beds for a morning nap.

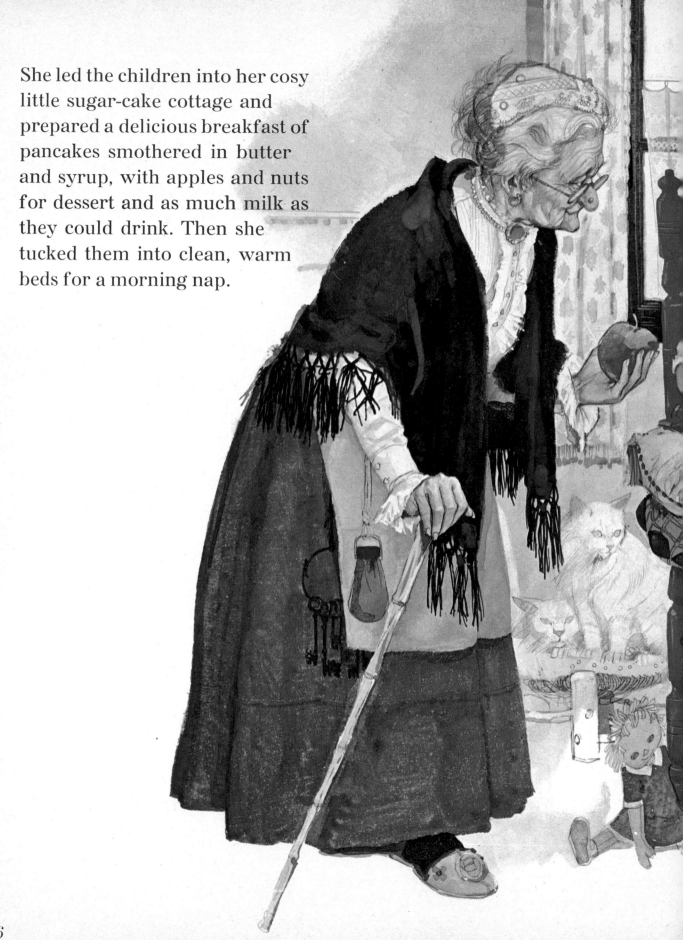

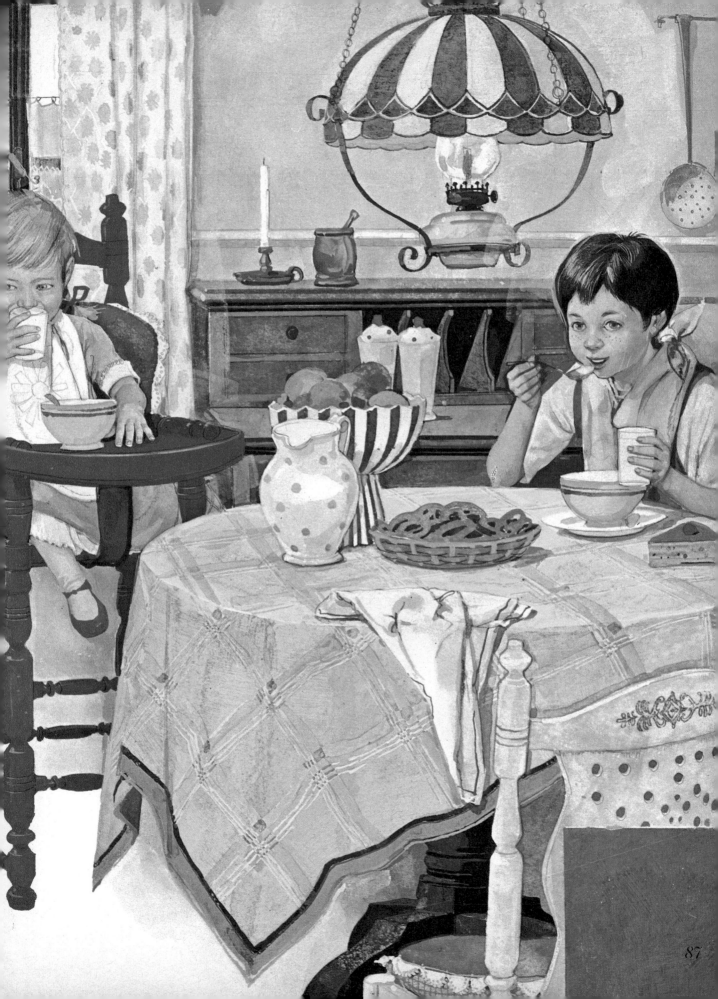

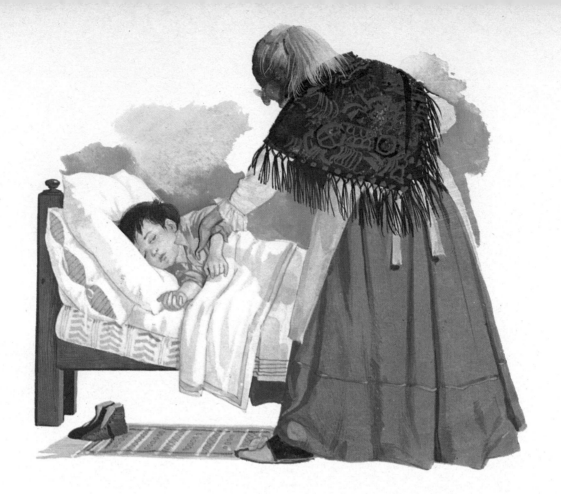

Feeling happy and safe at last, the children slept soundly, little knowing that the little old lady was really a witch who had built the delicious house covered with sweets to entrap little children.

When Hansel and Gretel awoke, instead of the kind old lady, they saw a fearful hag with a long hooked nose, cruel beady eyes, and scruffy hair. She grabbed Hansel and dragged him to her cellar, where she locked him in a cage and then ordered Gretel to bring him rich foods and lots of creamy milk to drink.

"Feed him well," cackled the witch. "And when he's nice and plump, I'll eat him for my dinner! As for you, dear child, bread and water is good enough until it's your turn to be fattened. No use wasting good food."

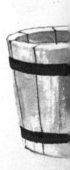

Every day the witch came to see how plump Hansel was getting.

"Are you fat enough yet, little boy?" she kept asking. "Stick out a finger and let me squeeze it."

But Hansel had a trick of his own. Knowing that the witch had poor eyesight, he stuck a dry bone through the bars of his cage, and she would squeeze the bone thinking it was one of his fingers.

"Curses!" the witch would scream. "This child gets thinner every day!"

Finally, one morning she lost her patience entirely and decided to eat Hansel that very evening.

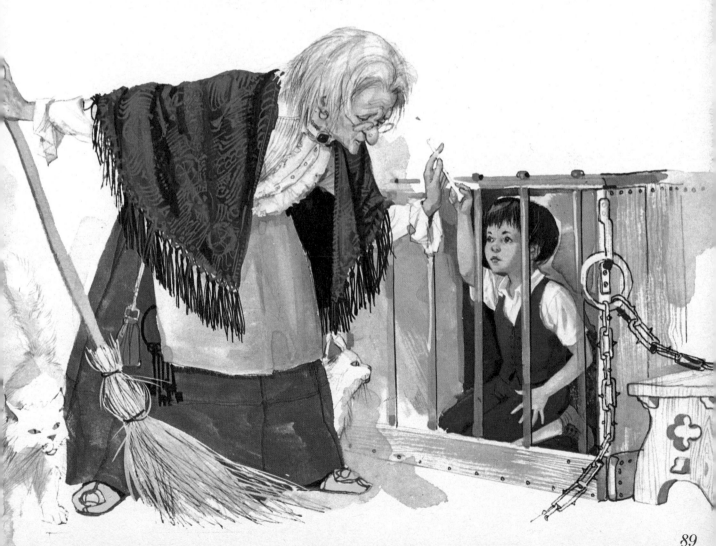

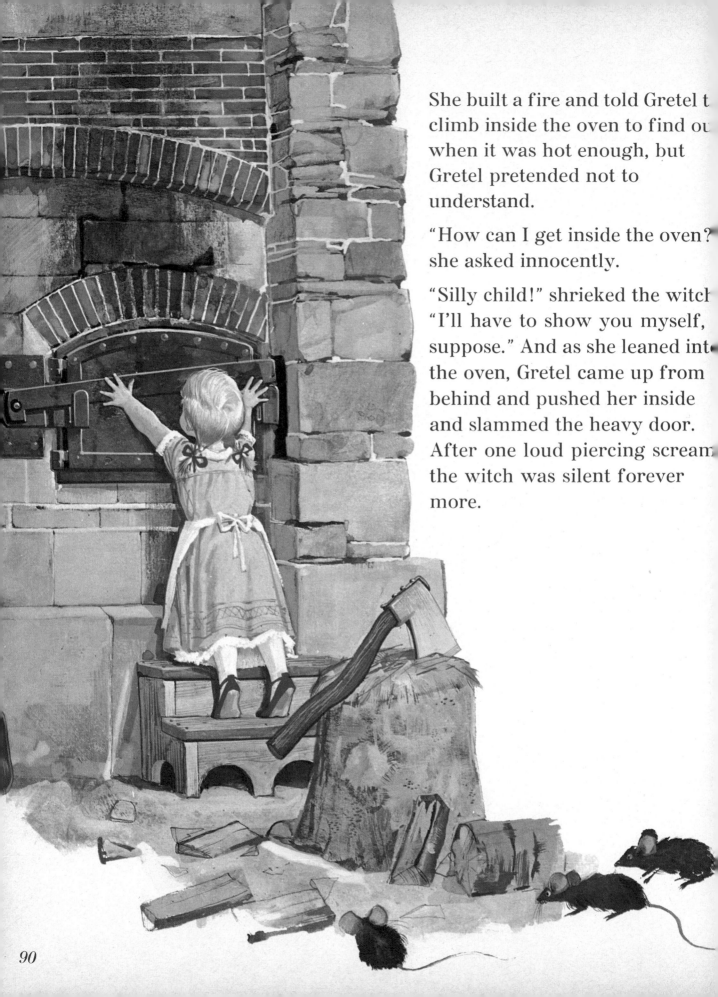

She built a fire and told Gretel t
climb inside the oven to find ou
when it was hot enough, but
Gretel pretended not to
understand.

"How can I get inside the oven?
she asked innocently.

"Silly child!" shrieked the witcl
"I'll have to show you myself,
suppose." And as she leaned int
the oven, Gretel came up from
behind and pushed her inside
and slammed the heavy door.
After one loud piercing scream
the witch was silent forever
more.

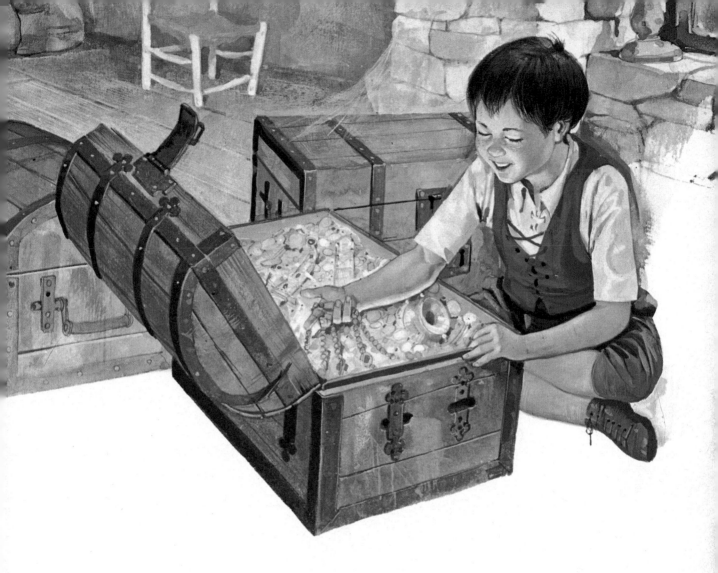

Quickly Gretel ran to the cellar to free her brother. They hugged each other joyfully and then ran through the house, searching for all the witch's treasure. In the attic were chests of gold and silver and caskets of jewels. Hansel stuffed his pockets, and Gretel filled her apron till neither could carry any more.

"Now we can go home to our beloved father," they cried happily to each other. "And we need never be hungry again."

Before they left the cottage, they peeked fearfully inside the oven. But all that was left of the wicked old witch was one big, hard-baked gingerbread cookie.

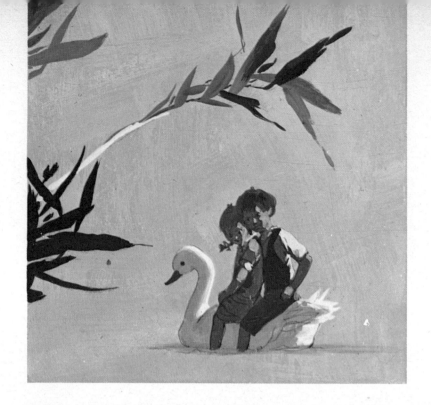

"We'd better get out of this enchanted forest before another witch or ogre catches us," said Hansel to Gretel.

They ran till they came to a broad lake where a white duck was swimming.

"Beautiful white bird," they cried, "will you carry us across?"

"Gladly," said the duck.

The children climbed on her back, and she took them to the other side of the lake, where they found a familiar-looking path. They rushed along the pathway and soon saw that it led straight to their father's cottage, much to their joy.

The poor woodcutter was astonished and happy to see his lost children once more, and since their cruel stepmother had died while they were gone, all of them could now live peacefully together. The gold and silver and jewels the children brought with them from the witch's house kept them in comfort for many years, and they were never hungry or cold or homeless again.

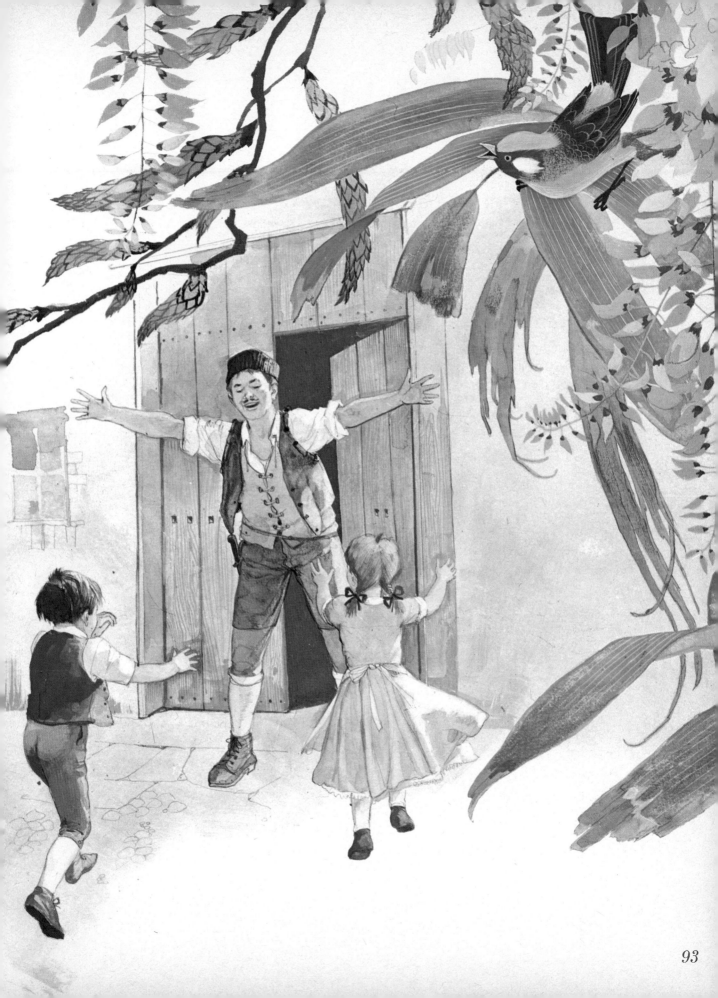

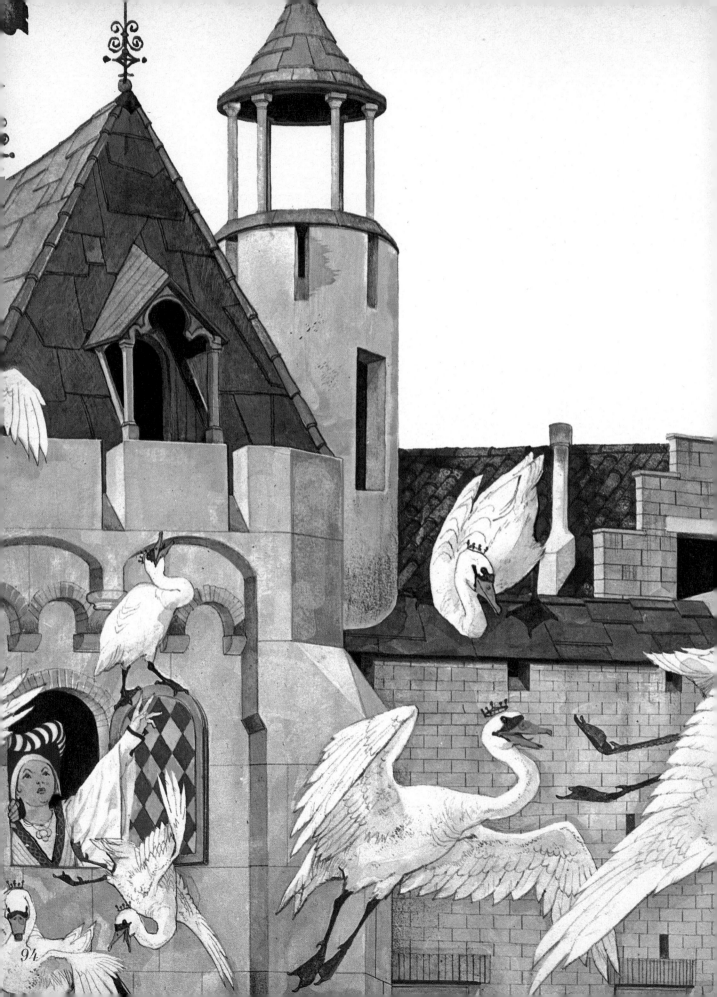

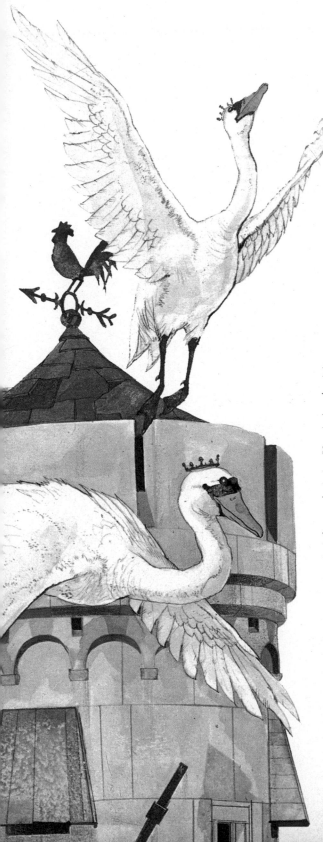

THE WILD SWANS

Once upon a time, in a faraway land, an aging king lived with his eleven sons and only daughter, Elisa. Although his queen had long since died, he tried to bring up the princes to be strong and fearless and the little princess to be kind and generous. They all lived together happily in their castle.

But one day the king married again, unaware that his new wife was a dangerous witch. From the very day of the royal wedding, the new queen hated her stepchildren and wanted only to be rid of them.

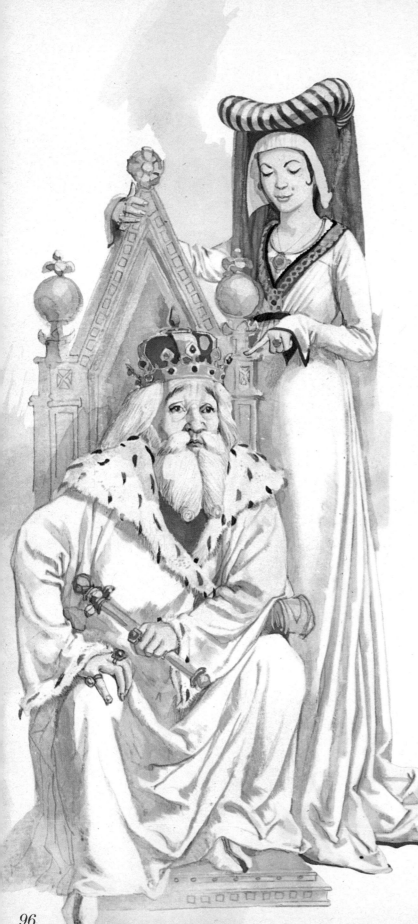

The evil queen soon devised a cruel spell and cast it over her eleven stepsons. Overnight they were changed into eleven wild swans wearing little gold coronets. But the queen was not satisfied at that.

"Fly away!" she shrieked. "I command you! Fly far beyond the borders of our kingdom and never come back!"

The eleven swans flew off, but the queen still was not satisfied until she had also banished the gentle Elisa to live with a poor woodcutter at the farthest edge of the forest. When the old king asked for his children, the wicked queen replied:

"Your sons are good-for-nothings and have gone off to find some mischief to do, and your daughter never wants to see you again."

Elisa lived for years with the woodcutter's family but never forgot her brothers. And when she was fifteen, she set off to search for them.

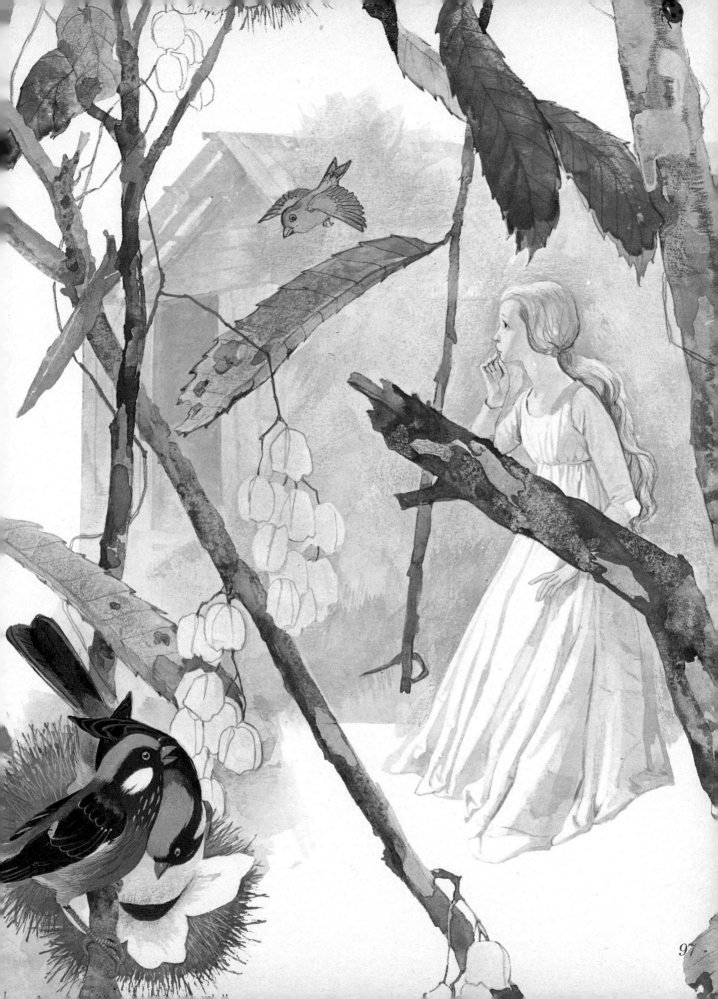

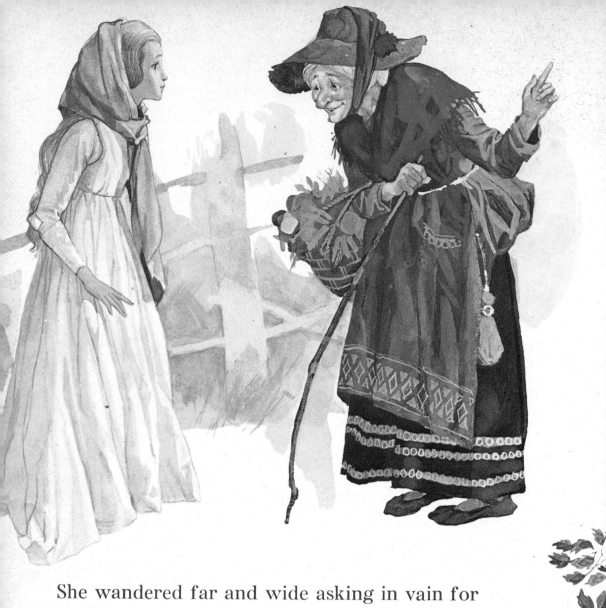

She wandered far and wide asking in vain for
her brothers, but one day she happened to ask
an old woman gathering herbs near the sea.

"I have not seen your brothers," the woman
replied. "But I have seen eleven wild swans with
golden crowns on their heads."

"Where? Oh, please tell me!" cried Elisa.

"There! On the beach," said the old woman.
"They come in from the sea every evening."

Elisa ran to the shore and sat watching the sky
till evening. Finally she heard a great fluttering
of wings, and toward her flew eleven wild swans.

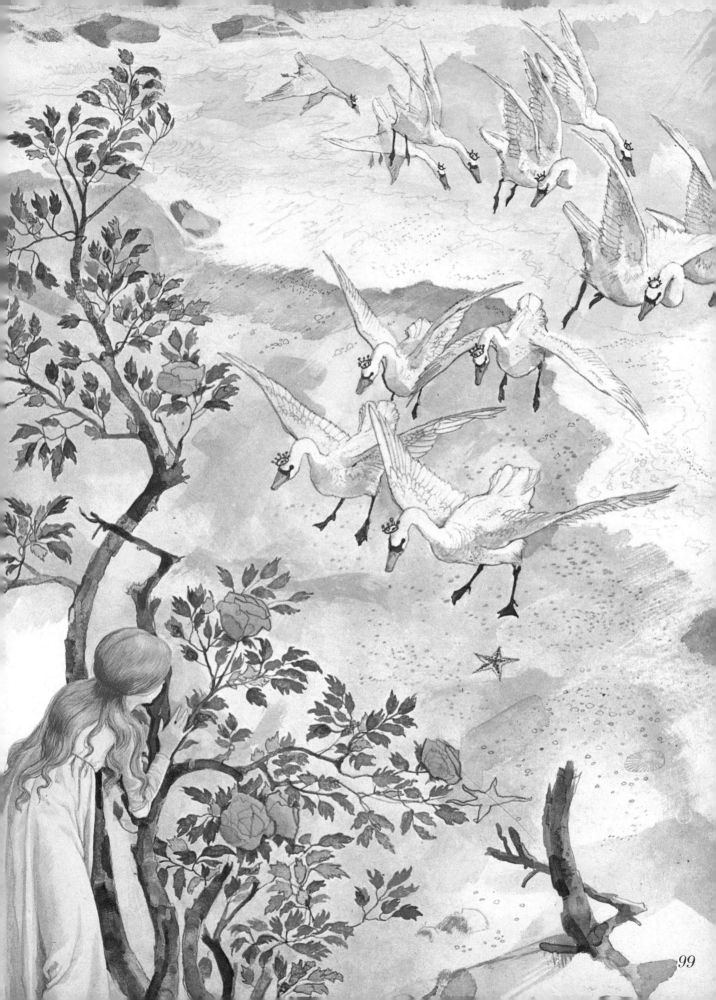

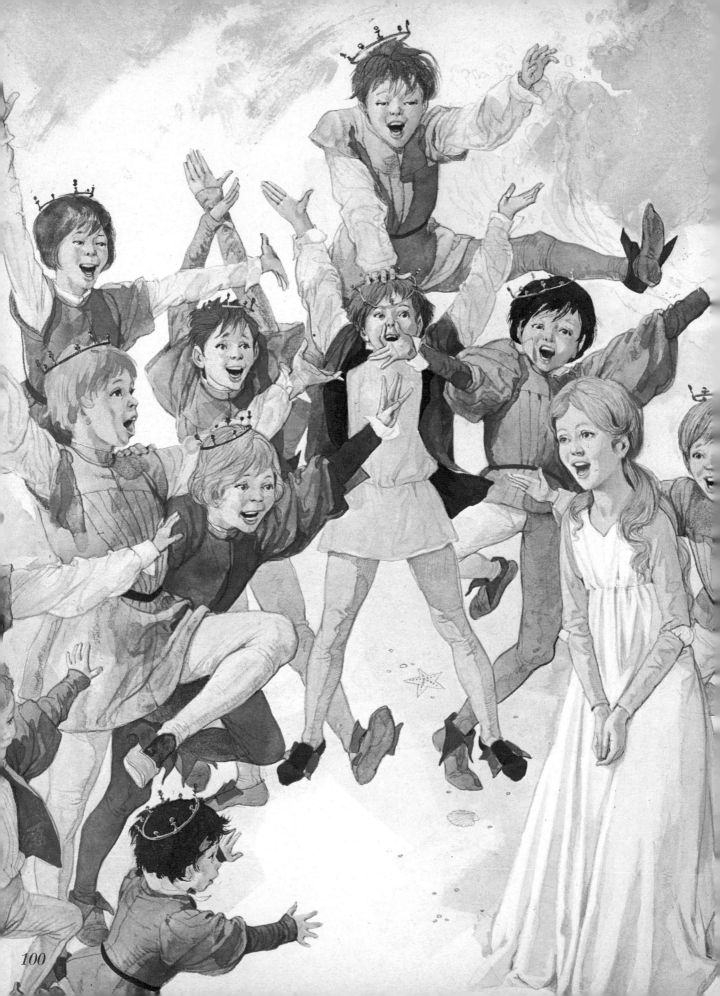

Elisa ran to them crying, "My brothers! I have found you at last!"

The swans joyfully recognized their sister, and just as the last rays of the sun disappeared they turned into the brothers she had loved so well.

"We must go about as swans from sunrise to sunset," they explained. "But after dusk we can again appear in our human form."

"Tell me everything," begged Elisa. "Where do you live?"

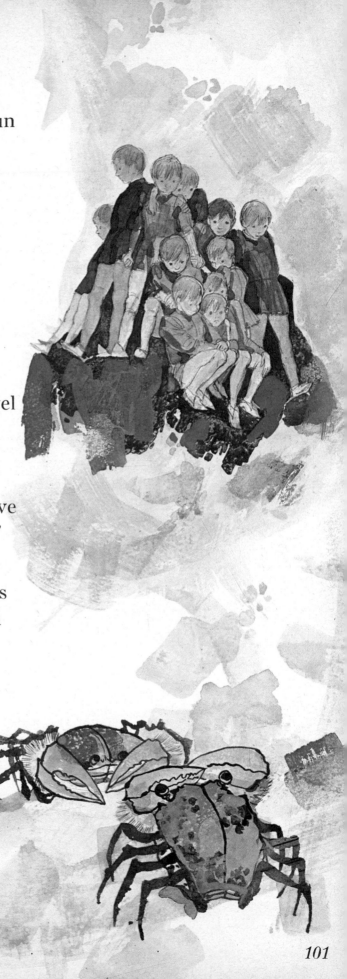

"Far away, dear sister," they answered. "To reach our new home, we must travel for two long days to the other side of the great sea. We rest for the night in our human shapes on a rock in the middle of the ocean, and the next day we fly on to our beautiful new homeland."

The brothers explained sadly that they were only allowed to visit their father's kingdom once each year, and only for a few days. Elisa wept when she heard that in just two days they must leave.

"Then take me with you," she sobbed.

At first her brothers refused her plea.

"It's too far," they said, "and too dangerous."

Finally Elisa persuaded them that, now that they had found each other at last, they must never be parted again.

"We'll make a net," they decided, "and carry her in it."

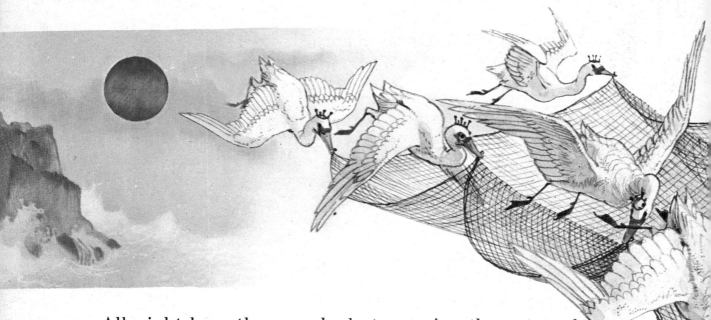

All night long they worked at weaving the net, and before dawn it was ready. At the first rays of sunlight, the eleven princes again became eleven swans. Elisa jumped into the net, and the swans flew off, carrying her with them high over land and sea. They crossed over oceans and rivers, castles and cities, and even flew across the marvelous realm of fairyland, where the good fairy Morgana was queen. Finally, they arrived at their distant homeland and gently laid Elisa down to sleep.

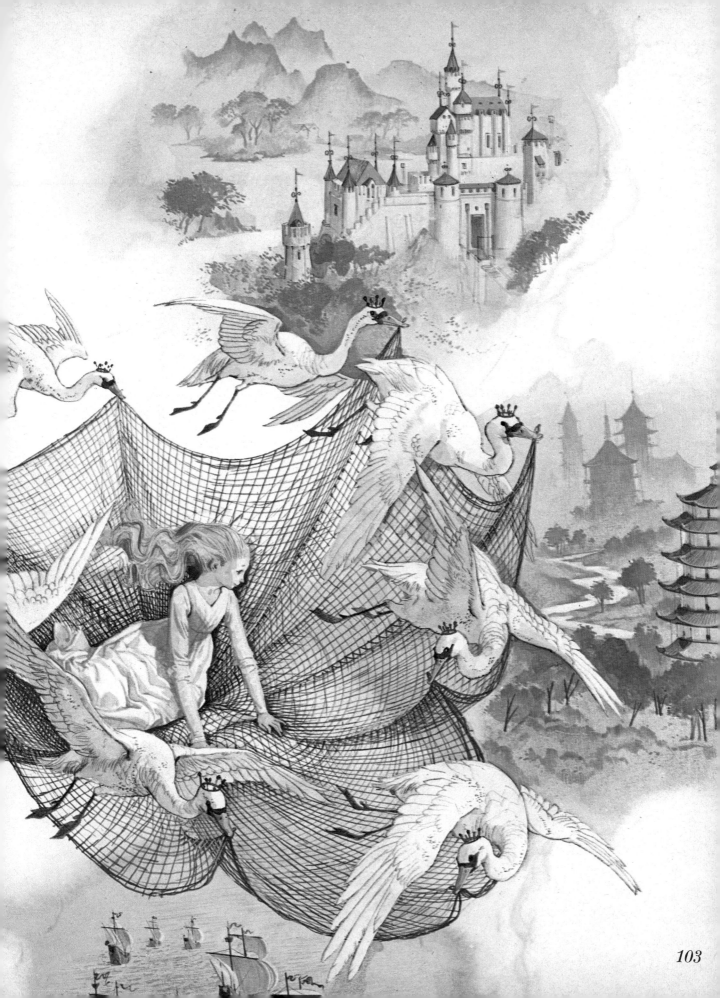

As Elisa slept, she dreamed she crossed the borders of fairyland once more and that Queen Morgana came to speak to her.

"I know, Elisa," said Morgana, "that your dearest wish is to release your brothers from the terrible spell cast over them."

"Oh, yes!" cried Elisa. "If I only knew how!"

"It will not be easy," answered the fairy queen. "You will have much pain and suffering before you succeed."

"I don't care how much I suffer," cried Elisa, "if I can free my brothers."

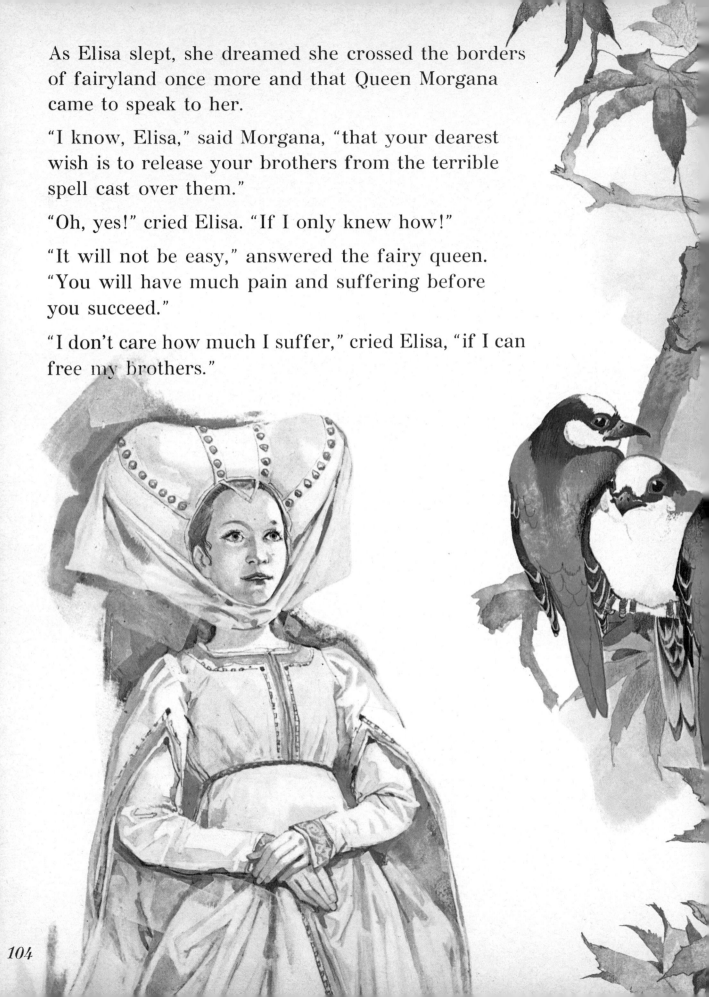

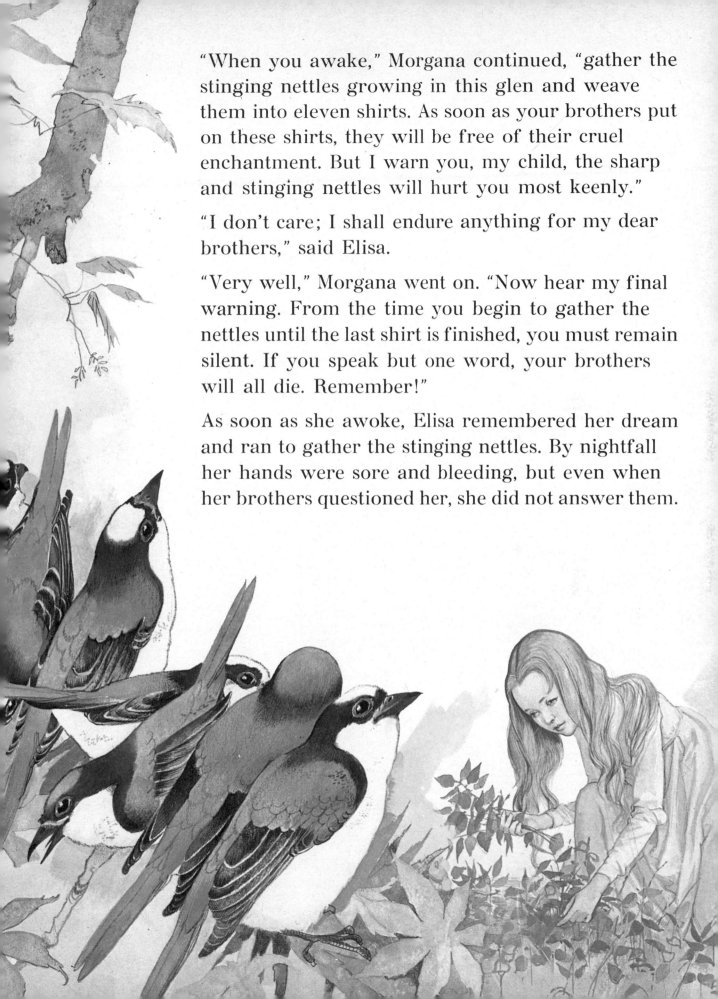

"When you awake," Morgana continued, "gather the stinging nettles growing in this glen and weave them into eleven shirts. As soon as your brothers put on these shirts, they will be free of their cruel enchantment. But I warn you, my child, the sharp and stinging nettles will hurt you most keenly."

"I don't care; I shall endure anything for my dear brothers," said Elisa.

"Very well," Morgana went on. "Now hear my final warning. From the time you begin to gather the nettles until the last shirt is finished, you must remain silent. If you speak but one word, your brothers will all die. Remember!"

As soon as she awoke, Elisa remembered her dream and ran to gather the stinging nettles. By nightfall her hands were sore and bleeding, but even when her brothers questioned her, she did not answer them.

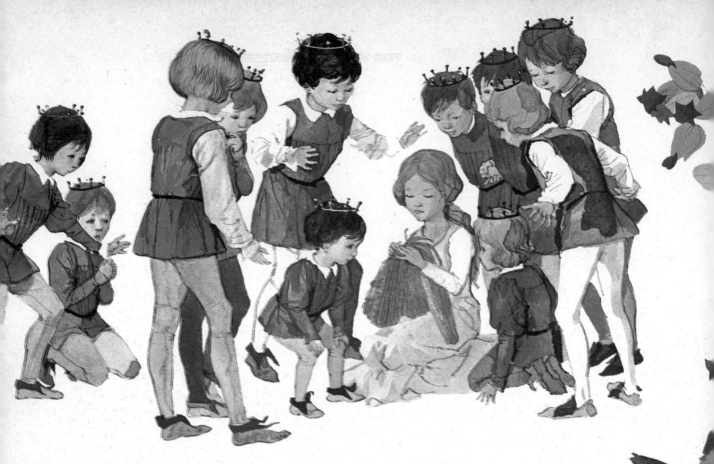

From that day on, not a single word passed Elisa's lips. In silence she gathered nettles and wove the shirts. Her hands were raw and bleeding, and she wept with pain—but she wept silently. Her brothers could not understand her behavior.

"Little sister," they pleaded, "speak to us."

But Elisa only smiled at them and kept on weaving.

One day the young king of the land came riding by with his hunting dogs. He stopped to question Elisa as she sat weaving. But when she did not answer, he became curious and stayed to watch her, enchanted by her beauty and gentleness. By the time his courtiers met up with him again, he was deeply in love with the mysterious young maiden.

"I will dress her in silks and velvets and put a crown on her head," he said to his chamberlain.

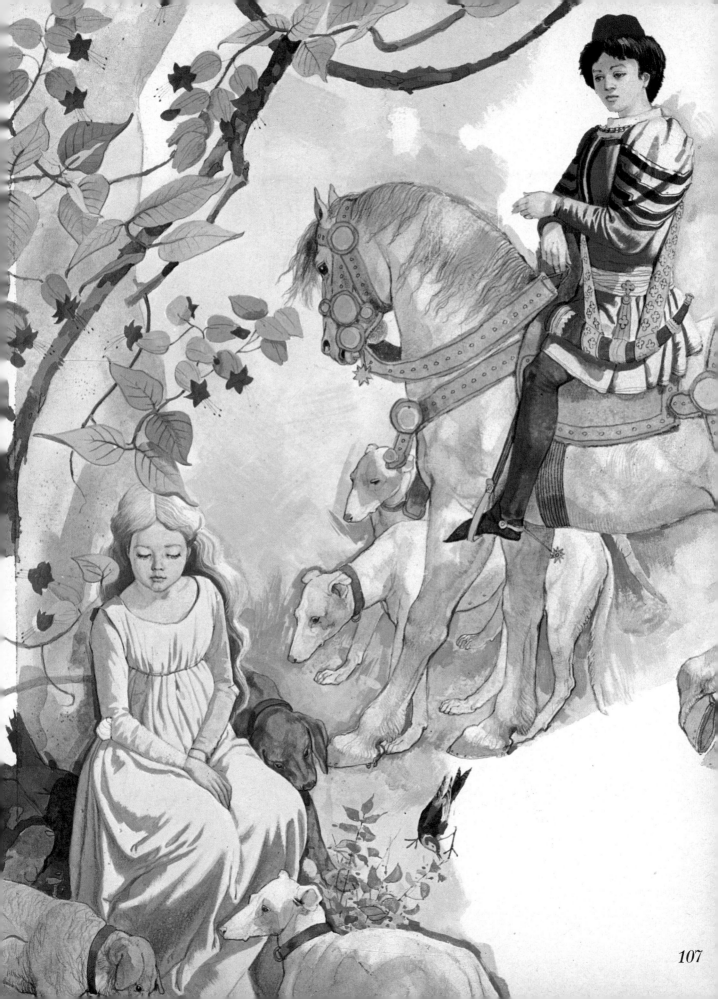

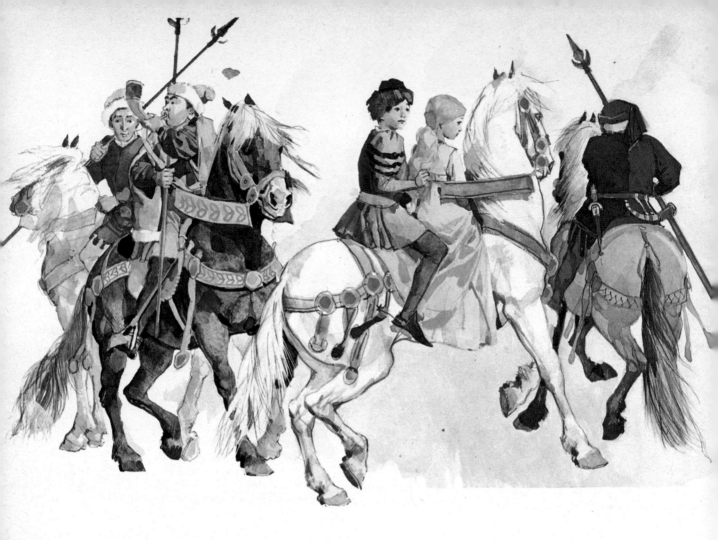

Although his chamberlain tried to dissuade him, the king put Elisa on his horse and led her back to his castle. Nor could Elisa break her silence to protest that she must stay in the glen to finish the shirts for her brothers. Unwilling and heartbroken, she rode off with the king. And though, back at the castle, the king showered her with rich gifts, Elisa never smiled. She sat in sadness through festive banquets and balls, never speaking or smiling.

The young king wished to make her happy, but he did not succeed until one day he returned to the glen where he had found her and brought back with him a bundle of nettles and the shirts she had been weaving. At last Elisa smiled and quickly began to work again.

Day after day she worked in silence, grieved that she was unable to reveal her secret to the young king, whom she now loved dearly. When the seventh shirt was finished, she needed more nettles to continue and remembered that the castle graveyard was the only place within the walls where they grew. That night, wrapped in a black cloak, she tiptoed there trembling with fear. The royal chamberlain, who had always believed the strange girl was a witch, saw her leave and ran quickly to the king.

"She's a witch, Sire!" he cried breathlessly. "I always suspected her, and now I can prove it."

"I don't believe it!" thundered the king.

"It's true, Sire! And one night you will see for yourself," replied the chamberlain as he left.

The king was deeply disturbed by this event, but he said nothing to Elisa.

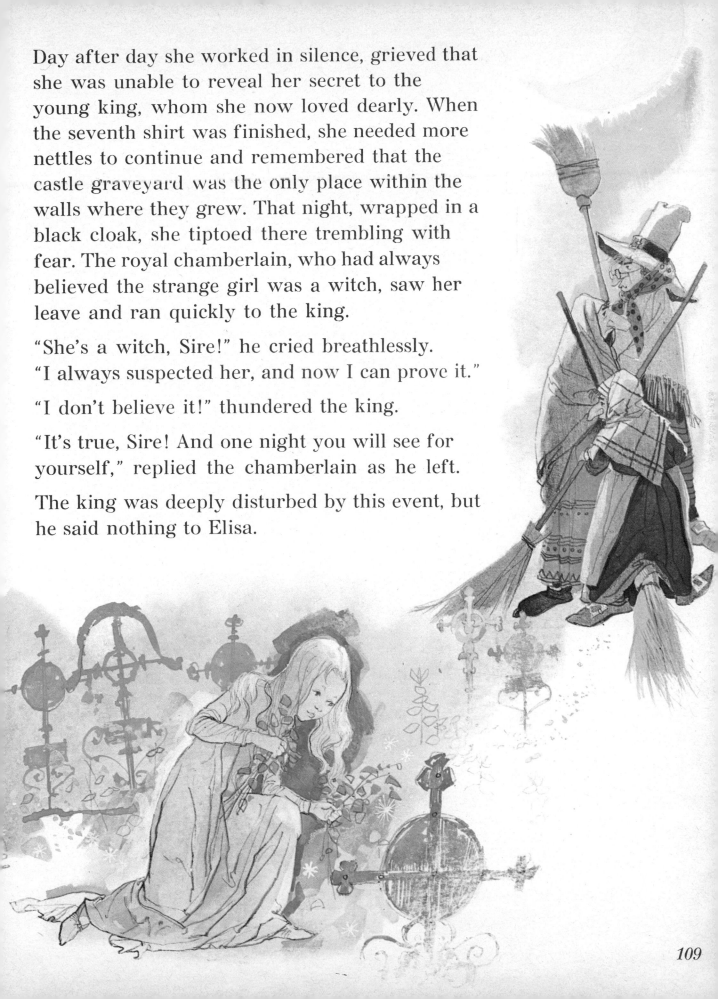

Finally ten shirts were done, but Elisa still needed more nettles to finish the last one. Once again she crept out to the graveyard, never suspecting that the king and his chamberlain were watching behind her.

"Now do you believe me, Sire?" whispered the chamberlain in triumph.

The king looked at Elisa as she knelt by a mossy tombstone, and his heart was broken. "I believe you," he said.

The next day he condemned Elisa to be burned as a witch within the week and imprisoned her in a terrible dungeon to await death. He took away her silks and velvets and made her wear the rough cloth she had woven of nettles. But she was happy, nevertheless, because she could finish the last shirt. When it was finished, she would die willingly, knowing that she had freed all her brothers.

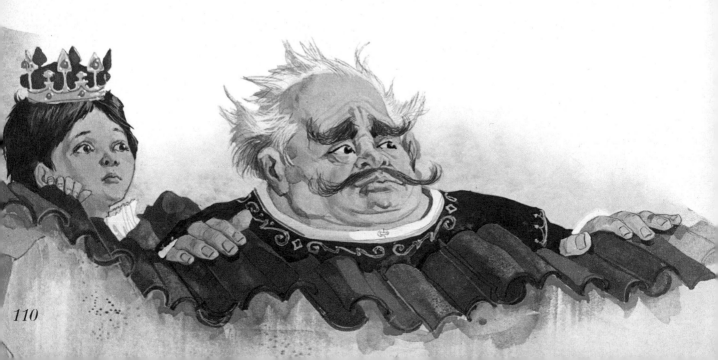

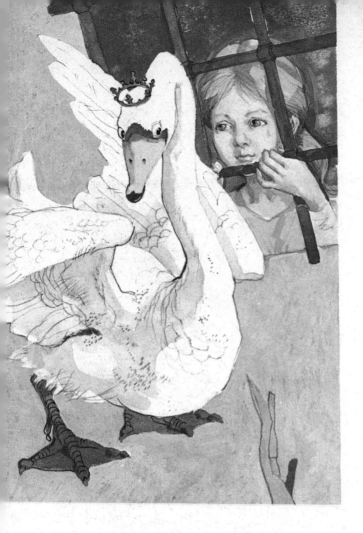

The night before Elisa was to die, a swan appeared at
her dungeon window. It was the youngest of the eleven
princes.

"Dear sister," he whispered, "we have been searching the
whole world for you. Be patient. I shall call the others,
and we shall come back to save you!"

But her brothers did not come, and the next morning
rough jailors took Elisa in a wooden cart, past the
crowds, to her place of execution. She did not look up
until she had sewed the last stitch on the last shirt. As she
broke off the final thread, there was a great noise in the
sky and eleven swans swooped down and gathered
beside her on the cart.

Elisa almost cried aloud, but quickly instead she threw
one of the nettle shirts over each of the swans.

Instantly, the swans became eleven princes again and embraced their sister.

"You have freed us!" they cried. "Now we shall free you!"

The crowd gasped in amazement at the miracle they had just seen. The young king came toward the cart and listened in wonder as the princes revealed their whole story.

"If only you had spoken!" the king said sadly to Elisa, as he begged her forgiveness.

"I dared not, Sire, but now I can speak of my love and I forgive you gladly."

The king clasped her hand and announced to his subjects that the generous and innocent girl would become his queen, and her eleven brothers would be princes of his realm. The very next morning the princes gave their sister's hand in marriage to the king, and there was general happiness in his kingdom that day and ever after.

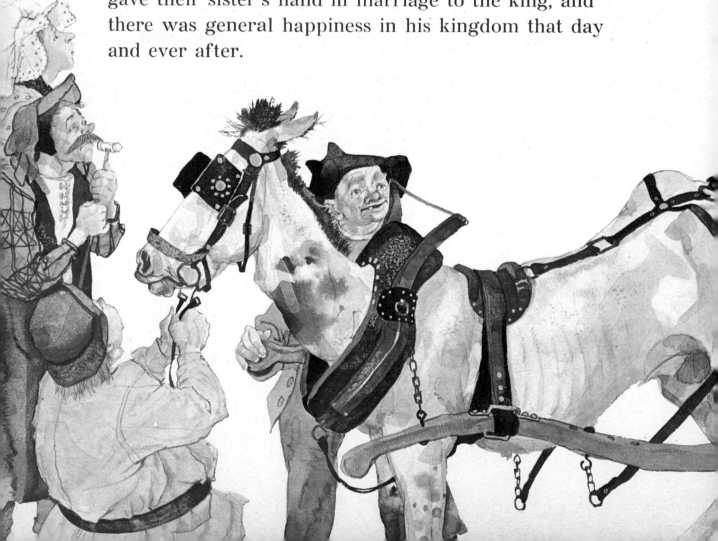

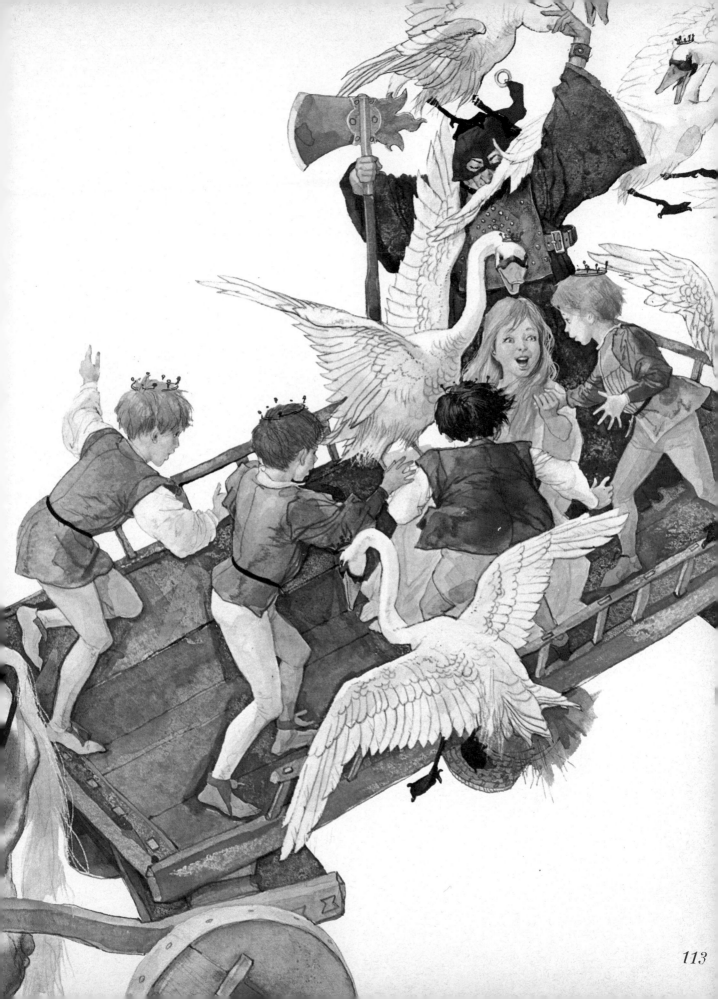

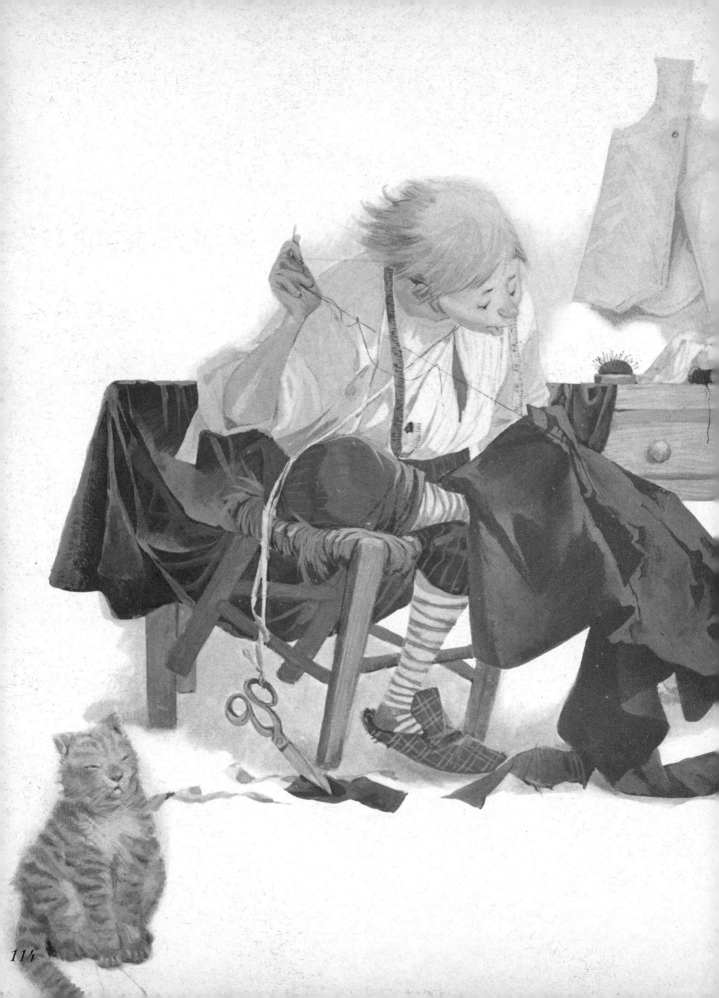

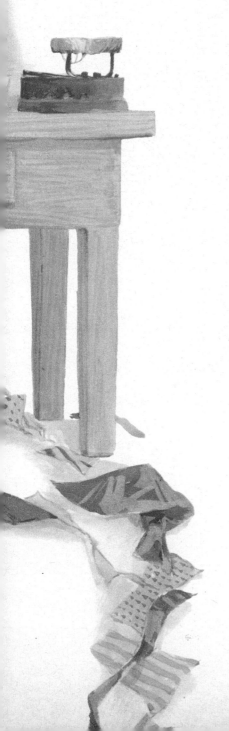

SEVEN IN ONE BLOW

Once upon a time, long ago, when giants still roamed the earth and terrified people, there lived a lively young boy named Bertram who worked as a tailor. He was a good tailor and sewed fine gowns and handsome jackets, but he would much rather have been out in the world seeking adventure. All day as he sat stitching in his shop, he dreamed of killing giants, fighting dragons, and rescuing lovely maidens. In his dreams he was always a great hero, of course, and much honored wherever he went.

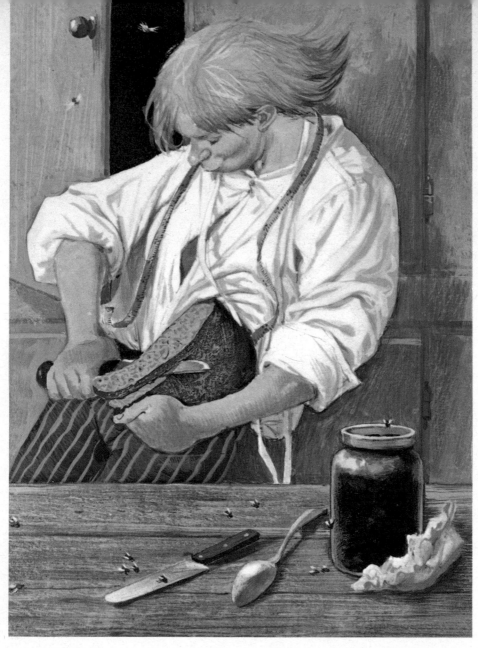

One morning Bertram felt particularly hungry, so before he started his sewing for the day he cut great slabs of black bread, covered them with creamy butter, and spread a thick layer of honey on top of it all. His snack looked so delicious that he couldn't wait to eat it. But it also looked delicious to the flies hovering outside his window. They swarmed in hungrily and soon covered Bertram's tasty snack completely. He swatted at them furiously with a towel, and with his very first swat he killed seven flies at once.

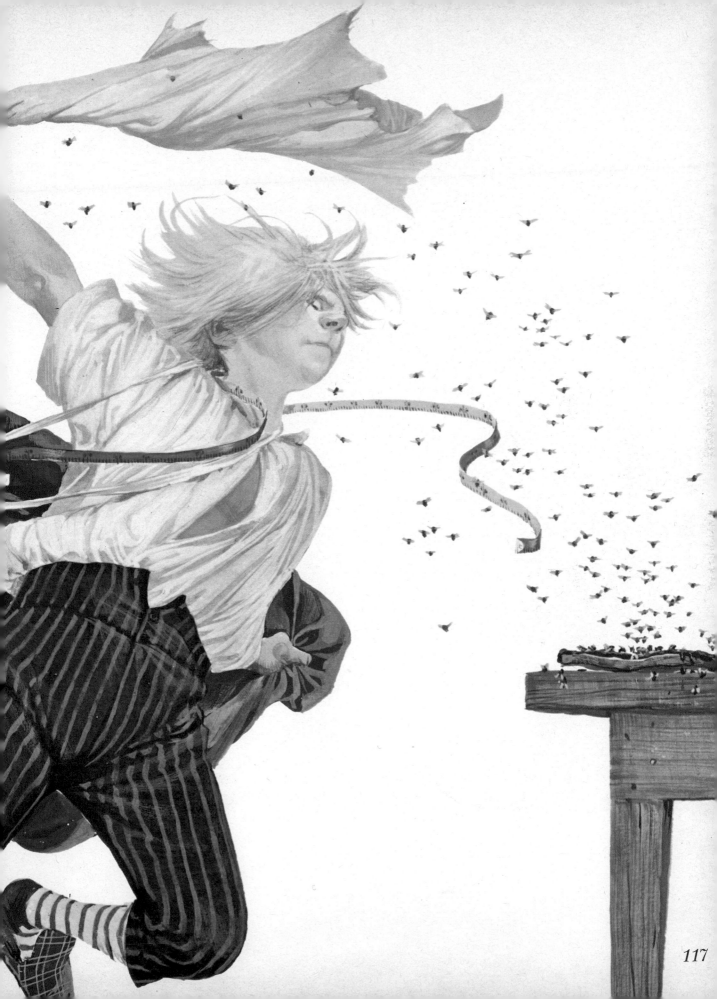

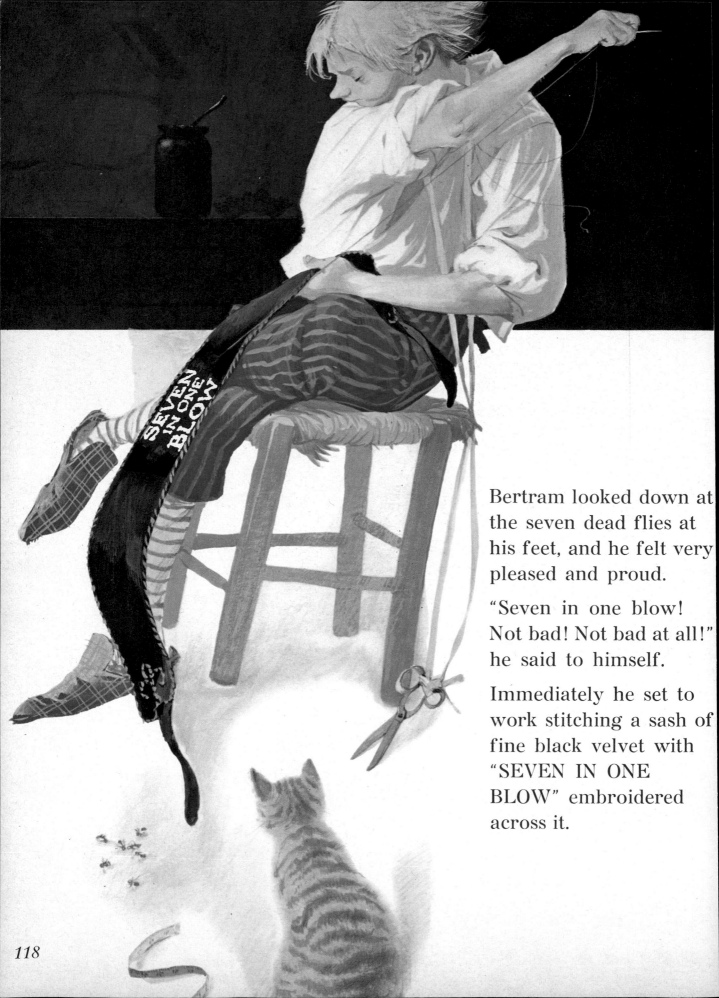

Bertram looked down at the seven dead flies at his feet, and he felt very pleased and proud.

"Seven in one blow! Not bad! Not bad at all!" he said to himself.

Immediately he set to work stitching a sash of fine black velvet with "SEVEN IN ONE BLOW" embroidered across it.

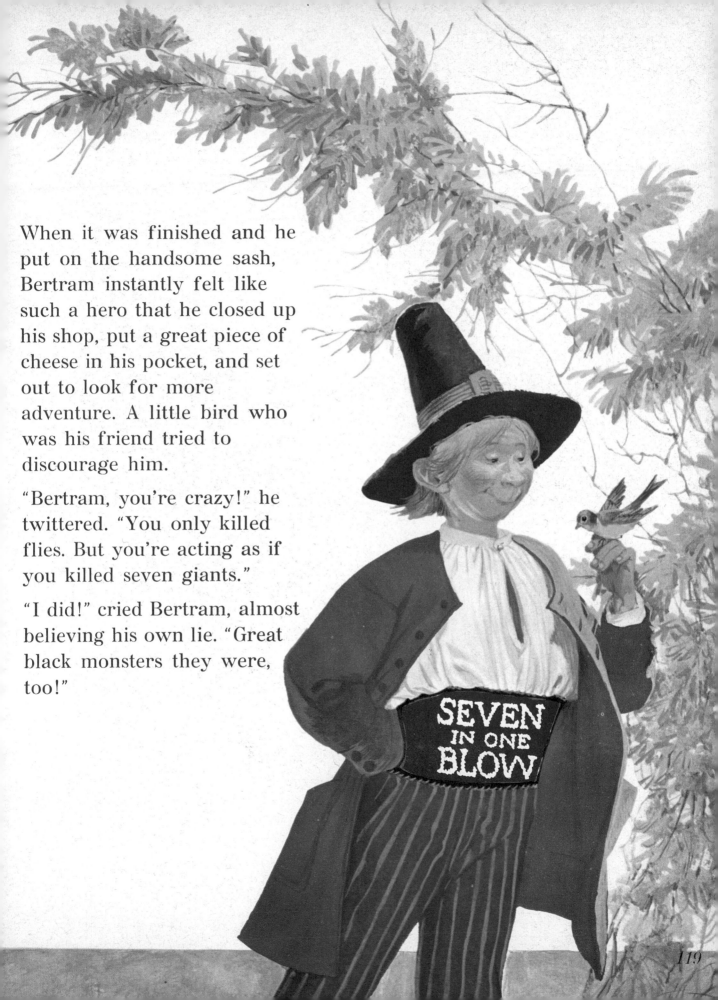

When it was finished and he put on the handsome sash, Bertram instantly felt like such a hero that he closed up his shop, put a great piece of cheese in his pocket, and set out to look for more adventure. A little bird who was his friend tried to discourage him.

"Bertram, you're crazy!" he twittered. "You only killed flies. But you're acting as if you killed seven giants."

"I did!" cried Bertram, almost believing his own lie. "Great black monsters they were, too!"

SEVEN
IN ONE
BLOW

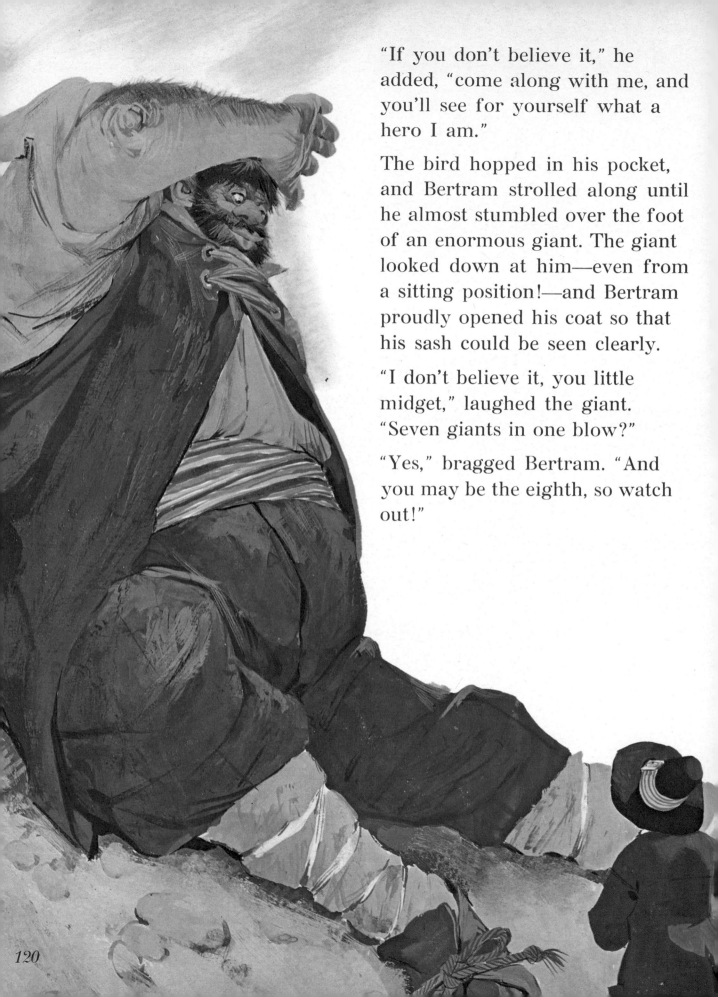

"If you don't believe it," he added, "come along with me, and you'll see for yourself what a hero I am."

The bird hopped in his pocket, and Bertram strolled along until he almost stumbled over the foot of an enormous giant. The giant looked down at him—even from a sitting position!—and Bertram proudly opened his coat so that his sash could be seen clearly.

"I don't believe it, you little midget," laughed the giant. "Seven giants in one blow?"

"Yes," bragged Bertram. "And you may be the eighth, so watch out!"

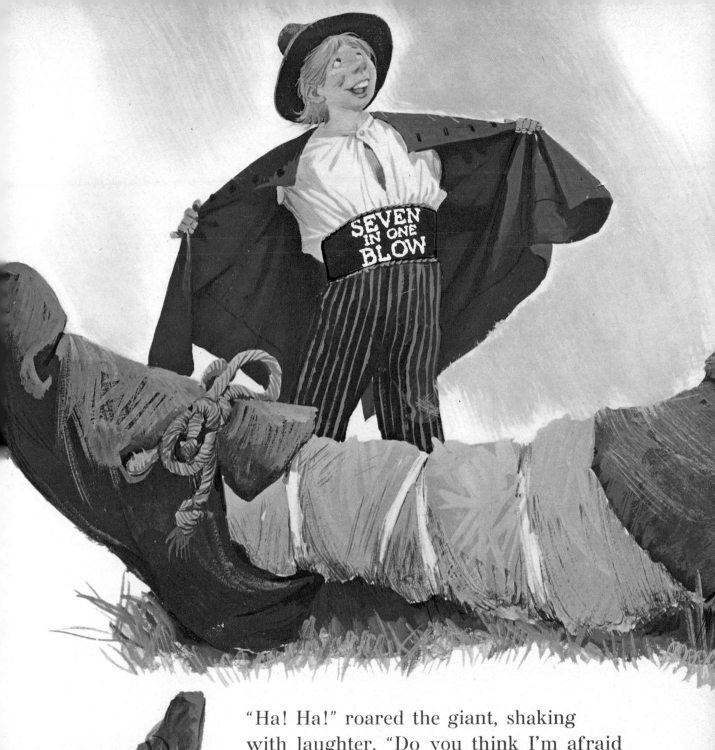

"Ha! Ha!" roared the giant, shaking with laughter. "Do you think I'm afraid of a little weakling like you? You just can't imagine how strong I am."

Then he looked around until he found a huge boulder stuck firmly in the ground.

"Now watch!" roared the giant. And with one great hairy hand he picked up the boulder as if it were a pebble and closed his fist tightly around it. The rock shattered into tiny fragments, and water poured out.

"Pooh! That's nothing. Watch me break my rock!" Bertram cried, pulling his big piece of cheese from his pocket and squeezing it tightly. The crumbly cheese seemed to shatter just like the rock, and milky water poured out of it. The giant was so near-sighted that he could not really tell the difference, and therefore he was quite impressed by the little man.

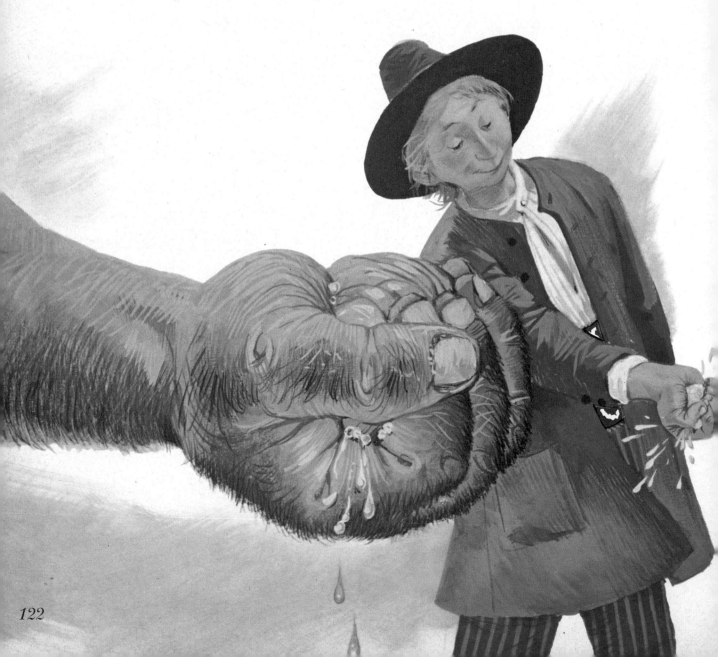

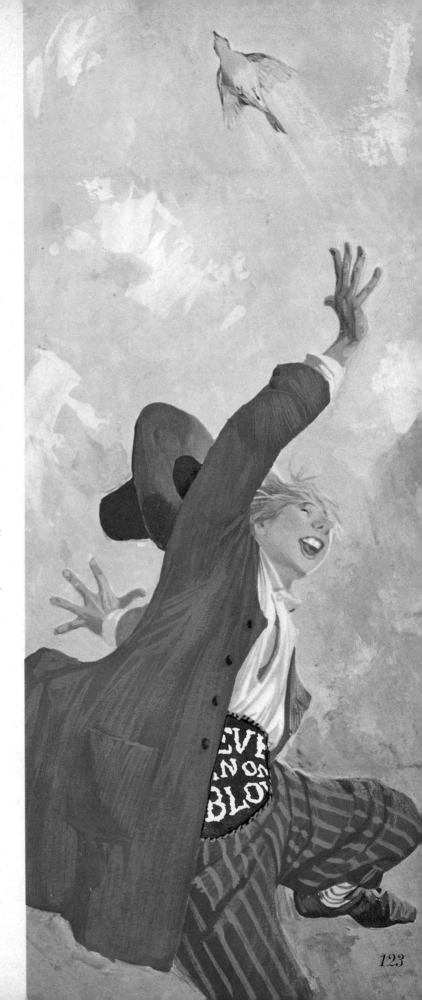

"Let's see how high you can throw a stone. I'll go first," the giant said next. Then he threw a stone so high into the air that it almost hit the clouds before it fell back to the ground.

"That's nothing. Watch this!" Bertram scoffed as he took his friend the bird out of his pocket and whispered to it to fly away. When the near-sighted—and dull-witted—giant did not see a stone fall to the ground, he thought Bertram had thrown it so high it had landed on the sun.

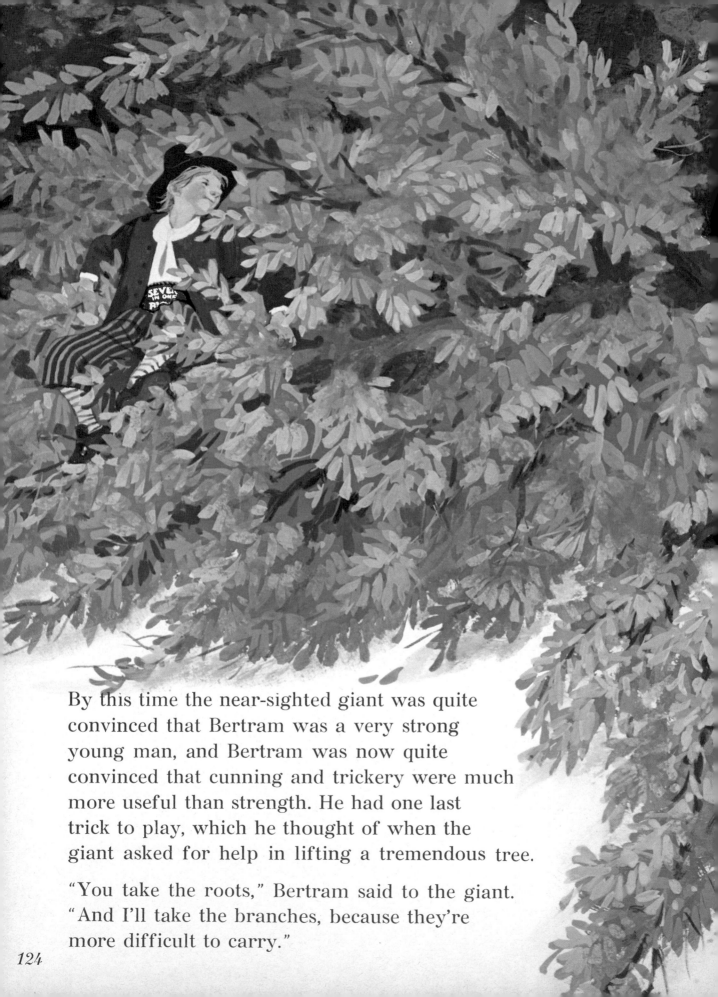

By this time the near-sighted giant was quite
convinced that Bertram was a very strong
young man, and Bertram was now quite
convinced that cunning and trickery were much
more useful than strength. He had one last
trick to play, which he thought of when the
giant asked for help in lifting a tremendous tree.

"You take the roots," Bertram said to the giant.
"And I'll take the branches, because they're
more difficult to carry."

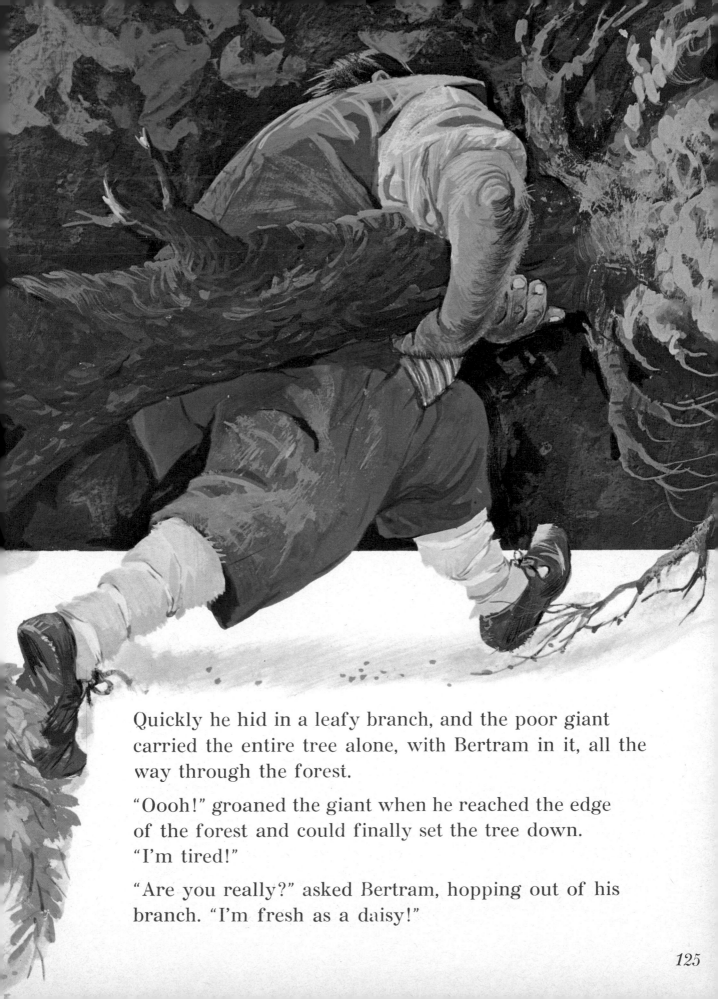

Quickly he hid in a leafy branch, and the poor giant carried the entire tree alone, with Bertram in it, all the way through the forest.

"Oooh!" groaned the giant when he reached the edge of the forest and could finally set the tree down. "I'm tired!"

"Are you really?" asked Bertram, hopping out of his branch. "I'm fresh as a daisy!"

Bertram went off feeling very pleased with himself, and more of a hero than ever. He was resting on the lawn near the royal palace when the king's High Chamberlain happened to pass by.

"Seven In One Blow?!" he exclaimed when he saw Bertram's sash. "You must be quite a hero, and our king is badly in need of heroes these days. I'll take you to him right away."

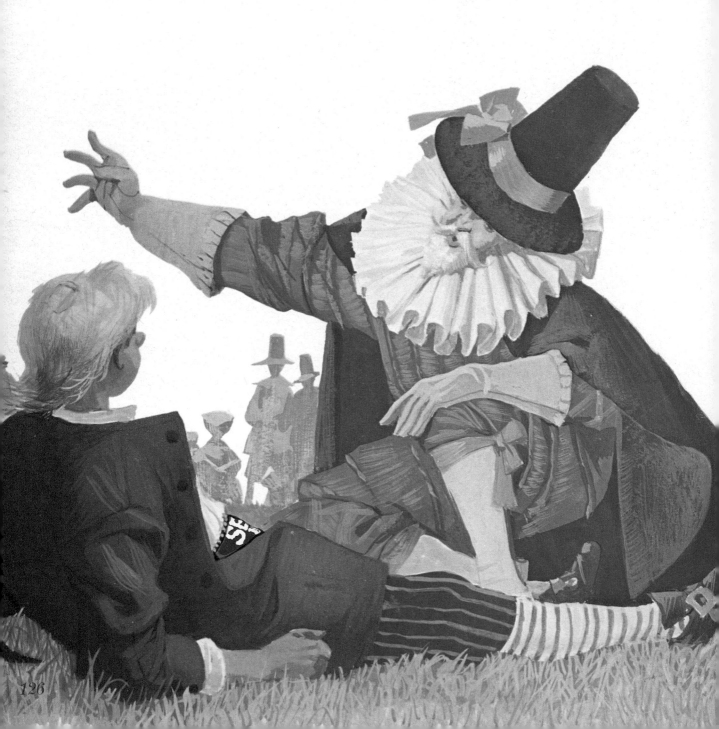

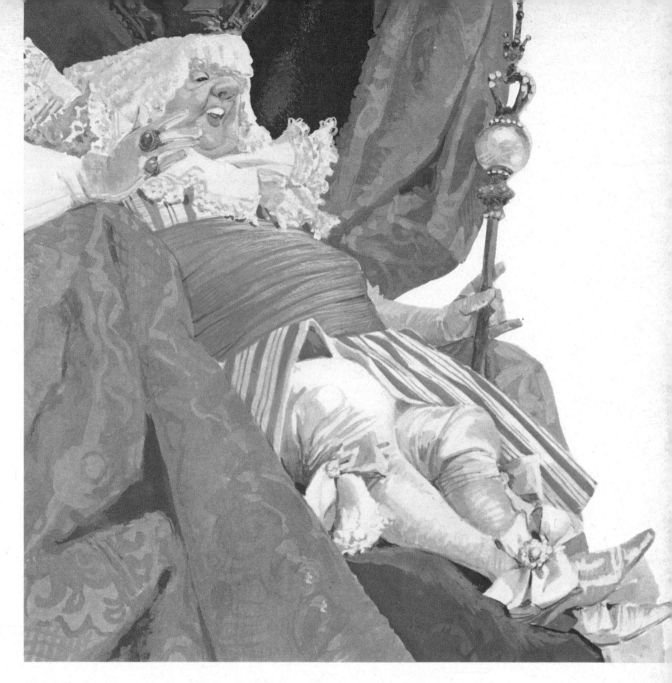

"I need a hero!" cried the king happily as Bertram knelt before him. "It's no fun being a king and ruling your realm any more. I'm always being threatened by assassins and rebellious subjects and giants."

"This great hero I bring you killed seven giants in one blow," said the chamberlain.

"And now I order him to kill two more," commanded the king. "They are Fiveton and Sixton, the wickedest of all giants in my kingdom."

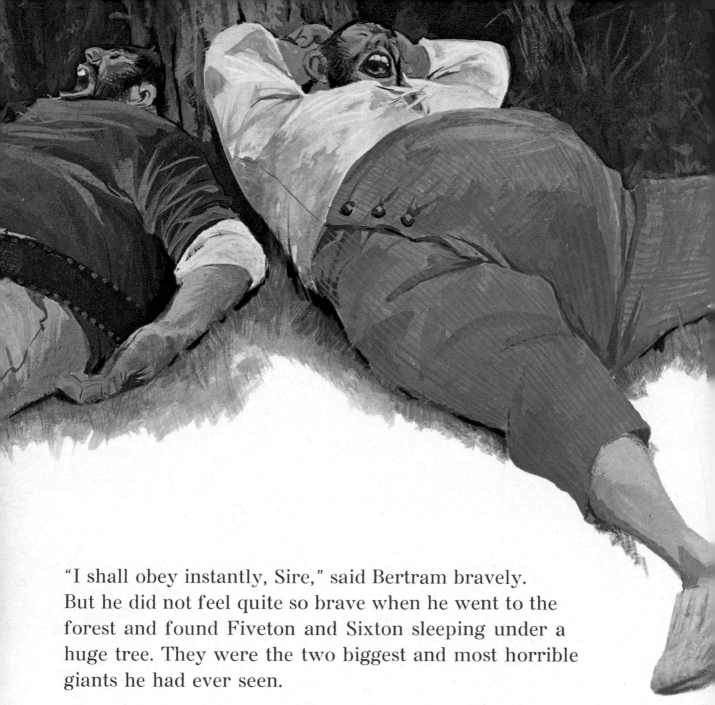

"I shall obey instantly, Sire," said Bertram bravely. But he did not feel quite so brave when he went to the forest and found Fiveton and Sixton sleeping under a huge tree. They were the two biggest and most horrible giants he had ever seen.

"Don't panic now! Remember you are the famous Seven-In-One-Blow," he said to himself. Filling his pockets with little stones, Bertram climbed to the top of the tree. When he was safely hidden way up in the branches, he took careful aim and fired a little pebble at Sixton's nose.

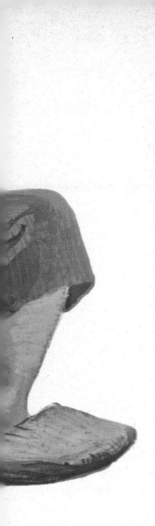

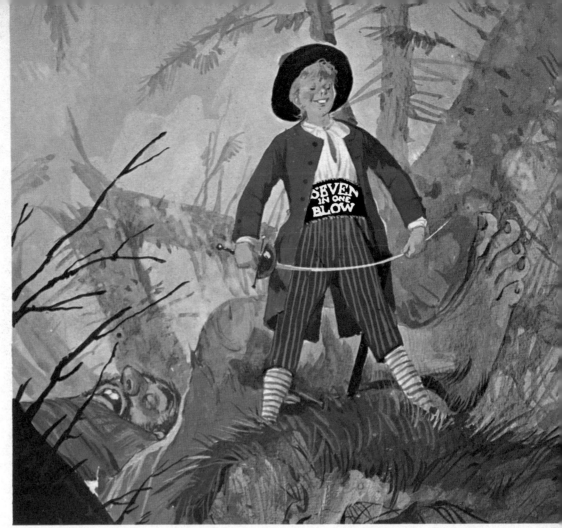

The giant woke and roared till the tree shook.

"You hit me!" he thundered at his brother.

"I did not. Go back to sleep," mumbled Fiveton.

But just at that moment a pebble hit him in the mouth, and Fiveton too began to roar with rage. Still unseen, Bertram hurled a few more pebbles, and in a minute the two giants were fighting each other furiously. First they kicked and bit and pulled each other's hair. Then they uprooted trees and began to club each other. Finally they broke open each other's skulls, at which point Bertram jumped out of his hiding place and stood victoriously over their dead bodies.

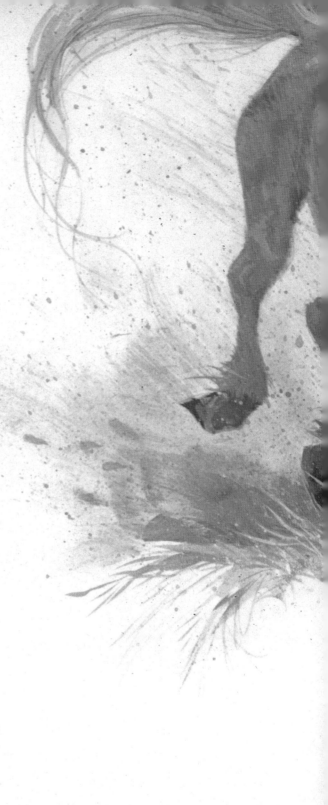

Proudly Bertram marched back to the castle to report to the king.

"There are two dead giants lying in the forest, Sire," he announced casually. "You'd better send someone out to clear them away."

The king was overjoyed at this news and was very impressed with Bertram.

"You've killed my very worst enemies," he cried gratefully. "If you can now subdue the fierce unicorn who has been terrorizing the countryside, I will give you my beautiful daughter as your bride."

Now Bertram had dreamed many dreams and invented many stories, but he had never in his wildest fantasies dared to imagine he might have a princess for a wife, or a king for a father-in-law. But he did like the idea very much, and so without stopping for a nap or a bite to eat he set out to conquer the terrible unicorn.

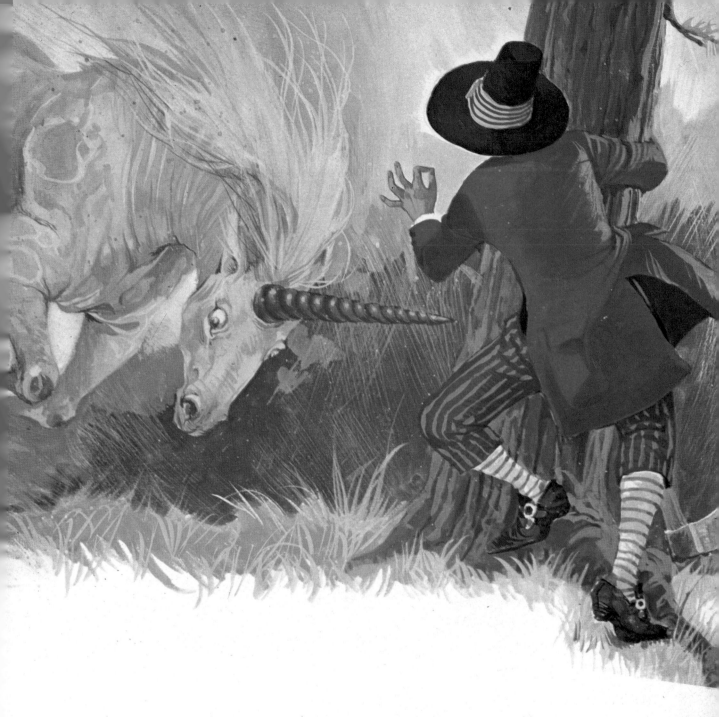

Bertram hid behind a tree till he heard a screaming
whinny, then a thunderous snort, and then the furious
pounding of hoofs. In a minute the fierce unicorn came
charging into the clearing with smoke pouring from
his nostrils and fire from his mouth. Bertram skipped out
from behind his tree and danced like a bullfighter in
front of the unicorn. The unicorn put his head down and
charged like a bull, aiming his single terrible horn
directly at Bertram's heart.

But before the horn could touch him, Bertram skipped behind the tree once again. The unicorn could not stop himself in time and charged right into the trunk, piercing it through with his horn. The furious animal almost knocked himself senseless and could not pull his horn from the tree in which it was stuck fast, so Bertram was able to rope and tie him easily. Then he freed the unicorn by cutting the end of its horn off, and led the animal meekly back to the palace, right to the throne room. There Bertram and the unicorn knelt humbly before the king.

His Majesty kept his promise, and in two days Bertram had a princess for a wife and a king for a father-in-law. One day he would become king himself, and ever after his subjects would enjoy retelling stories of his heroic deeds—and even inventing new ones. Bertram himself never needed to invent another one again.

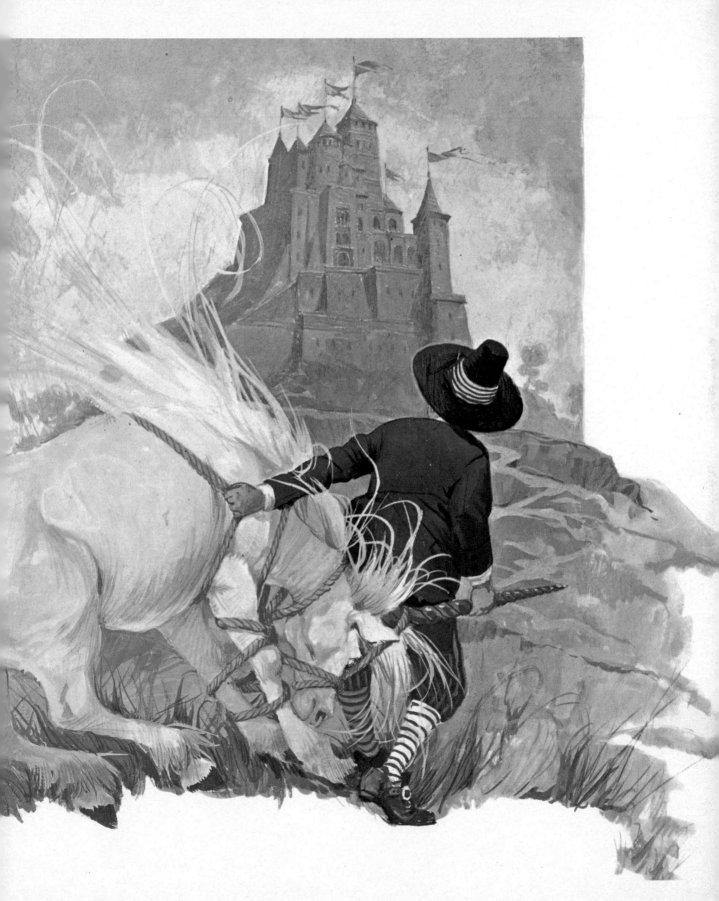

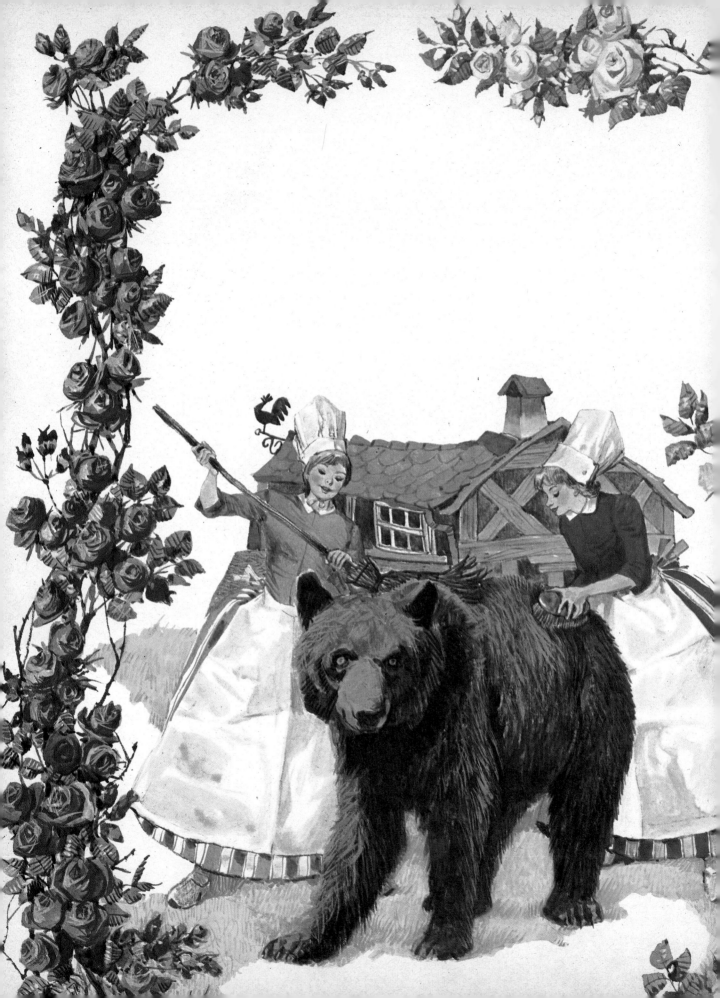

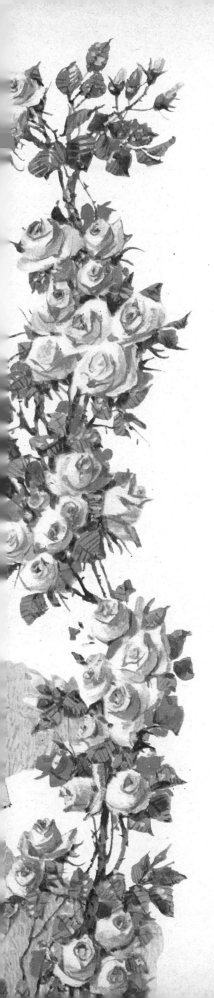

SNOW WHITE AND ROSE RED

Once upon a time, close by a great forest, there was a little cottage with two rosebushes growing beside it. One had blossoms of purest white, and the other had blossoms of deepest red. In the cottage lived a poor widow whose two daughters were as beautiful as the roses, so she called them Snow White and Rose Red. Both her daughters were as good as they were beautiful, and they willingly helped their mother clean house and tend the garden.

The two sisters loved each other deeply and often went to the forest hand-in-hand to pick berries or gather nuts. All the wild creatures trusted them; the rabbits ate out of their hands, and birds sang special songs to them.

In summer, Rose Red always put two fresh roses—one white and the other red—in a bowl by her mother's chair. In winter, Snow White kept the fire blazing and always had water boiling for a hot cup of tea.

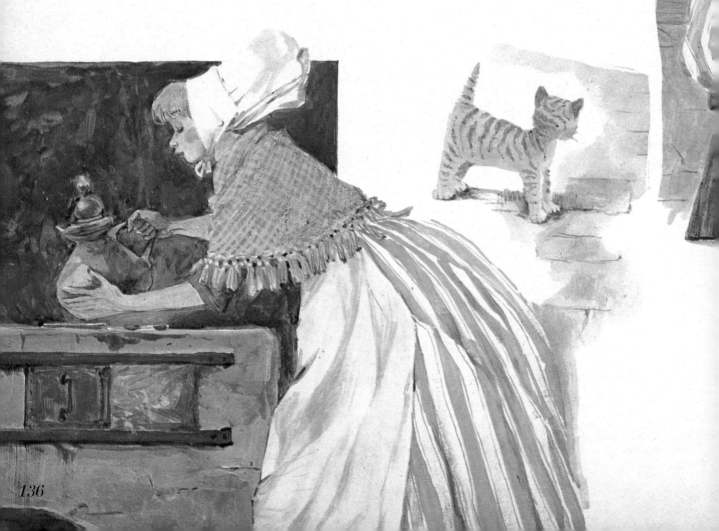

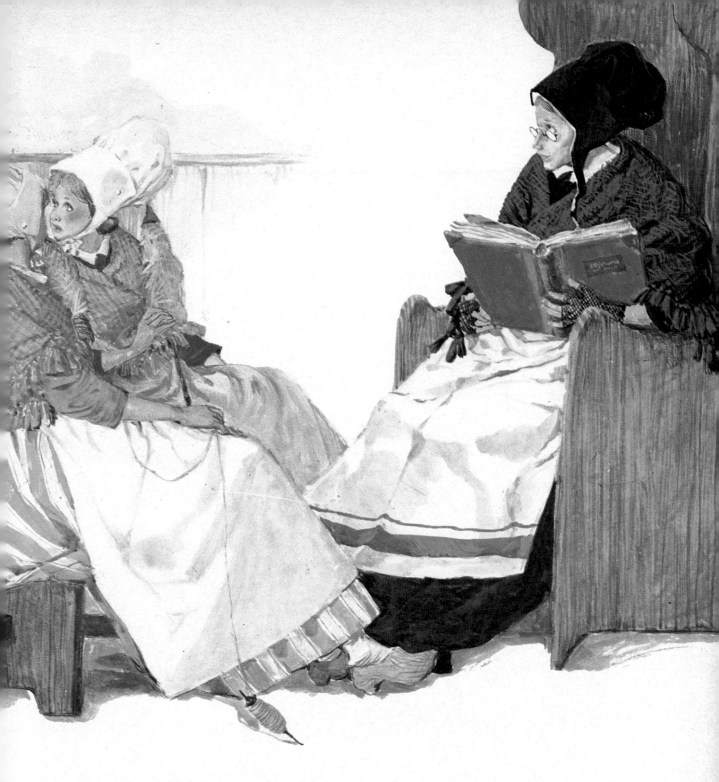

On cold winter evenings, their mother read from a great book while her daughters spun thread by her side. One stormy night they heard a soft knocking at the door. Snow White and Rose Red hid in fear behind their mother.

"Don't be frightened," she said. "It is surely some poor traveler lost in the storm and in need of our help."

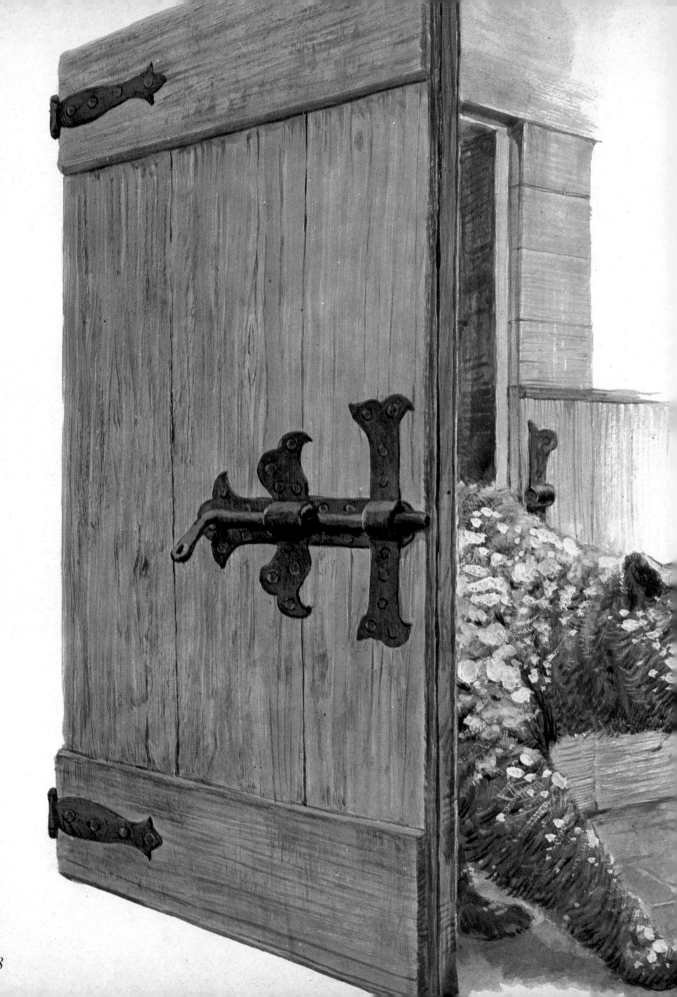

She drew back the heavy iron bolt, and when she opened the door, her daughters screamed and hid under their bed, because in walked a great shaggy bear.

"Don't be afraid, my pretties," said the bear very gently. "I won't hurt you. I'm frozen and only want to warm myself by your fire for a moment."

"Poor thing," said the mother. "Come right in and lie down at our hearth."

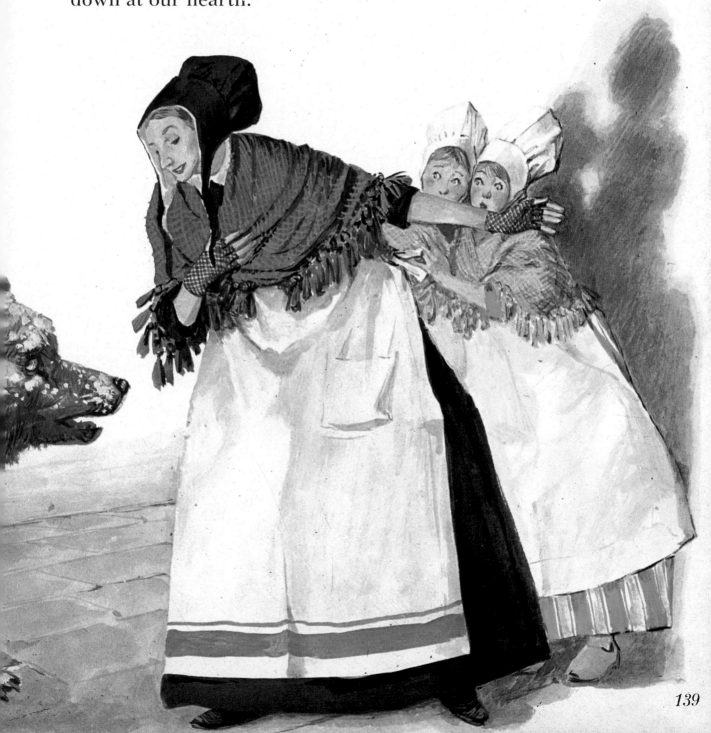

Snow White and Rose Red, no longer afraid, came out to make friends with their guest and to offer him tea with honey. Soon they began to play with him as if he were a huge furry toy. They pulled at his fur, rode on his back, and tickled him till he pretended to growl fiercely.

The next morning the bear went off, but every evening through the long winter he knocked on the cottage door at sunset and came in to enjoy the fire and more hot tea with honey. Snow White and Rose Red never bolted the door for the night until their shaggy friend was safely inside.

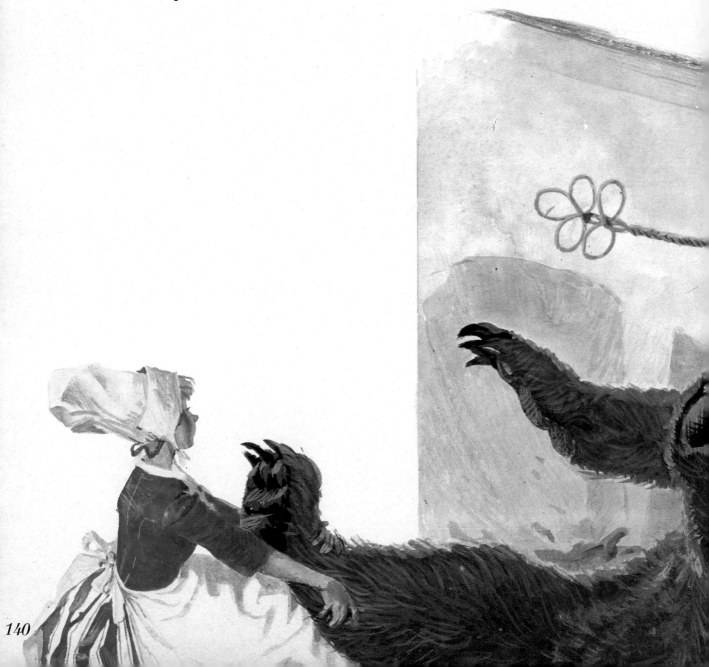

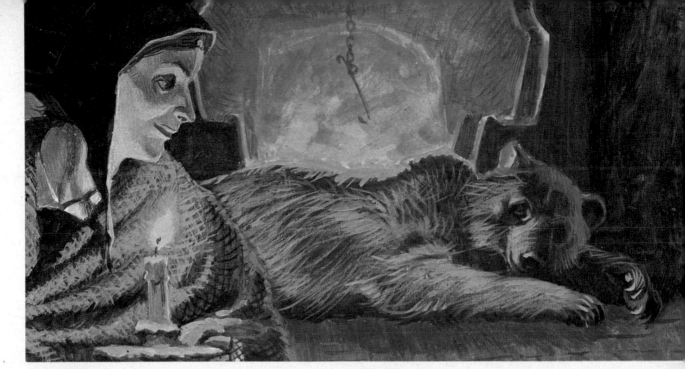

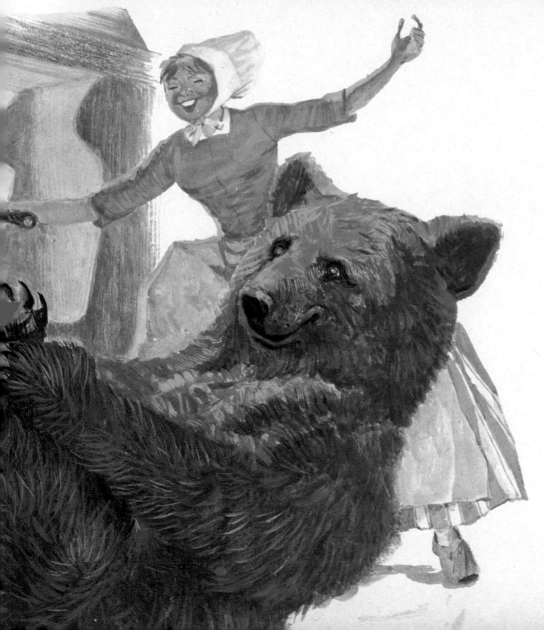

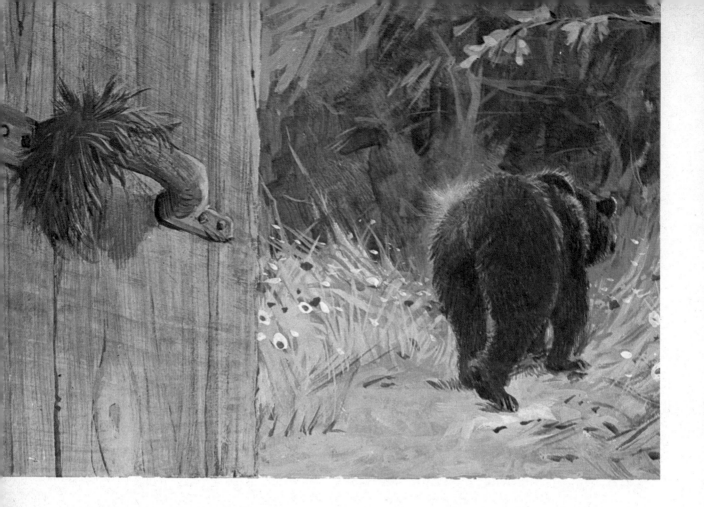

But when spring came, the bear had to say goodbye.

"I must stay in the forest now and guard my treasure against the wicked dwarfs," he explained. "They are locked under the frozen ground all winter, but when the warm spring comes they escape and are free to run about the forest stealing everything they find."

As the bear walked through the door, his coat caught on the big latch and a clump of his black fur was left behind.

But the bear did not seem to notice and continued on his way.

Snow White said to her sister, "How strange! I thought I saw a flash of gold on our bear's back. But perhaps I was mistaken."

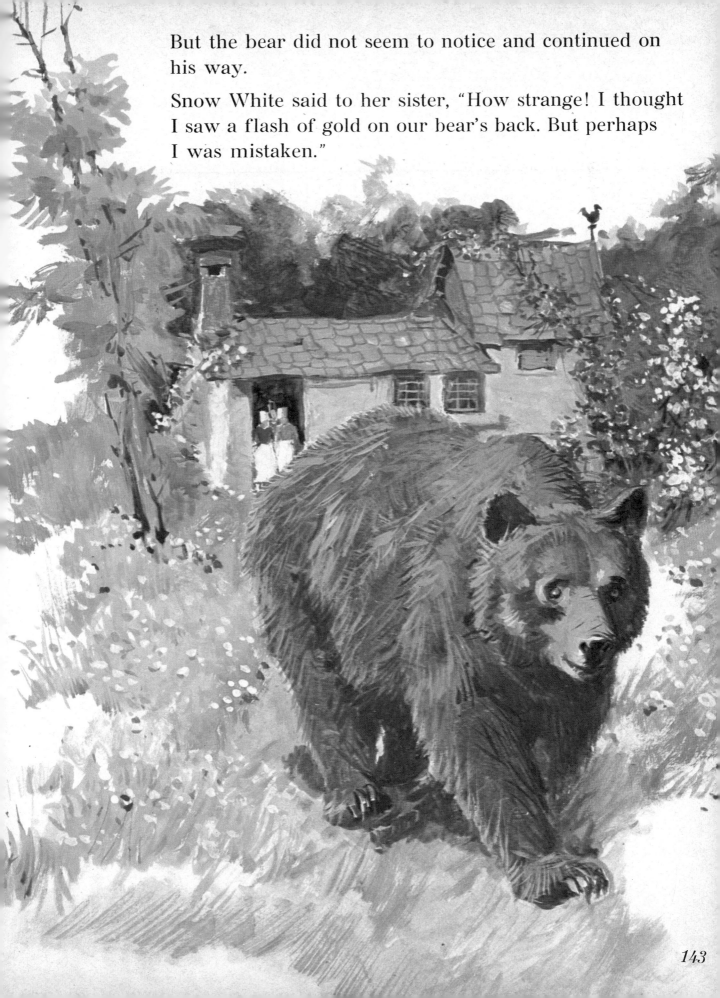

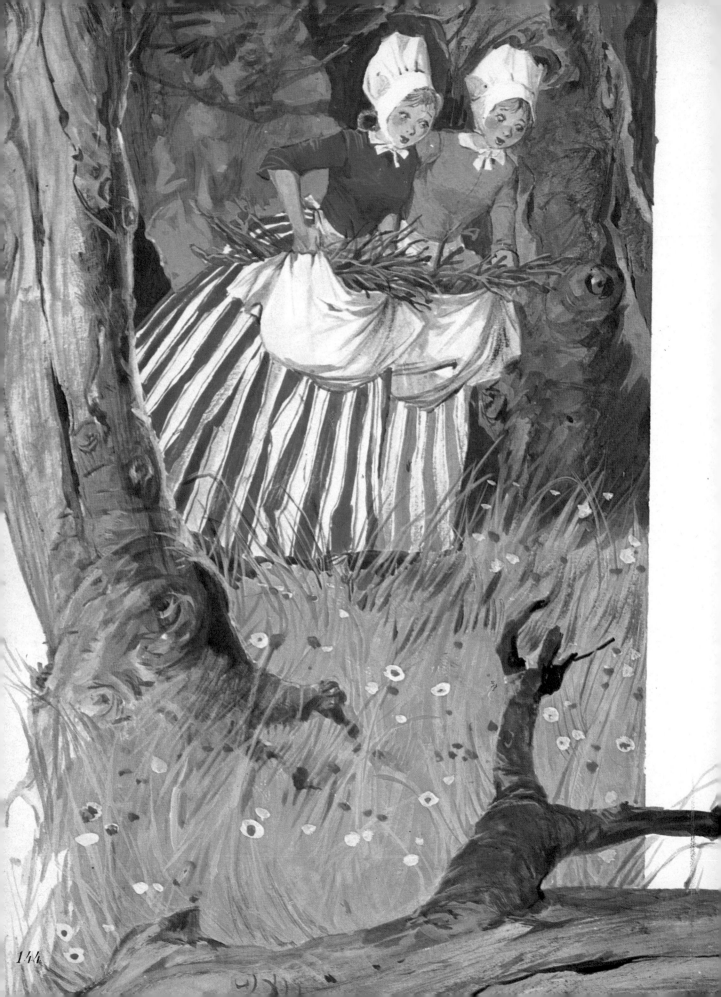

One day shortly after the bear had left, while gathering firewood the sisters came to a fallen tree, beside which a funny little creature danced up and down. When they got closer, they saw a tiny dwarf with a shriveled old face and a beard at least a yard long. The end of his beard was caught in a crack in the tree trunk, and he bounced up and down in rage.

"Help me, you silly girls!" he shrieked.

"Willingly, sir. But how?" answered Snow White politely.

"Are you dummies? Can't you see my beautiful beard is stuck? Do something!" he screamed louder than ever.

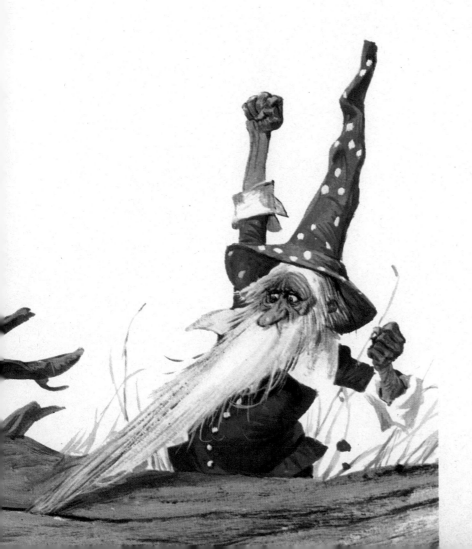

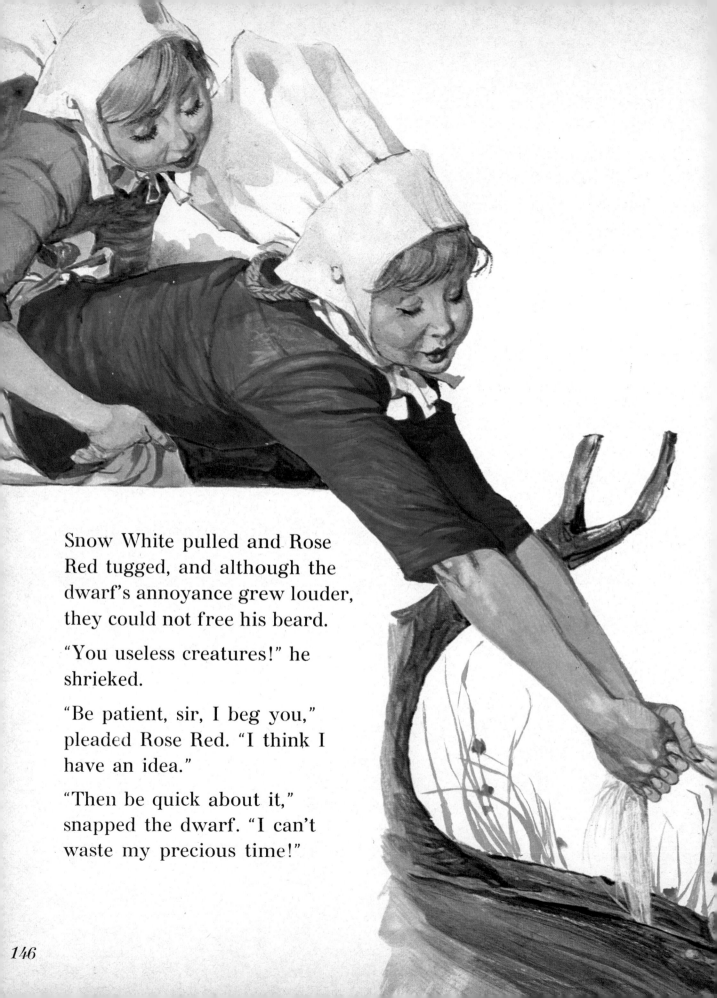

Snow White pulled and Rose Red tugged, and although the dwarf's annoyance grew louder, they could not free his beard.

"You useless creatures!" he shrieked.

"Be patient, sir, I beg you," pleaded Rose Red. "I think I have an idea."

"Then be quick about it," snapped the dwarf. "I can't waste my precious time!"

While he kept scolding, Rose Red pulled a pair of sharp scissors from her pocket and quickly snipped off the end of his beard. The dwarf was freed at last but showed no gratitude.

"My beard, my beard! What have you done to it, you worthless ninnies?" he shouted and, snatching up a bag of gold lying nearby, ran off without a word of thanks

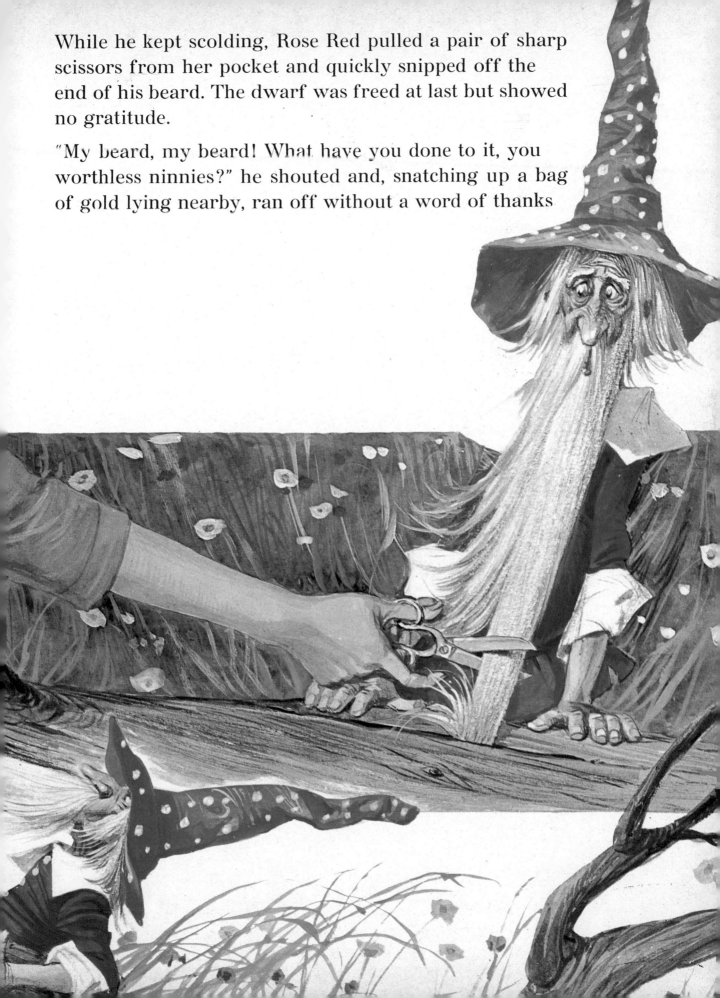

Snow White and Rose Red thought him very rude but quickly forgot about him, until one day their mother sent them to catch some fish for dinner. As they approached their favorite stream, they thought they saw a great grasshopper jumping up and down on the bank; but when they came closer, they found it was the dwarf, just as angry as ever.

"Help me, you useless creatures!" he screamed when he saw them. "Do something!"

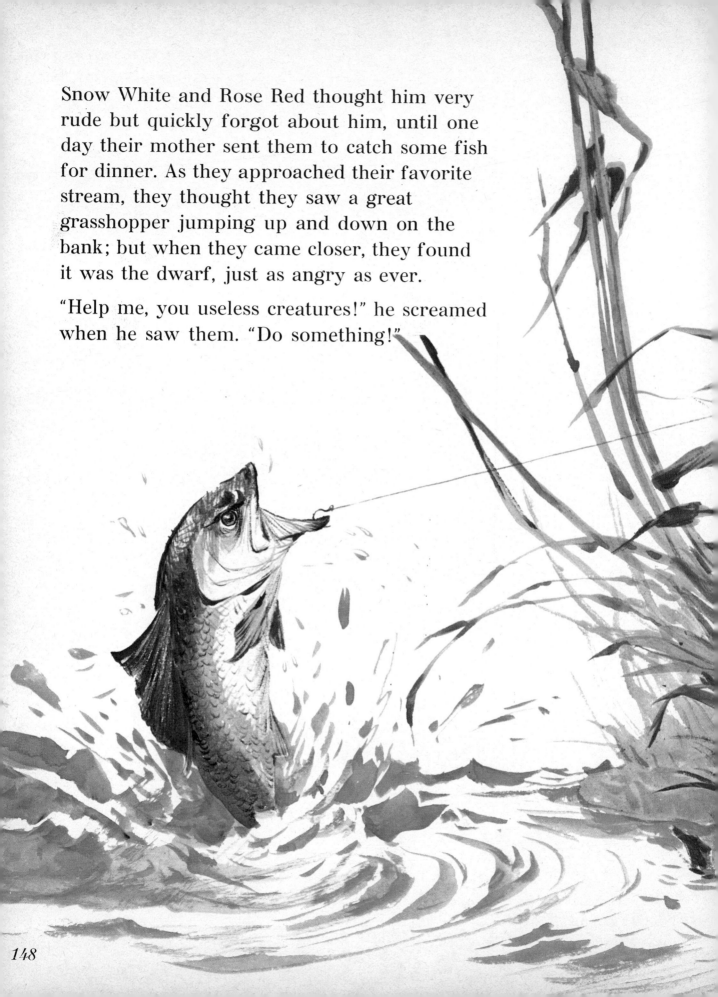

The dwarf had caught a great fish, but his beard had become tangled in his fishing line, and the fish was pulling him into the water. This time Rose Red knew what to do immediately. She pulled out her scissors and cut off a tiny bit of the long beard, and the dwarf was free again.

"Useless foul baggage!" he shrieked. "Have you no sense!" And once again, without a thank-you, he snatched up a sack of pearls lying on the bank and ran off.

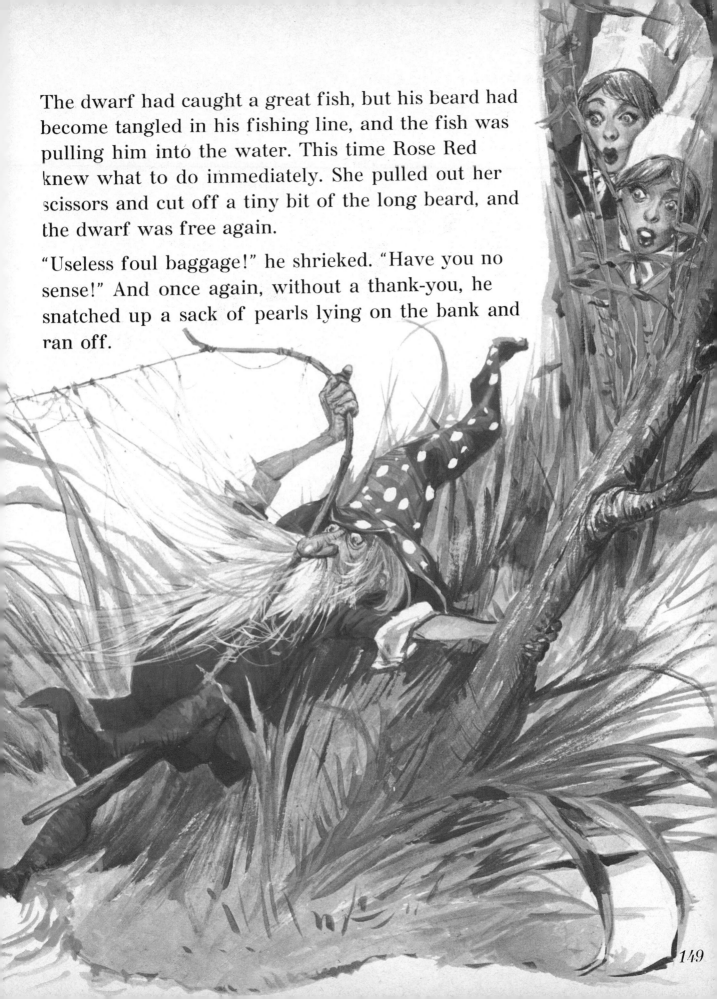

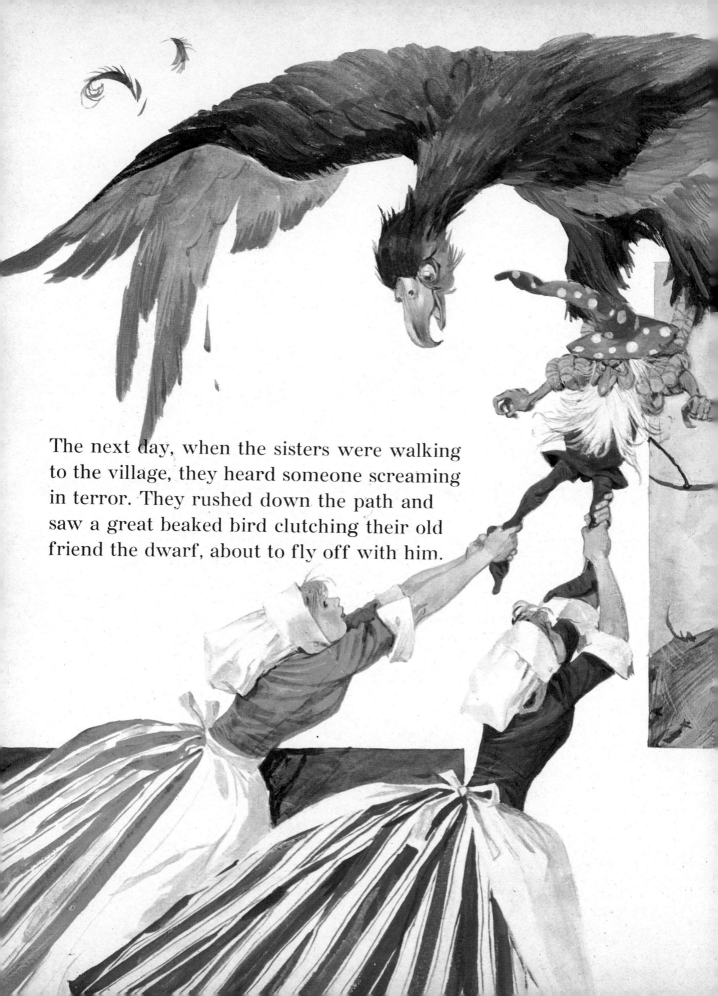

The next day, when the sisters were walking to the village, they heard someone screaming in terror. They rushed down the path and saw a great beaked bird clutching their old friend the dwarf, about to fly off with him.

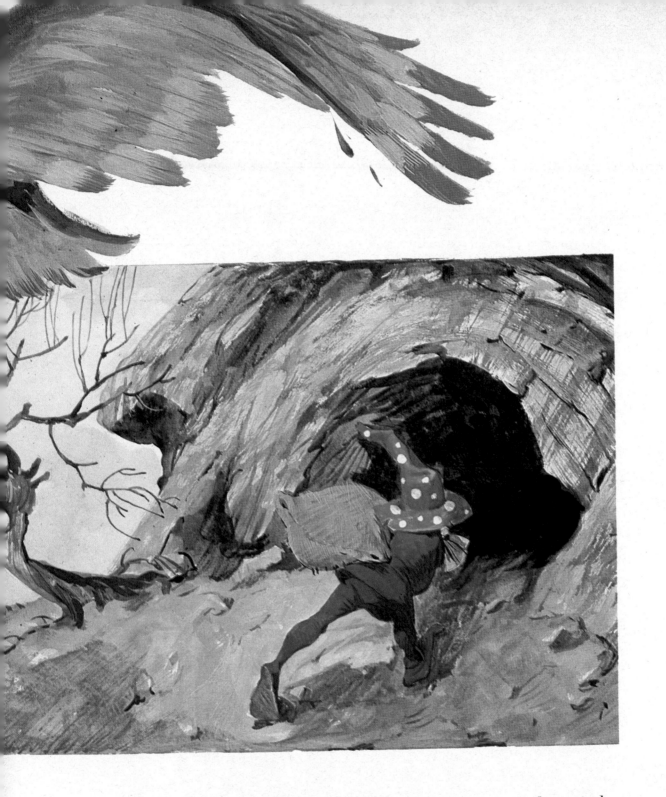

Quickly, Snow White seized the dwarf by one leg and
Rose Red caught him by the other. They pulled and
tugged and finally freed the dwarf. This time the sisters
knew what to expect and were not surprised when the
dwarf cursed them furiously, grabbed his sack of
jewels, and ran off to his cave.

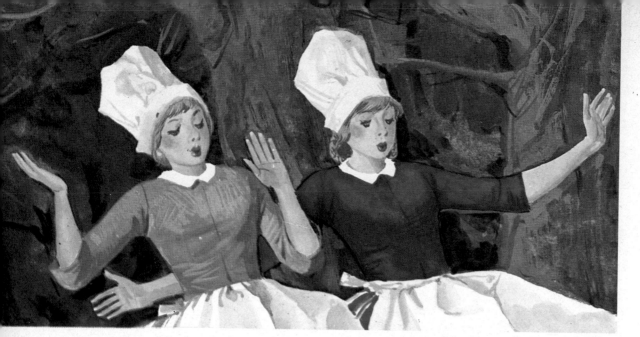

On their way home from
the village the sisters found
the dwarf again, not in
trouble this time but
sitting and gloating over
hundreds of precious jewels
strewn around him. When
he saw Snow White and
Rose Red admiring his
treasure, he attacked them
with his familiar fury.

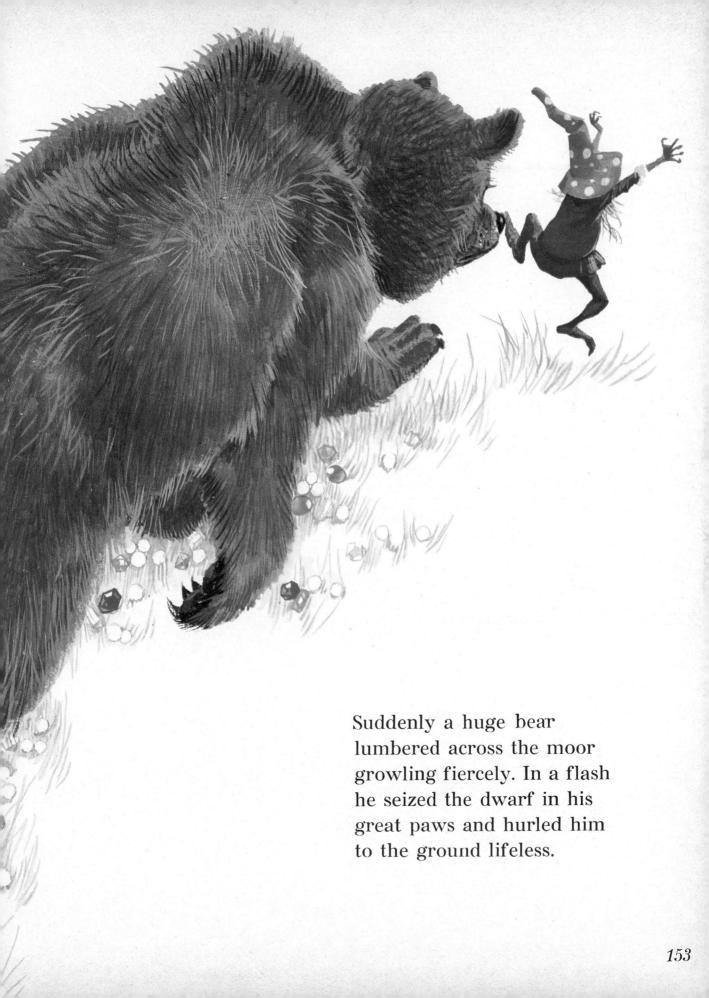

Suddenly a huge bear lumbered across the moor growling fiercely. In a flash he seized the dwarf in his great paws and hurled him to the ground lifeless.

Snow White and Rose Red were terrified of the beast until they heard a kind and familiar voice. They recognized their own beloved bear, and as they ran to embrace him, his shaggy fur fell off, and there before them stood a handsome figure dressed in cloth of gold.

"I am a prince," he said. "But, after stealing most of my wealth, that wicked dwarf put a curse on me and changed me into a bear. His death has set me free at last."

The sisters were overjoyed, and before long Snow White married the prince, and Rose Red married his brother. Their widowed mother came to live with them, bringing with her the two rosebushes which every year bore lovely roses of purest white and deepest red.

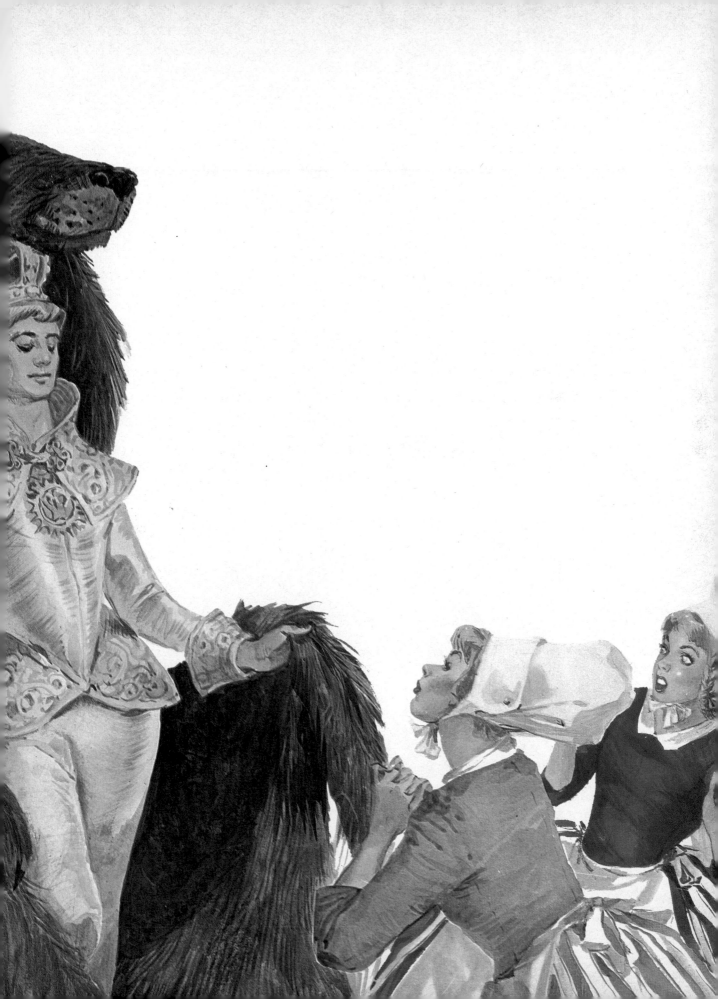

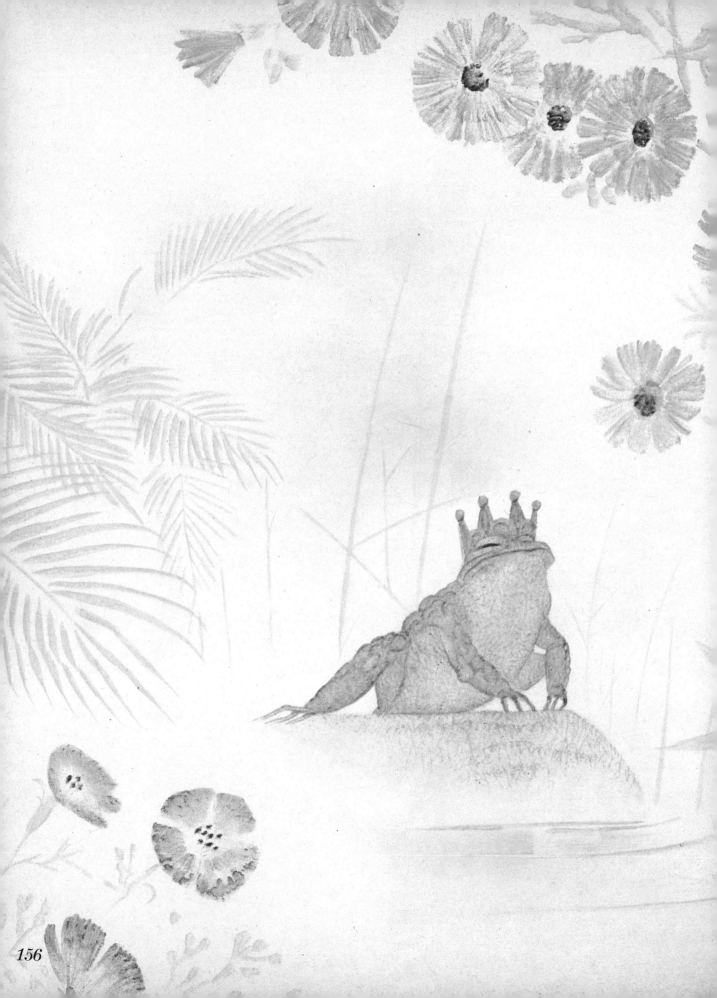

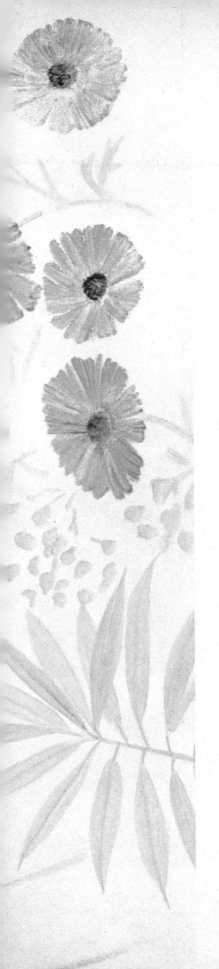

THE FROG PRINCE

Once upon a time there was a spoiled little princess who had too many toys to play with, too many beautiful dresses to wear, and too many delicious things to eat. Therefore, nothing pleased her, and she was always restless and annoyed and dissatisfied.

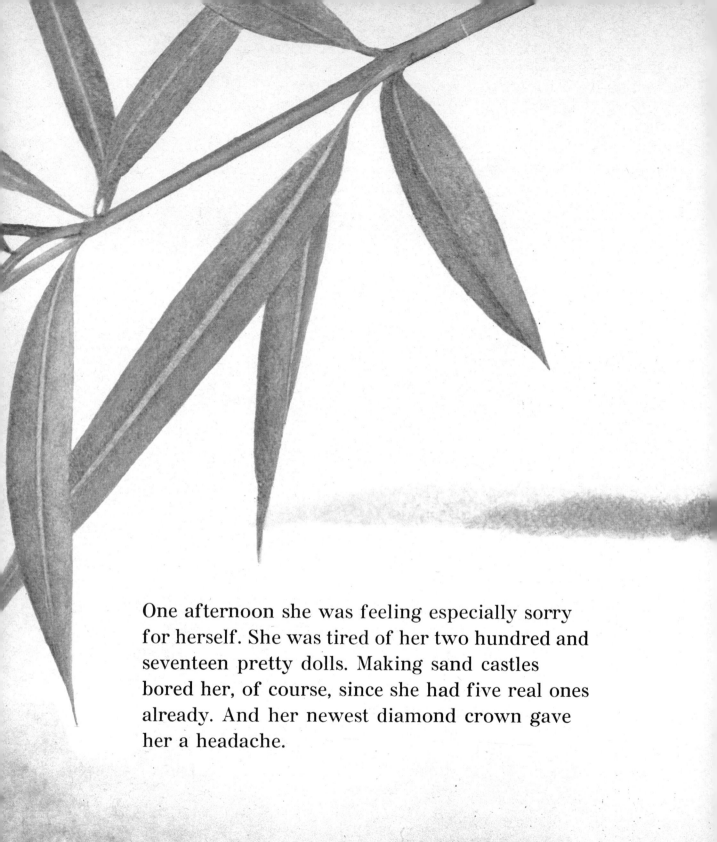

One afternoon she was feeling especially sorry
for herself. She was tired of her two hundred and
seventeen pretty dolls. Making sand castles
bored her, of course, since she had five real ones
already. And her newest diamond crown gave
her a headache.

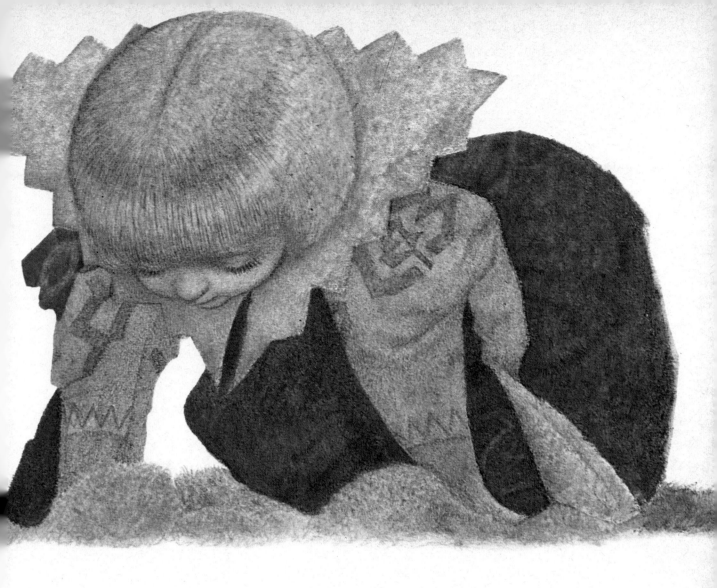

She sat irritably rolling a golden ball by her lily pond. Now, since playing ball near the water is not a very sensible idea, it was not long before the ball bounced out of her hands and deep down into the pond.

The ball was made of purest gold and was naturally very heavy, so it sank right to the bottom immediately. This sent the cranky little princess into a royal tantrum.

"Oh!" she screamed. "I'd do anything to get my beautiful golden ball back!"

"Would you really?" croaked a voice by her side.

"Ugh! How disgusting!" shrieked the princess when she saw a giant frog sitting near her.

"I may not be so beautiful," replied the frog, "but I do dive beautifully. If I find your ball, would you really do anything I ask?"

"Why yes!" cried the princess.

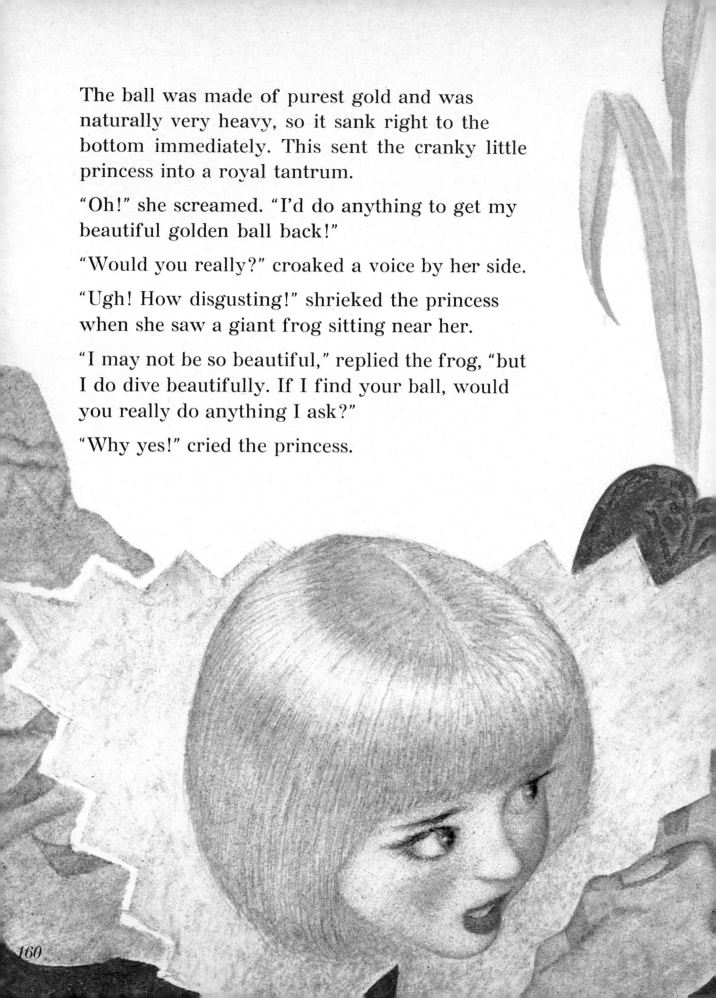

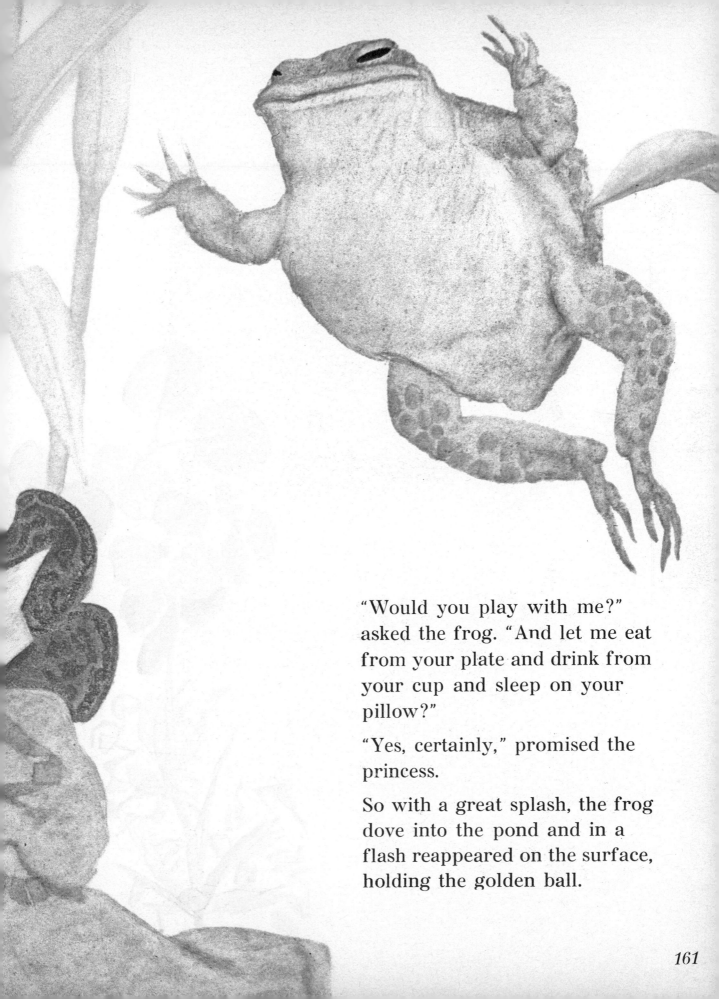

"Would you play with me?" asked the frog. "And let me eat from your plate and drink from your cup and sleep on your pillow?"

"Yes, certainly," promised the princess.

So with a great splash, the frog dove into the pond and in a flash reappeared on the surface, holding the golden ball.

The princess was delighted to have her golden ball again and immediately started to run back to her castle.

"Wait a minute!" croaked the frog. "What about all your promises?"

"WHAT promises?" the princess called back over her shoulder as she kept on running.

"I have my golden ball back," she said to herself. "I really don't have to worry about those silly promises to that disgusting frog now."

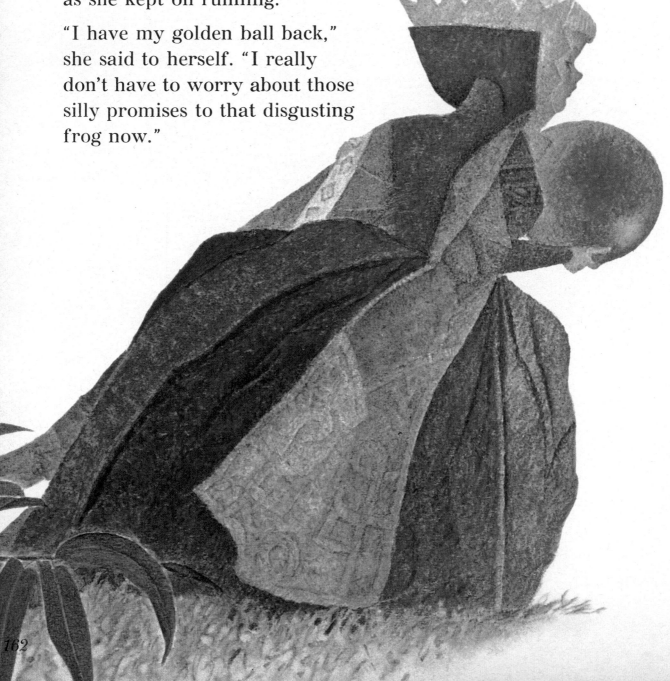

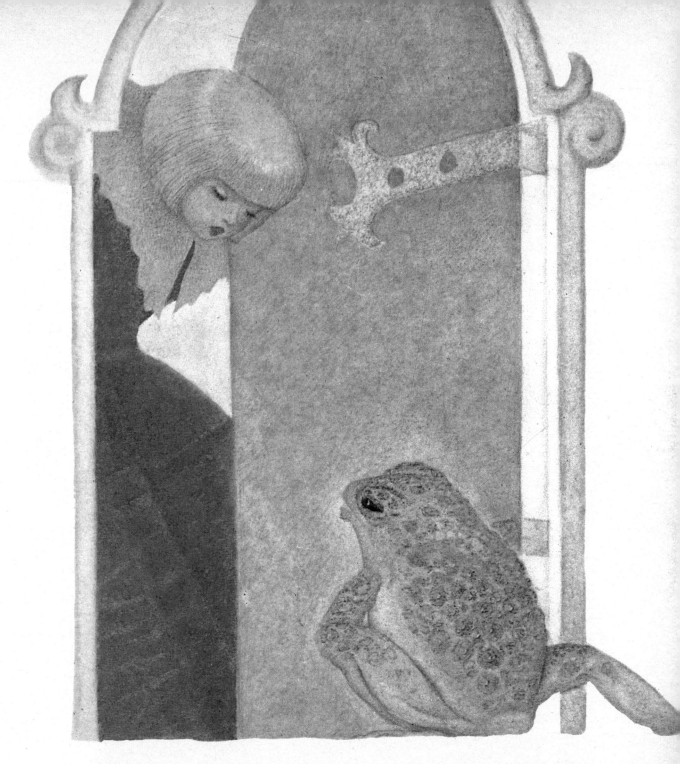

The following day, when she and her father the king
were eating their royal luncheon, they heard strange
footsteps outside the dining hall—splashy, wet footsteps
on the marble stairs. Next there came a splashy, wet
tapping at the door. The princess opened it and found
the big frog squatting outside.

She slammed the door quickly, but the king noticed that she seemed upset and ordered her to tell him what had happened. Now, even a princess may not disobey a king, especially her own father, so she had to tell the whole story.

"Did you actually make all those promises to that kind frog?" asked the king sternly.

"Yes, Sire," answered the princess in a very meek voice.

"Have I not tried to teach you that a true princess must always keep her promises?" the king went on.

"Yes, Father," whispered the willful little princess.

"Then you know what you must do, don't you?" said the king, gently but firmly.

"Yes, Sire," she answered, knowing that she must obey her father. She opened the door, and immediately the frog padded into the dining hall.

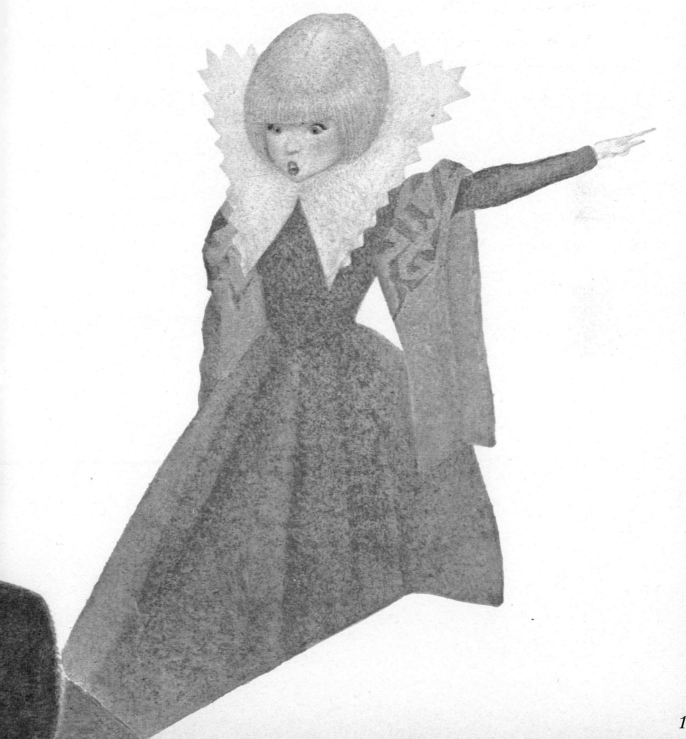

The ugly frog took one great leap and, with a wet plop, landed on a satin chair right next to the princess.

"Now," he croaked happily, "may I eat from your plate and drink from your cup as you promised?"

The princess looked at her father with a pitiful expression, but the king only stared back sternly.

"Please do!" she forced herself to say politely, then turned her head away and shivered.

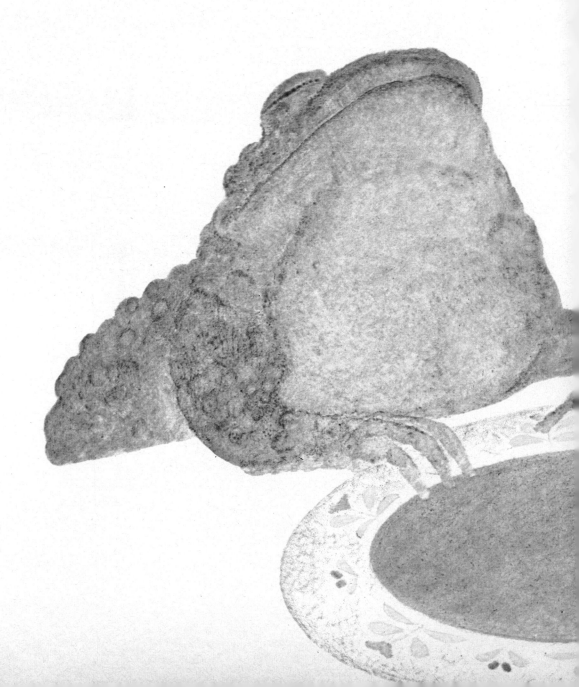

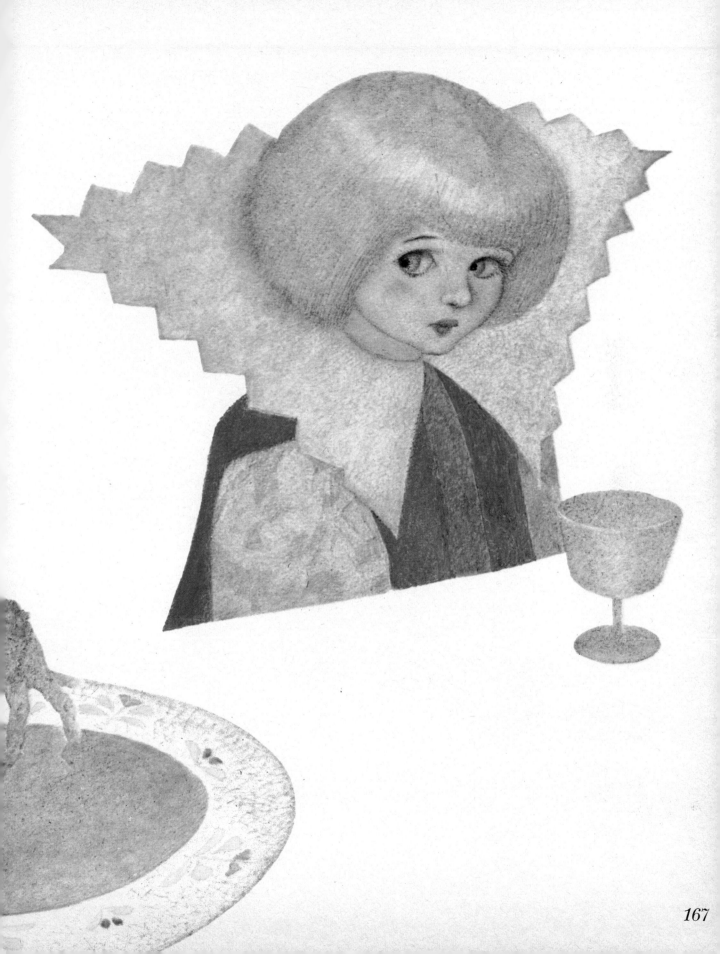

The princess could not eat a morsel herself, but the frog ate and drank heartily. Furious at her predicament, the princess gnashed her teeth and schemed at how she would get even with the annoying frog later. When he was finished, the slimy old frog yawned and stretched his flippers.

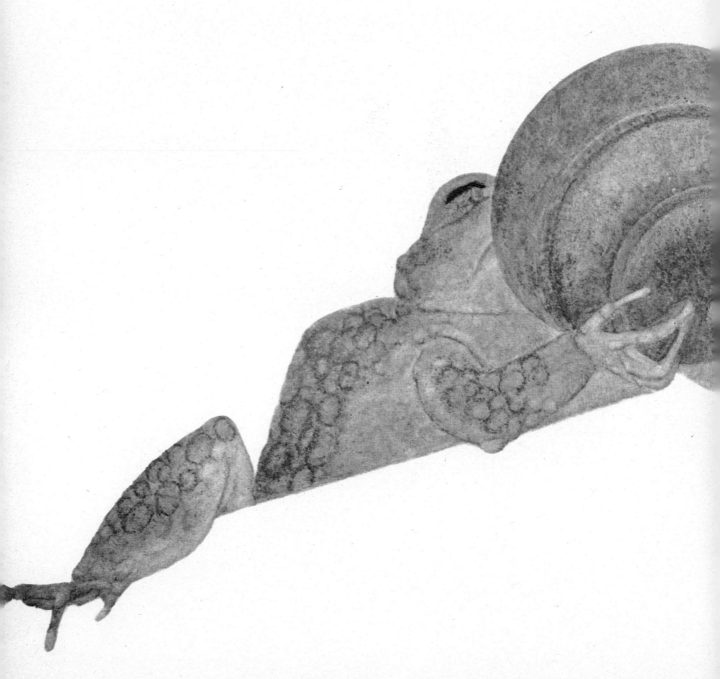

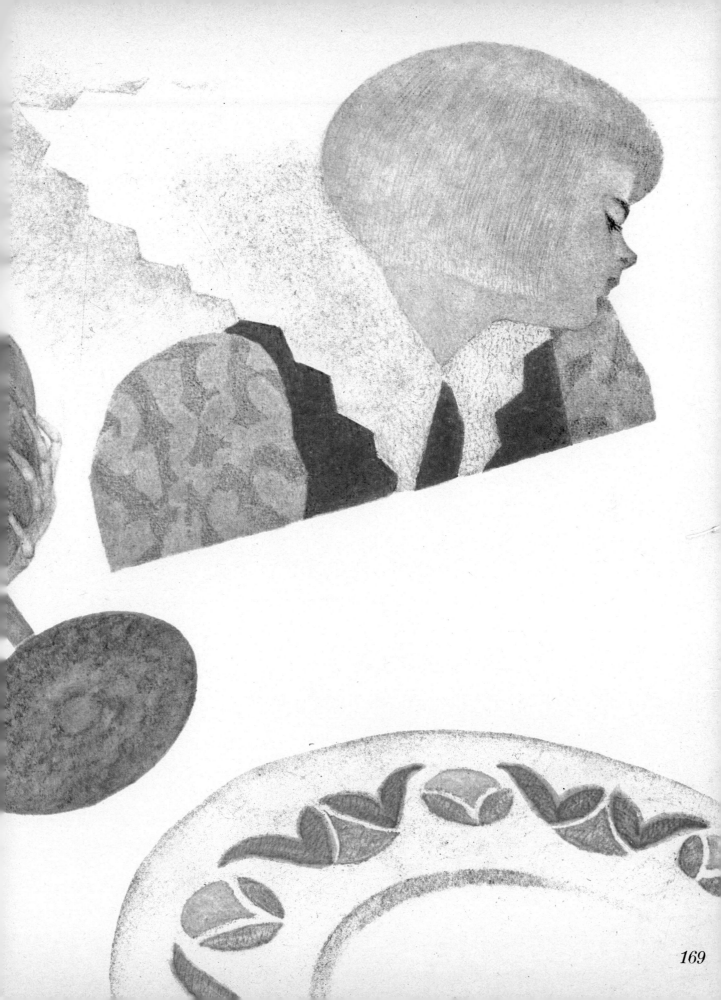

"Will you let me sleep on your satin pillow now, as you promised?" he croaked sleepily.

Again the princess looked helplessly toward her father, but again the king only frowned at her.

"Of course," she said obediently, then carried the frog to her bedchamber and let him sleep on her satin pillow.

For three days and three nights the frog continued to eat from her plate, drink from her cup, and sleep on her pillow. The princess herself hardly ate or drank or slept at all.

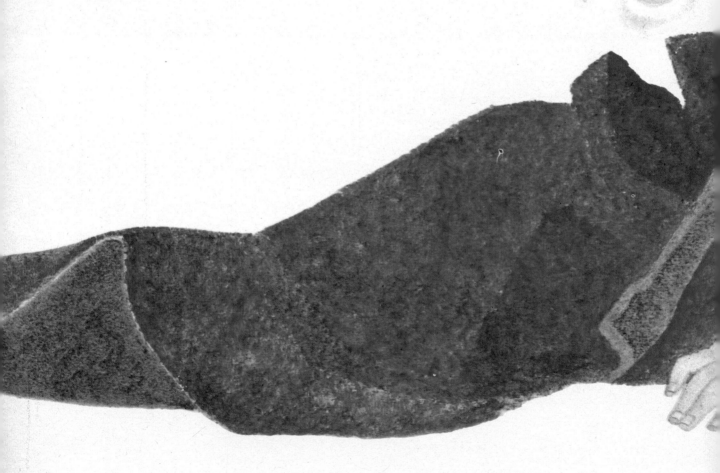

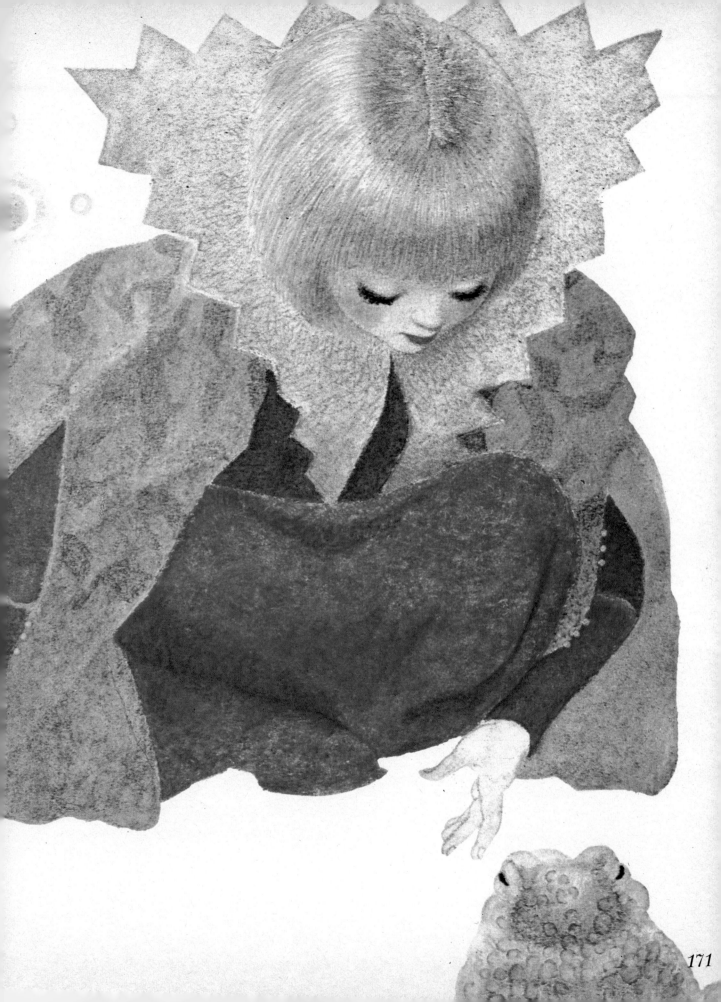

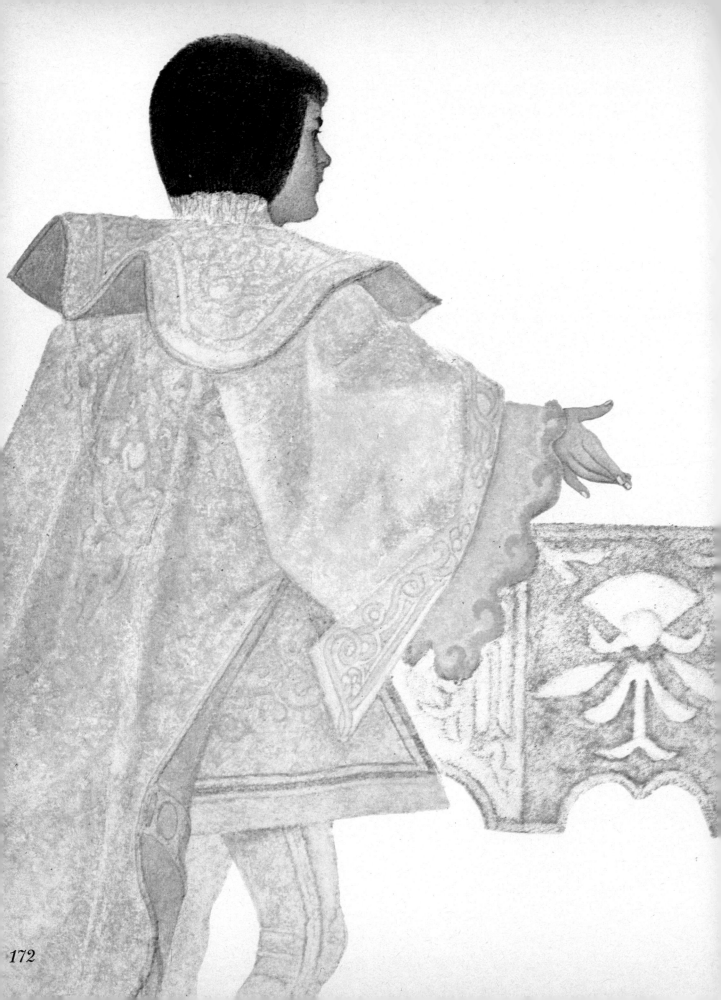

On the third night, completely
exhausted, the princess finally
fell asleep. And when she
awoke, the frog was gone;
instead, near her pillow stood a
prince dressed in gold velvet
and brocade. She listened in
wonderment as he explained
that a spiteful fairy had turned
him into a frog and had forced
him to live in the lily pond until
a beautiful princess would
allow him to eat from her
plate, drink from her cup, and
sleep on her pillow for three
days and three nights.

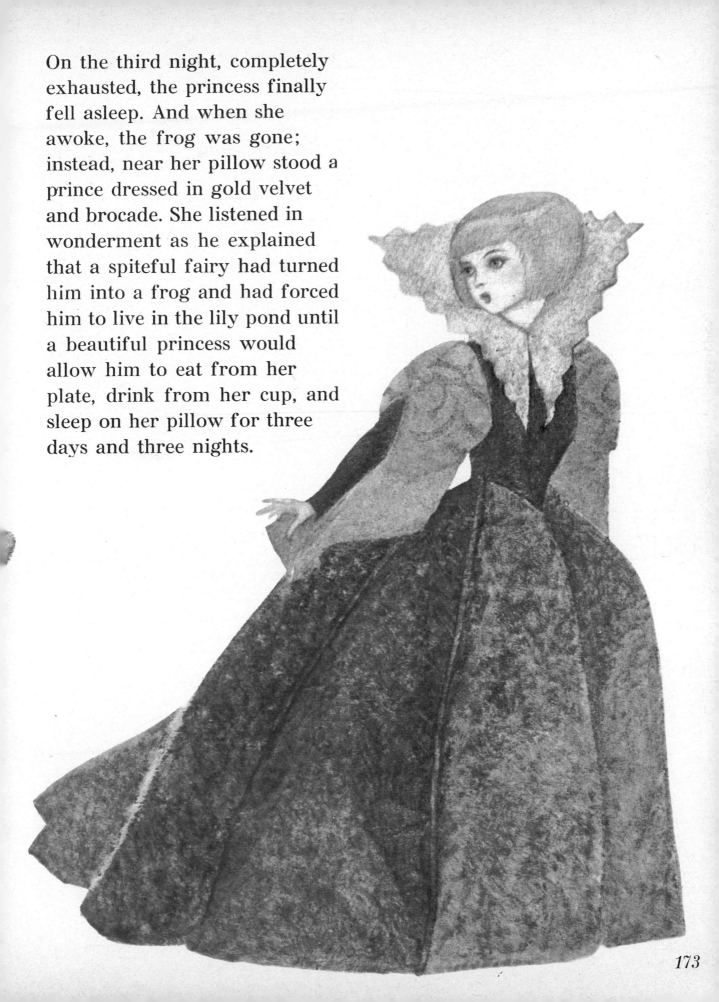

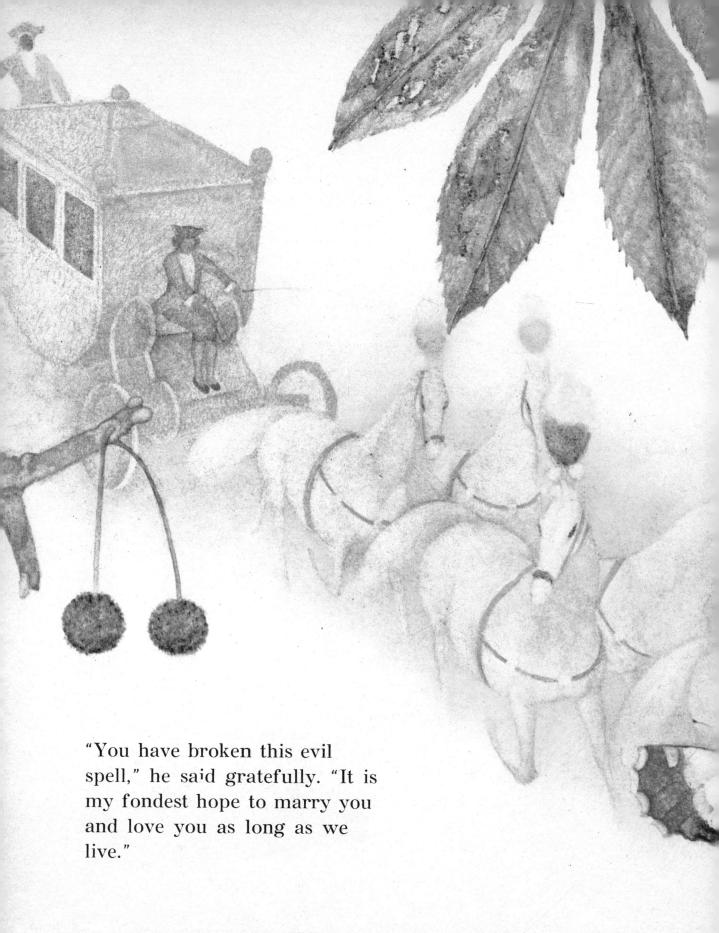

"You have broken this evil spell," he said gratefully. "It is my fondest hope to marry you and love you as long as we live."

Already in love with the handsome young prince, the princess did not hesitate and quickly promised to be his bride. The king was delighted with the match, and soon a splendid coach drawn by eight white horses with golden harnesses appeared to carry them away. And so the prince and his bride returned to his own wonderful kingdom, where they began a long, happy life together.

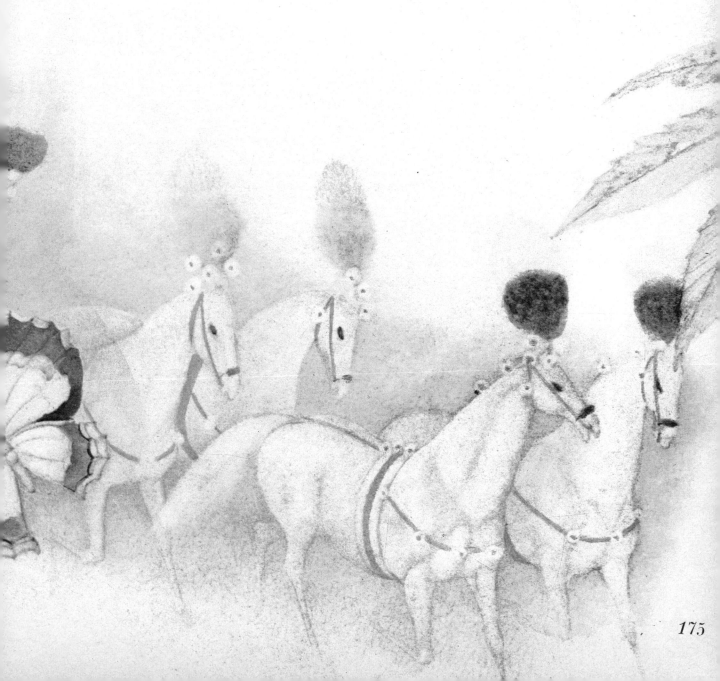

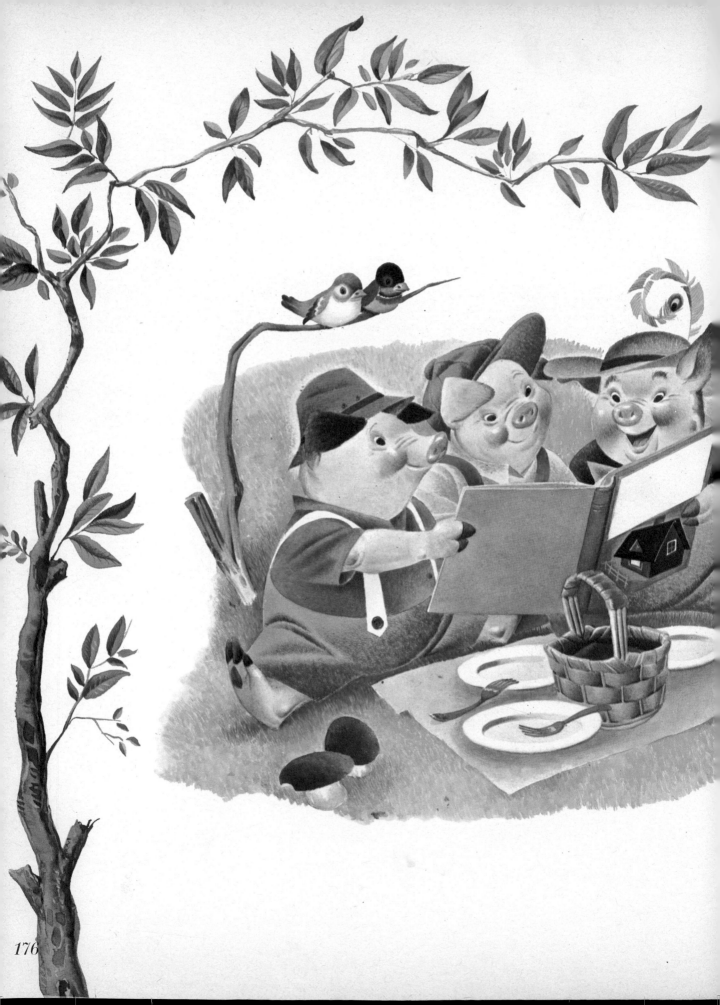

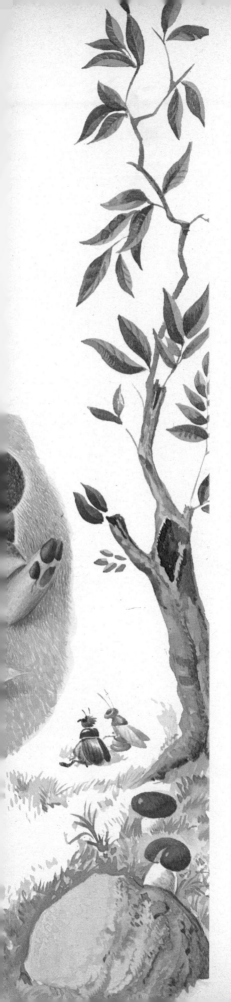

THE THREE LITTLE PIGS

Once upon a time, there were three little pigs who lived happily with their mother until it was time for them to leave their pleasant sty and make their way in the world by themselves. They loved romping through the green fields, but they could not really enjoy themselves freely because they were always afraid of the big bad wolf, a nasty creature who preferred tender little pig to any other wolf-food. One day they solved their problem.

"We'll each build a wolf-proof house," they decided.

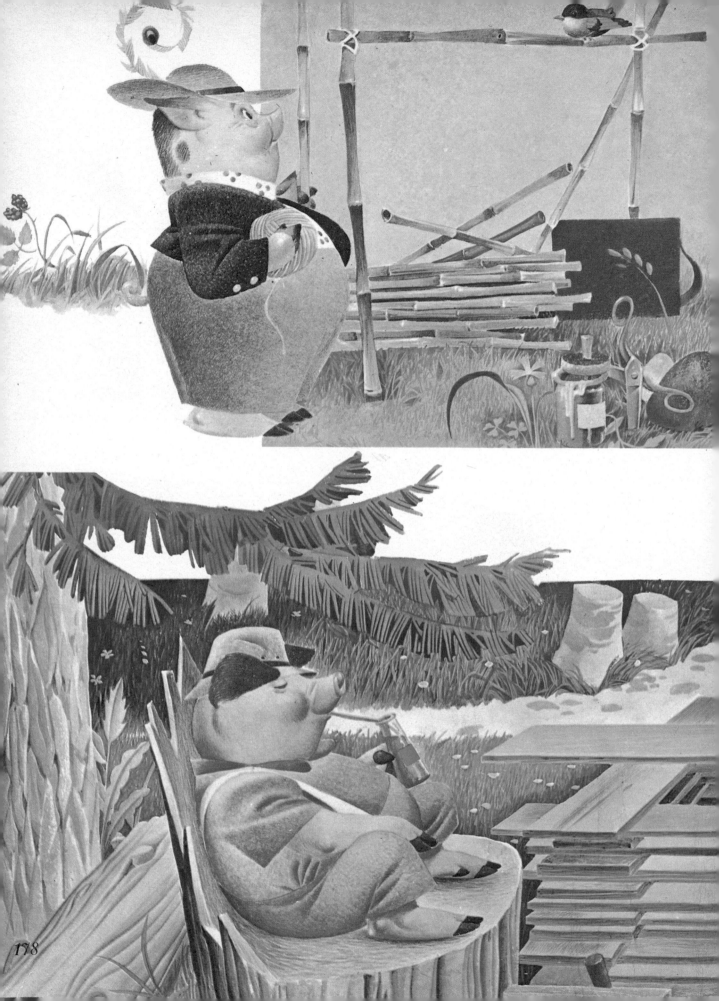

They read books on how to make wolf-proof houses and consulted other creatures who were expert builders; they looked at birds' nests, checked beehives, and studied beaver dams. Finally they were ready.

The first little pig built himself a pretty little house of bamboo poles, and his brother built a handsome little house of wood. They both felt very safe, but the third little pig warned his brothers that their houses were not strong enough to be wolf-proof.

But the other two would not listen, and so the third brother stopped arguing with them and built his own house of bricks and mortar. His house was the strongest and sturdiest and even had a tall chimney, locks on the windows, and bolts on the doors.

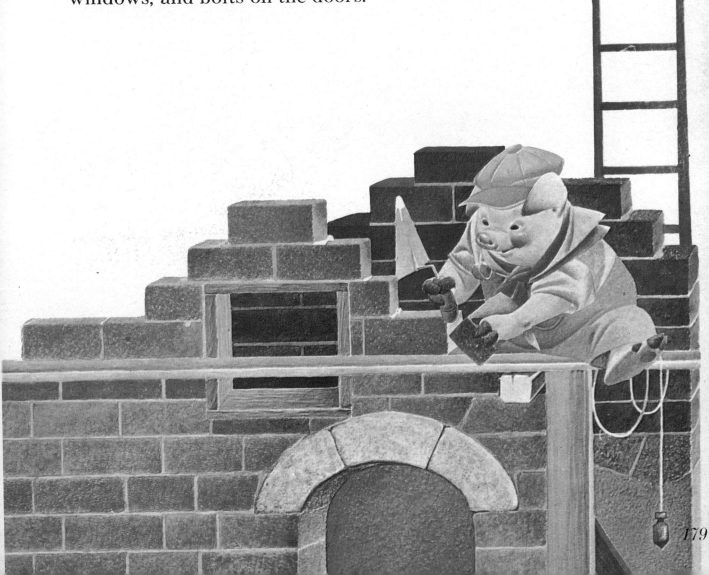

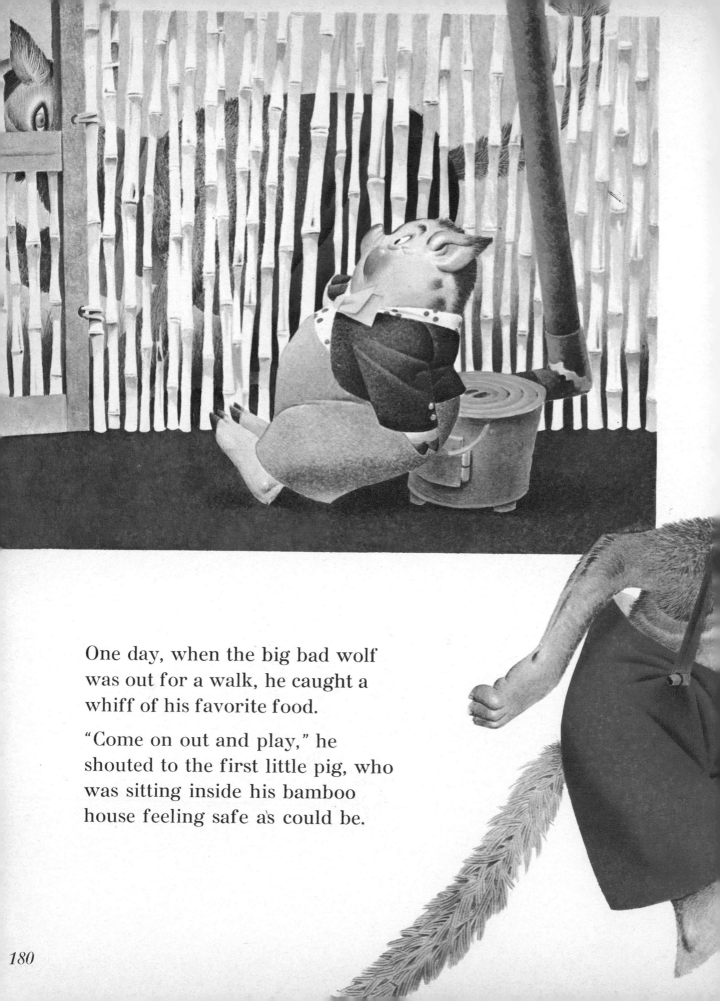

One day, when the big bad wolf was out for a walk, he caught a whiff of his favorite food.

"Come on out and play," he shouted to the first little pig, who was sitting inside his bamboo house feeling safe as could be.

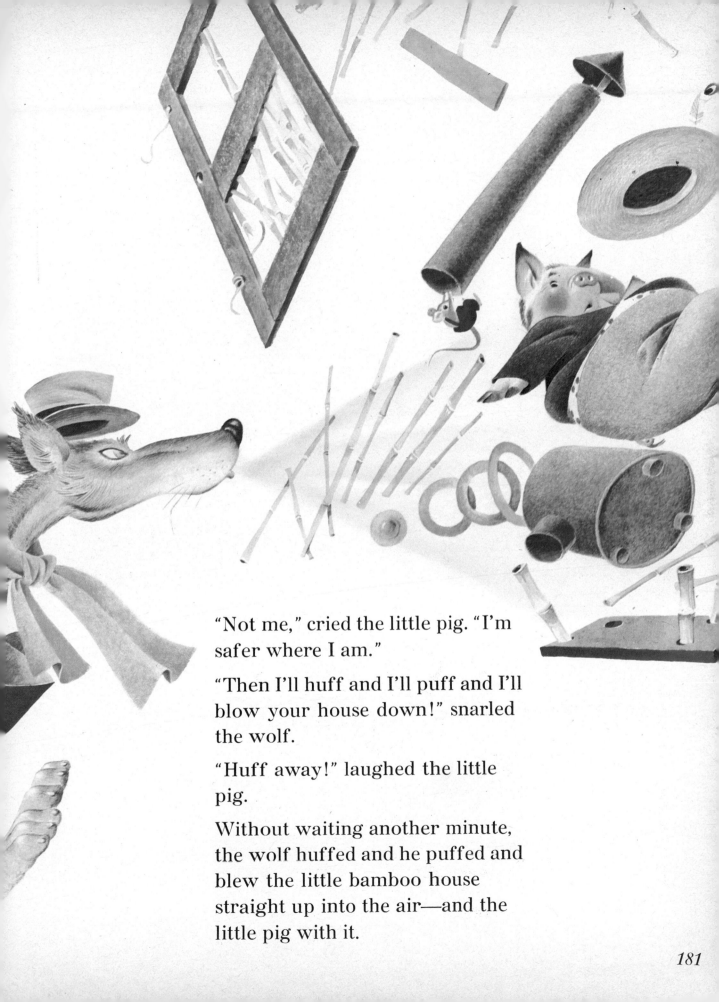

"Not me," cried the little pig. "I'm safer where I am."

"Then I'll huff and I'll puff and I'll blow your house down!" snarled the wolf.

"Huff away!" laughed the little pig.

Without waiting another minute, the wolf huffed and he puffed and blew the little bamboo house straight up into the air—and the little pig with it.

He was blown right across the meadow and landed on his brother's doorstep. The two little pigs locked themselves inside, and both felt safe in the handsome little house of wood. When the wolf came loping by, the smell of his favorite food made him hungrier than ever.

"Come out and play—I'm lonely," he called, knowing there were little pigs inside.

"Not us!" the little pigs called back and giggled and chuckled because they felt so safe in their cosy little wooden abode.

"Then," growled the wolf fiercely, "I'll huff and I'll puff and I'll blow your house down!"

He sucked as much air as he could into his lungs and then blew one of his famous blasts, the most powerful one ever.

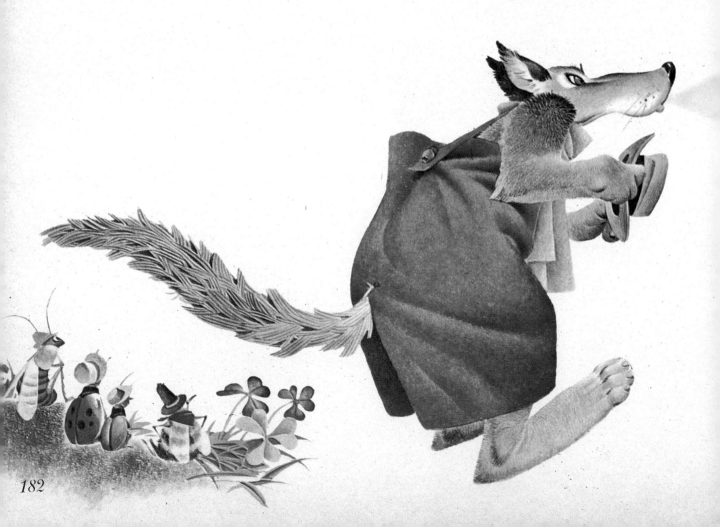

The handsome little wooden house collapsed, and the roof was blown straight up into the air with the two little pigs clinging to the rafters.

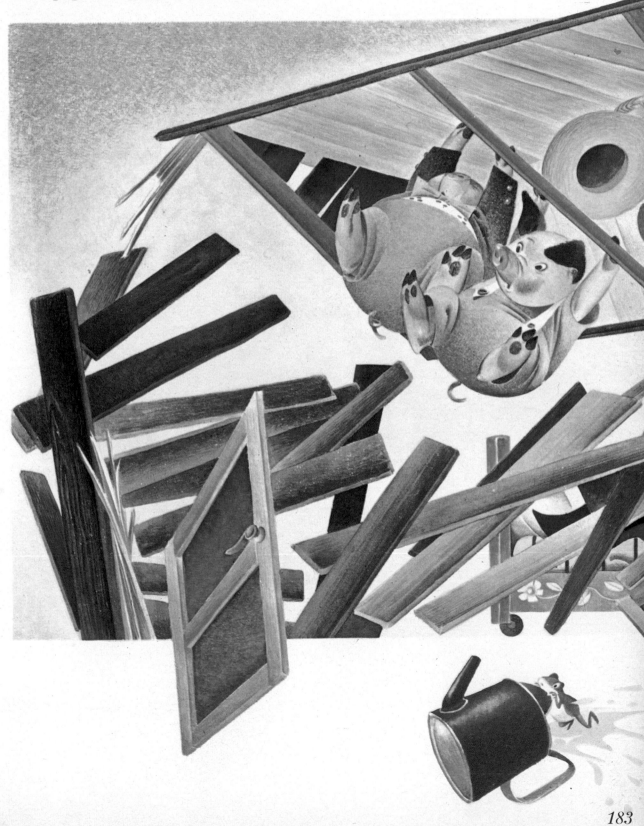

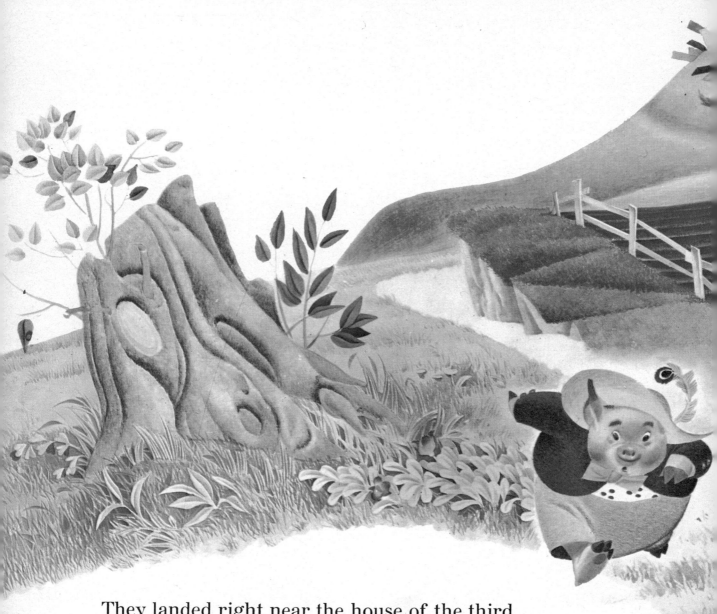

They landed right near the house of the third
little pig and ran lickety-split to his door, with the
wolf trailing right behind them. Their brother
called to them from the window that his door was
open, so they rushed inside and slammed it shut.
Quickly they bolted the bar across the door
and locked the locks on the windows. Then, safe
and sound, they waited inside the little house of
bricks and wondered what the big bad wolf
would do next.

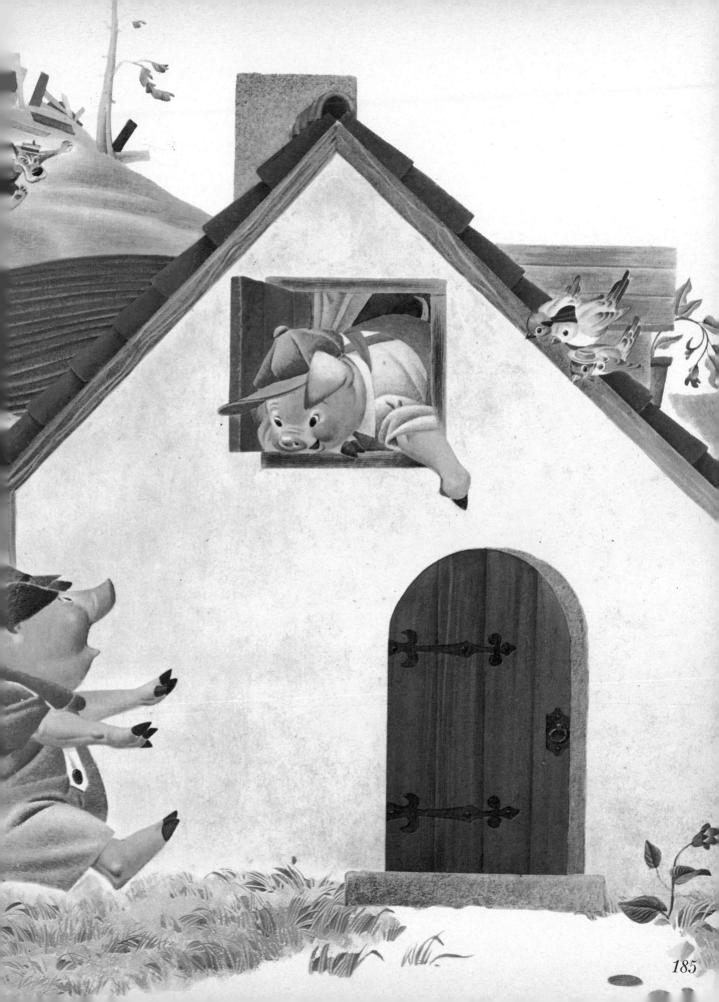

By this time, the big bad wolf was hungrier than ever and even more tempted by the smell of his favorite food. He was furious because the first two little pigs had escaped him, and this time he was determined to eat all three for his dinner. He knew just what to do, of course.

"I'll huff and I'll puff and I'll blow your house down!" he roared to the brothers inside.

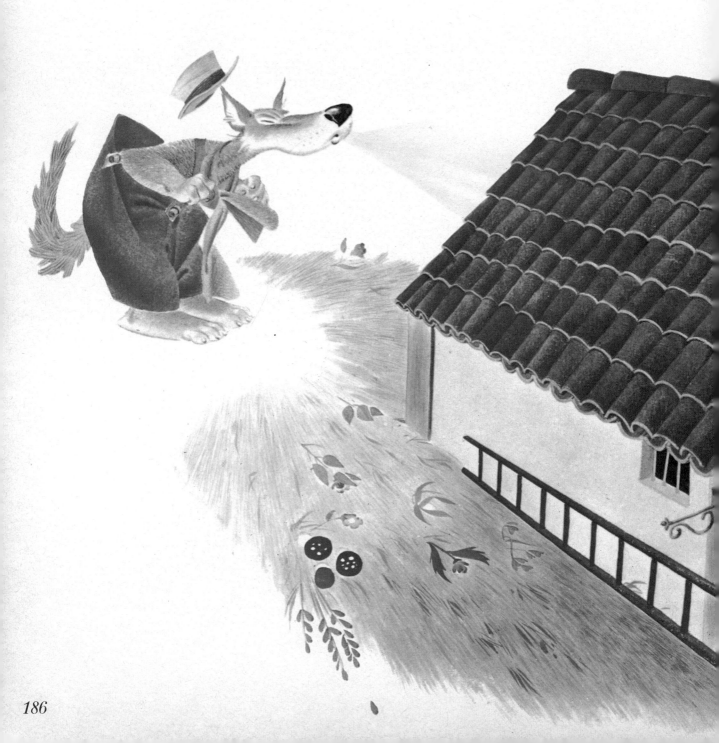

He drew in all the air he could hold and blew it out in one of his famous blasts. But nothing happened. The strong little house stayed firm and sturdy. He blew another blast, and chairs flew into the air, along with brooms, spades, barrels and everything else, but the little house still did not budge an inch. The little pigs giggled happily, safe inside.

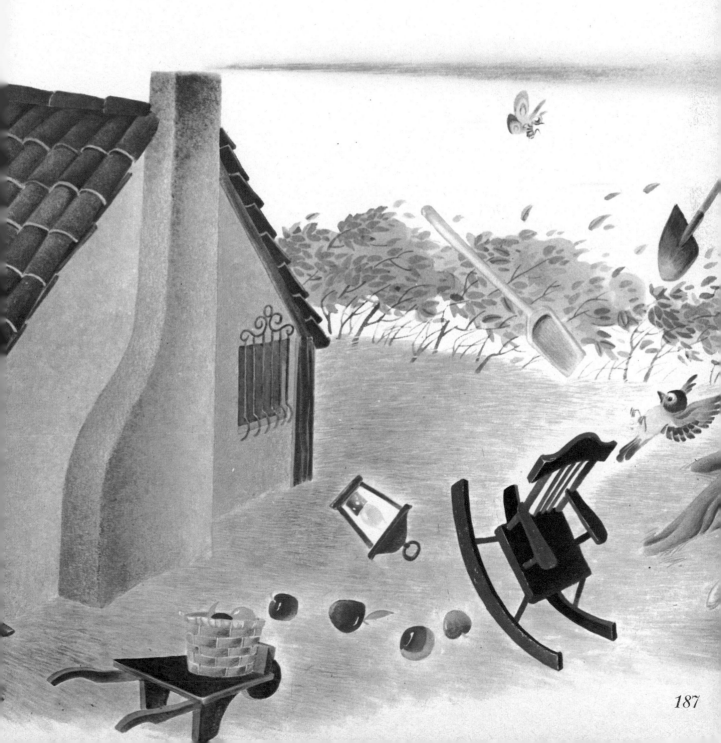

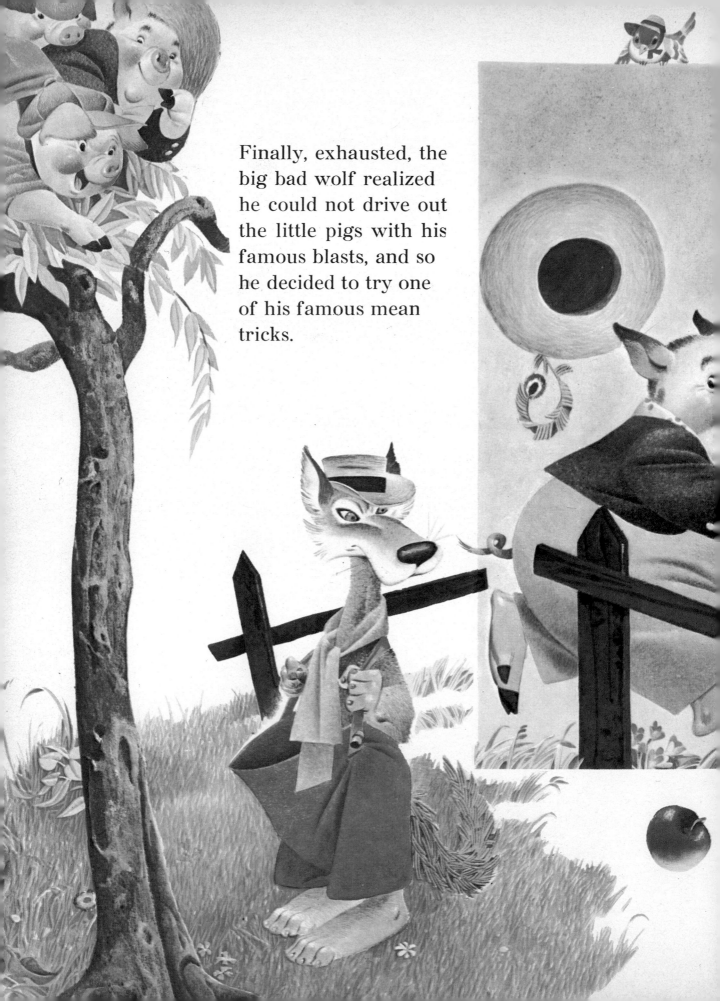

Finally, exhausted, the big bad wolf realized he could not drive out the little pigs with his famous blasts, and so he decided to try one of his famous mean tricks.

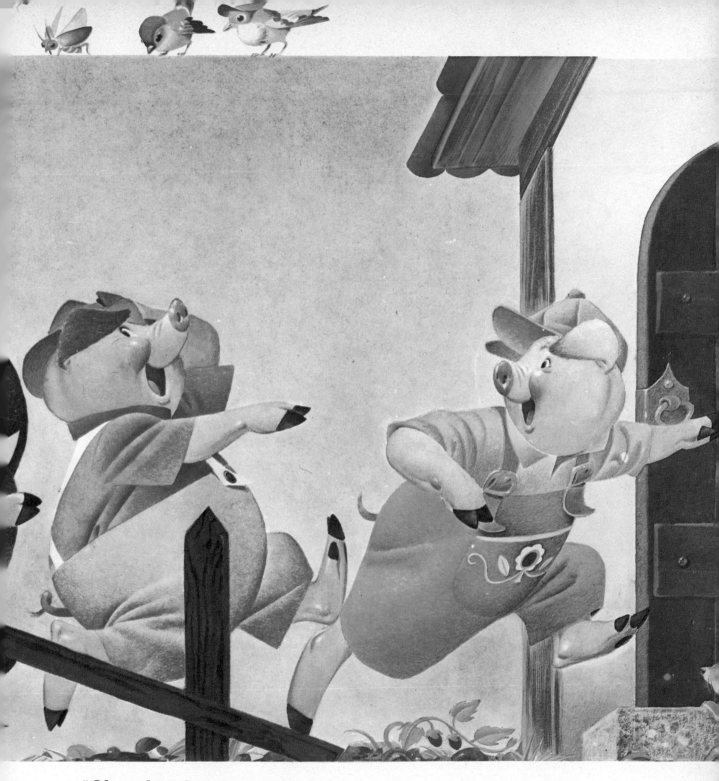

"Oh, what lovely apples you have in your tree!" he called out sweetly. "Let's pick them together and share them," he went on in a friendly voice.

But the little pigs could not be tricked. They climbed into the tree from the roof and threw apples down at the wolf. Then, when his back was turned, they jumped from the tree and rushed right back into their little house.

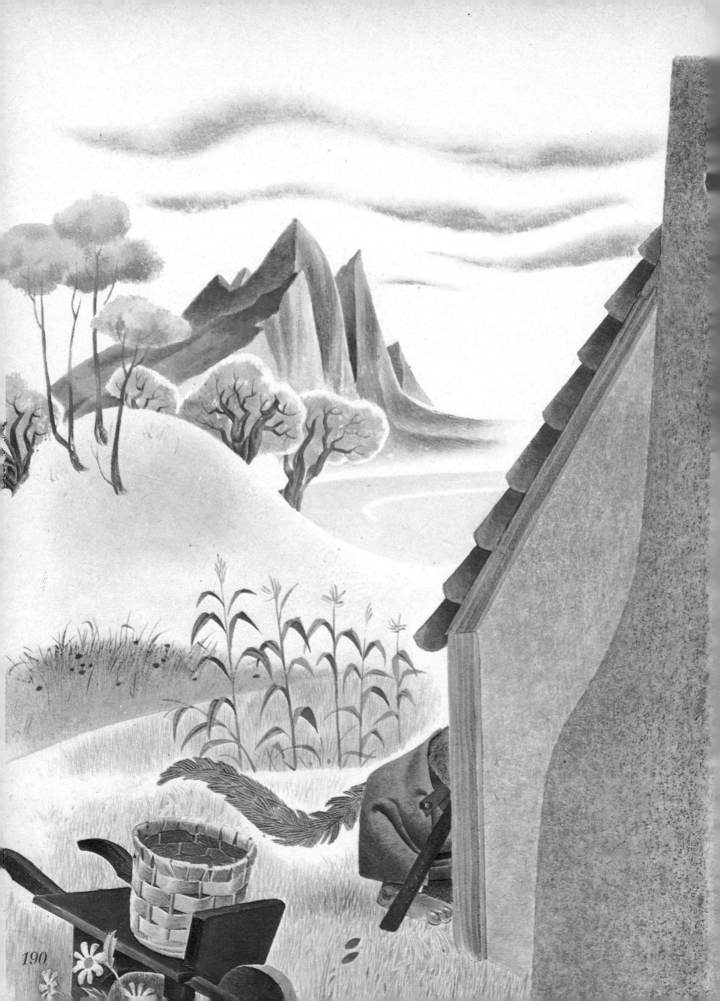

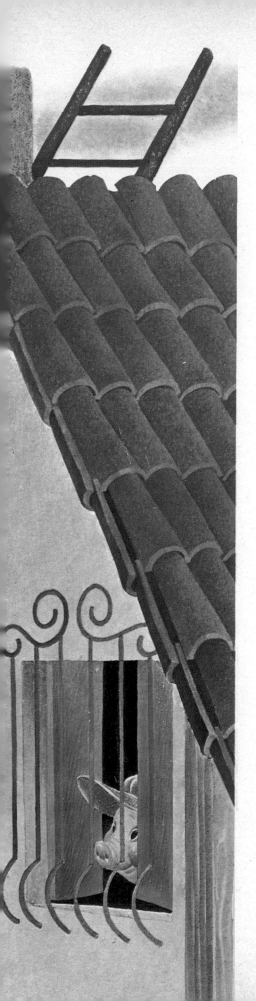

When the wolf realized that the three little pigs had tricked him and were once again safe inside their sturdy little brick house, he was angrier than ever—and hungrier as well. His famous blasts had failed, and so had his famous trickery. He had to invent a new plan! He found a long red ladder and very, very quietly, so that the little pigs would not hear him, propped it up behind the house and climbed to the roof.

"This time I'll really catch them and have myself a fine dinner," he chuckled to himself. "I'll slide down their chimney and pounce on them like a hawk. They'll never know where I came from."

But the shrewd third little pig had been watching from the window, and while the big bad wolf was climbing onto the roof, the three little pigs had time to think up a plan of their own.

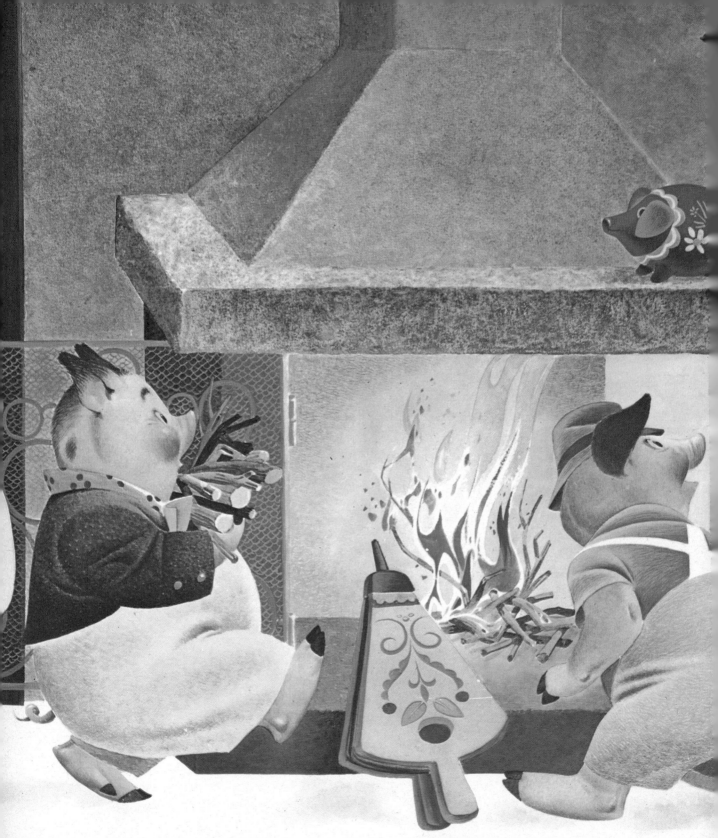

"I know what we'll do," said the third little pig calmly.

"Abandon the house!" squealed one brother.

"Hide in the forest!" whimpered the other.

"No, you two sillies," laughed their brother.

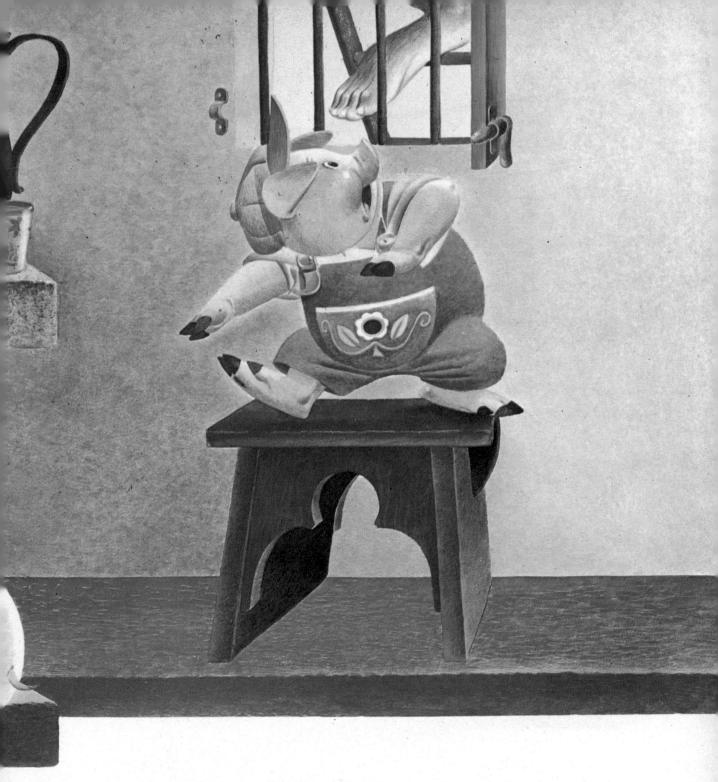

"We'll build a great hot fire in the hearth, and when the wolf comes down the chimney he'll get a warm welcome. Come on, help me!"

Quickly the three got to work and laid a huge pile of logs in the hearth and set them ablaze. Great flames shot up the chimney just as the wolf started down tail-first.

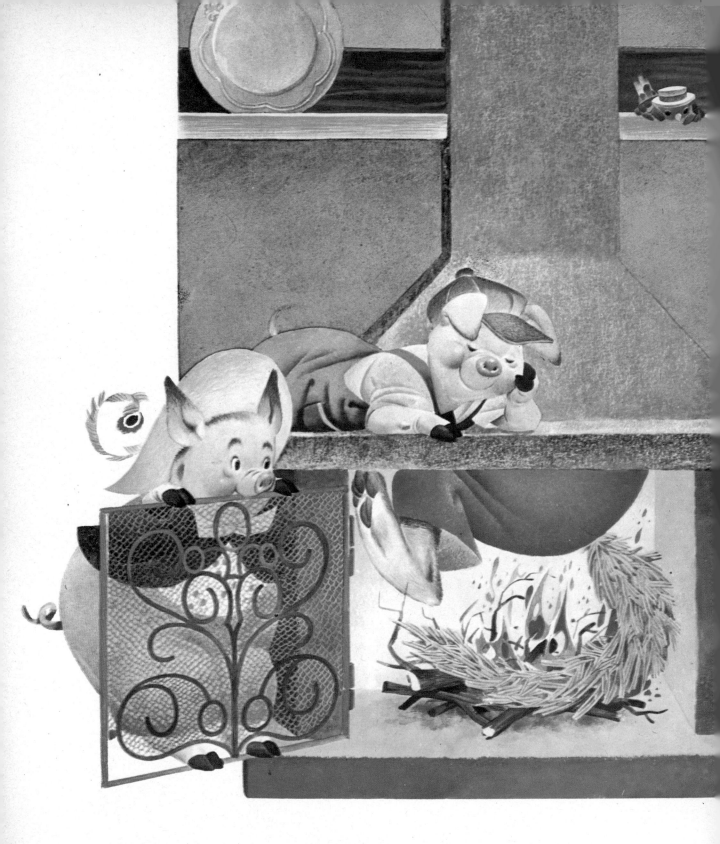

Instantly his great hairy tail was aflame, but he
could not stop sliding and fell straight onto the
burning logs.

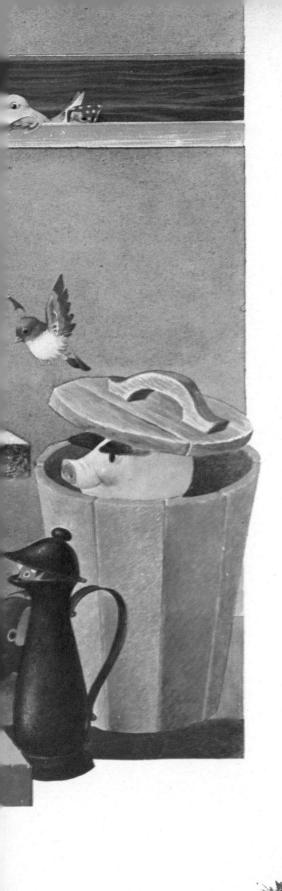

"Help! I'm burning up!" he roared as he rushed out of the fireplace. "Let me out!" he shrieked, screaming with pain and running round in circles.

The first little pig opened the door, and the fiery wolf dashed outside. He ran across the meadow in great leaps and bounds and was never heard of again. After this, the three little pigs built another sturdy house of bricks, big enough for all of them, and lived there happily ever after, safe from the big bad wolf and any other enemies.

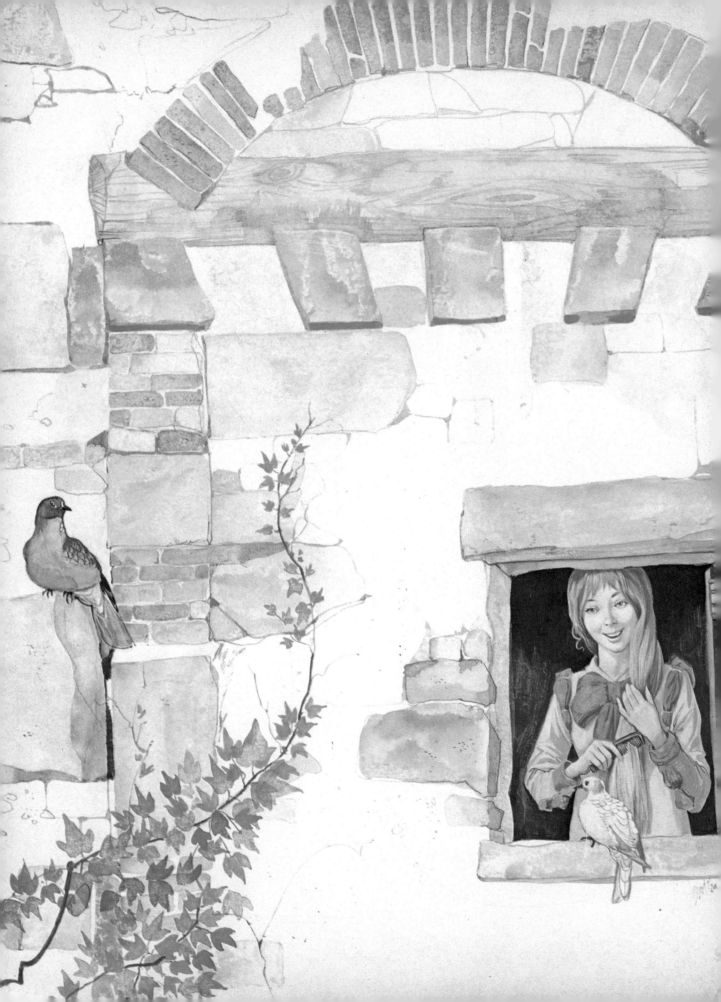

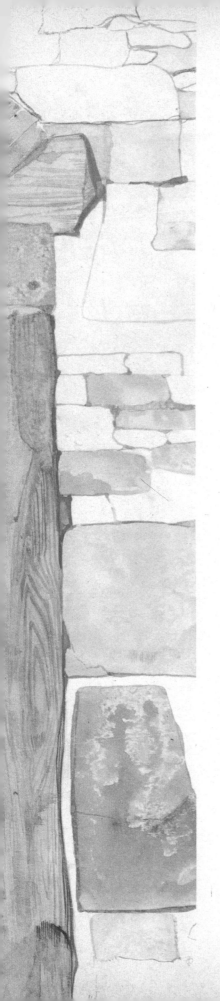

RAPUNZEL

Once upon a time, in a tiny cottage near the forest, there lived a young woodcutter and his beautiful wife. They were happy with each other and never lonely. A big, honey-colored dog, a mother hen, and three chicks kept them company. But they were even happier when they found out that they were soon to have a baby. The young husband was overjoyed that they would soon have a child of their own. He did everything he could to help his wife and to prepare for the baby's arrival. He swept the house, gathered the eggs, and carried water. Every night he worked long hours carving a cradle just the right size for a new baby.

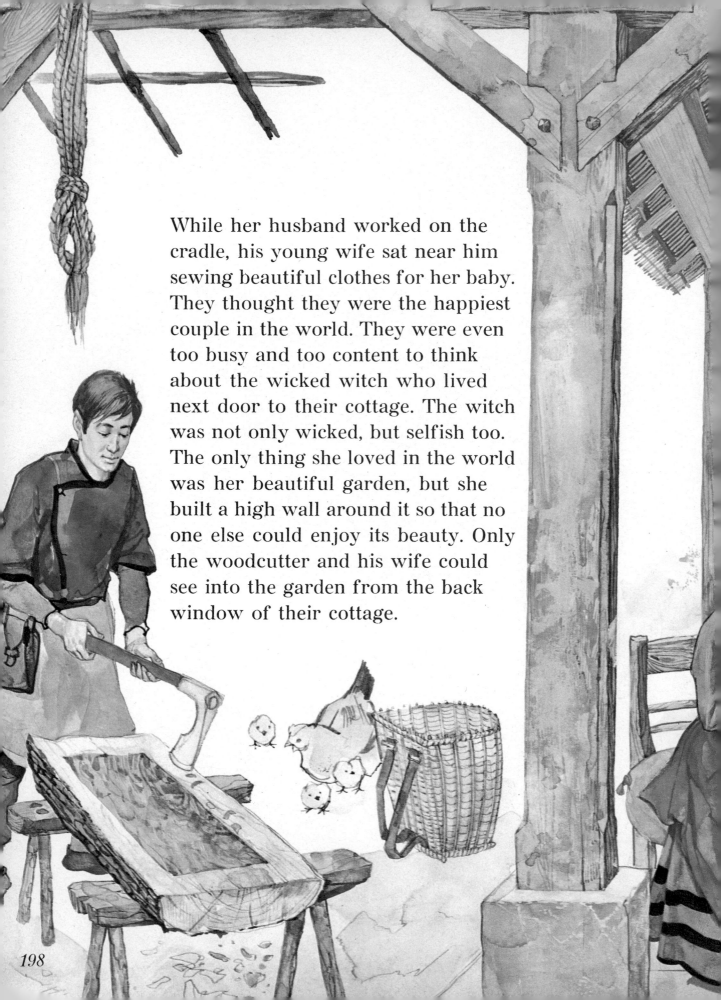

While her husband worked on the cradle, his young wife sat near him sewing beautiful clothes for her baby. They thought they were the happiest couple in the world. They were even too busy and too content to think about the wicked witch who lived next door to their cottage. The witch was not only wicked, but selfish too. The only thing she loved in the world was her beautiful garden, but she built a high wall around it so that no one else could enjoy its beauty. Only the woodcutter and his wife could see into the garden from the back window of their cottage.

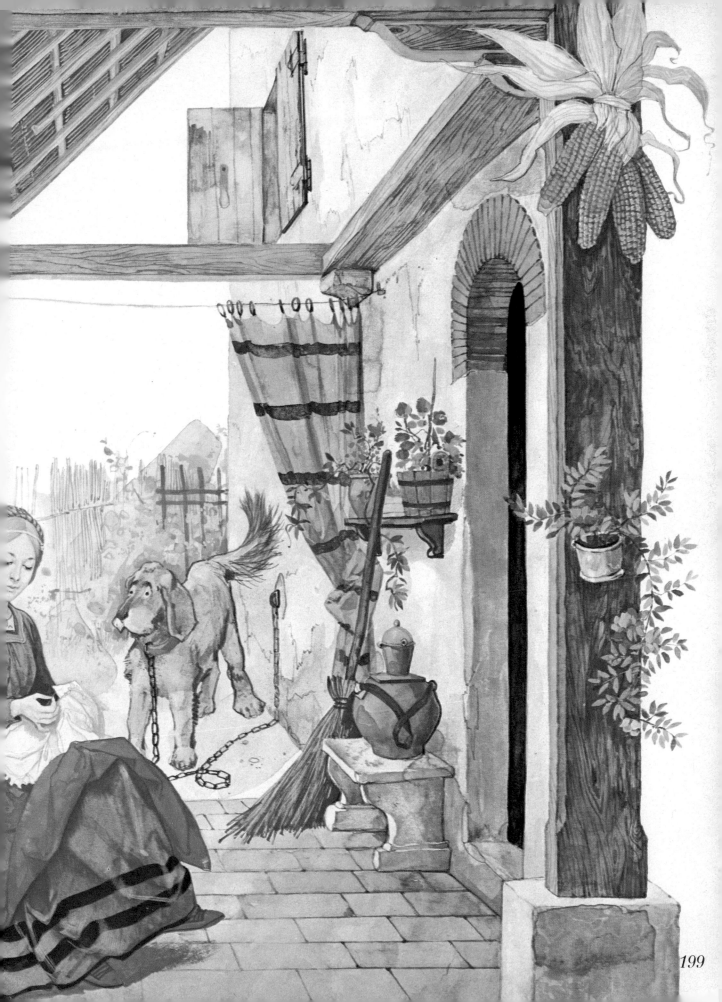

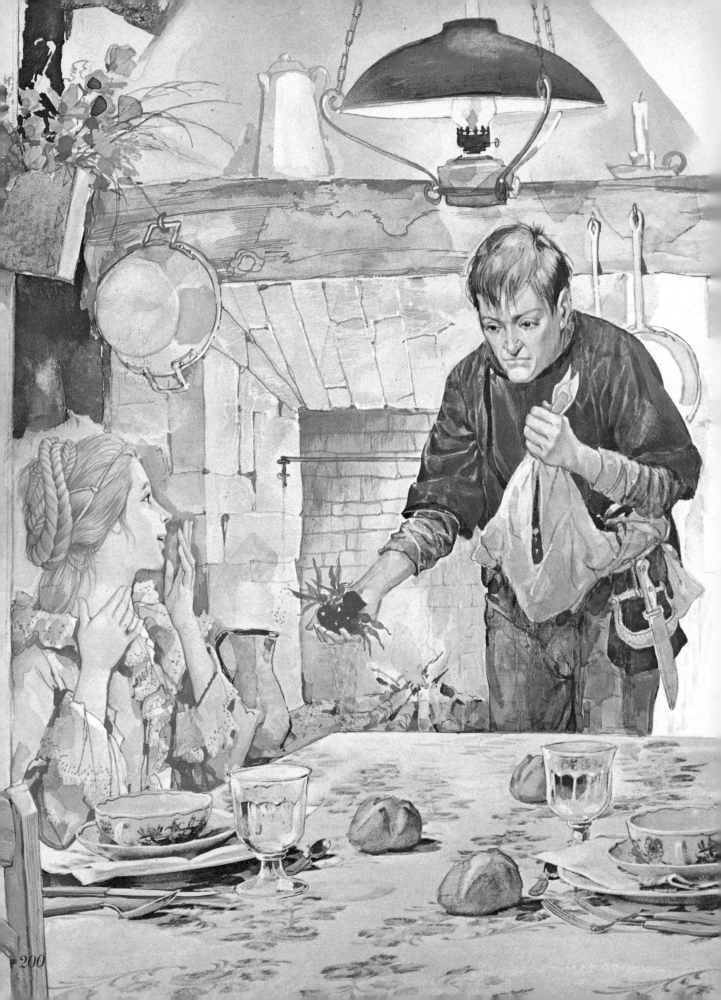

One morning shortly before their baby was to be born, the young wife stood at the window and looked into the beautiful garden.

"Oh," she sighed, "what beautiful radishes! How tender and fresh they look! How I would love to eat some right now!"

The young husband was horrified.

"How can you hope to eat anything from the witch's garden?" he asked. "You know she never gives anything to anyone."

"I know," sighed his wife sadly. But she could not stop thinking about the radishes. For days she refused to eat anything until, finally, because he loved her so much, her husband decided that she should have what she desired so greatly. That night when all was still, he climbed carefully over the high garden wall and gathered the fattest, reddest radishes he could find.

"They're just as delicious as they look!" his wife cried happily, as she ate every last one.

Every night after that, her husband climbed into the garden and stole more of the witch's radishes.

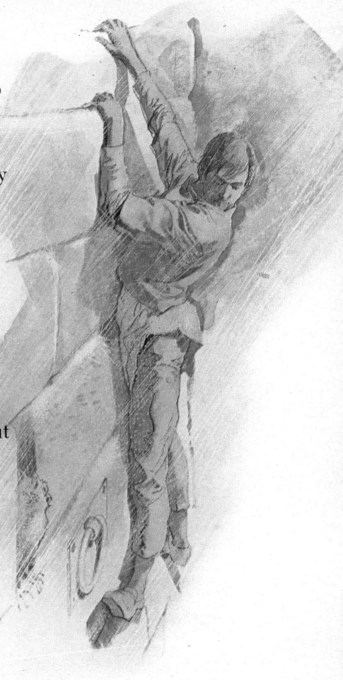

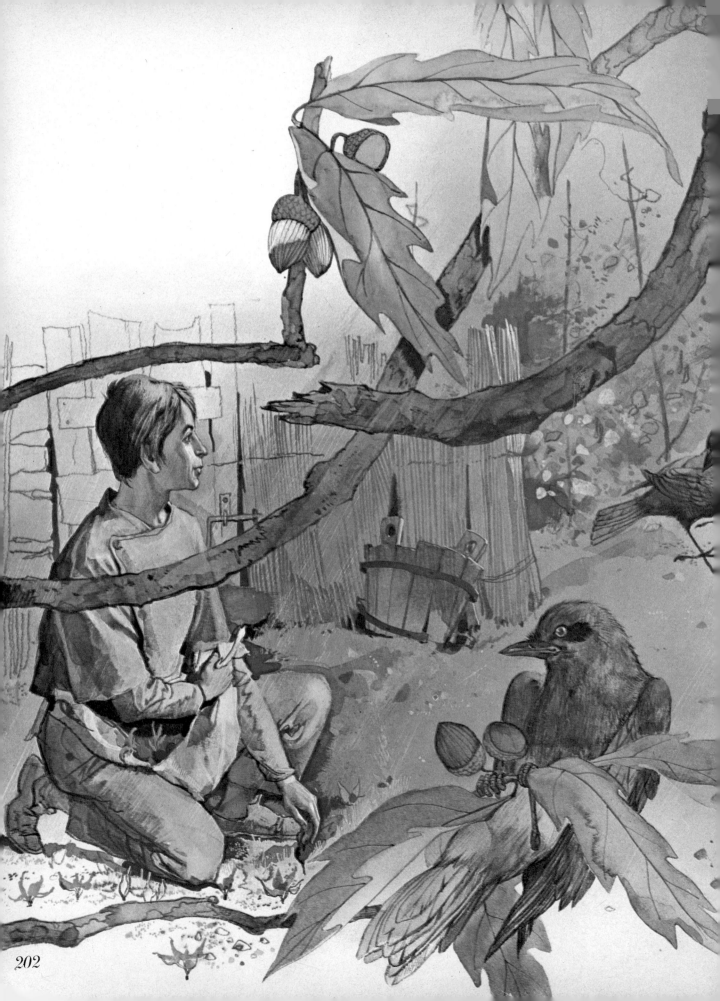

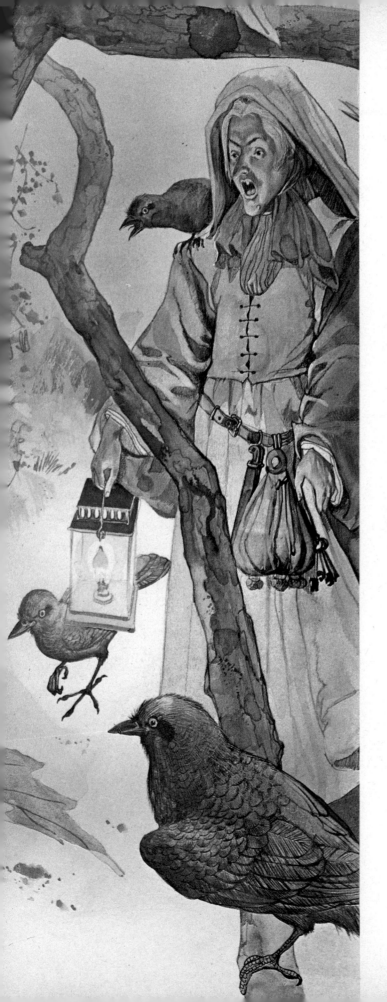

But one night, as the woodcutter climbed over the wall, the terrible witch was lying in wait for him, surrounded by her black screeching ravens.

"How dare you be so bold to intrude into my garden like a thief and rob me of what is mine! You have taken something precious from me!" she raged. "And soon, in return, I shall take something precious from you. I shall take away your baby and raise her as my own child."

She refused to hear any more of the poor man's tearful pleas concerning his wife's condition and dismissed him harshly.

When their baby daughter was born, there was no joy in the woodcutter's cottage. There was only sadness. In vain the young couple pleaded for the old witch's forgiveness, but she would not listen. She would not forgive the husband's intrusion.

"Your child is my child now," cackled the witch as she snatched the baby from the arms of the weeping parents. "I shall call her Rapunzel."

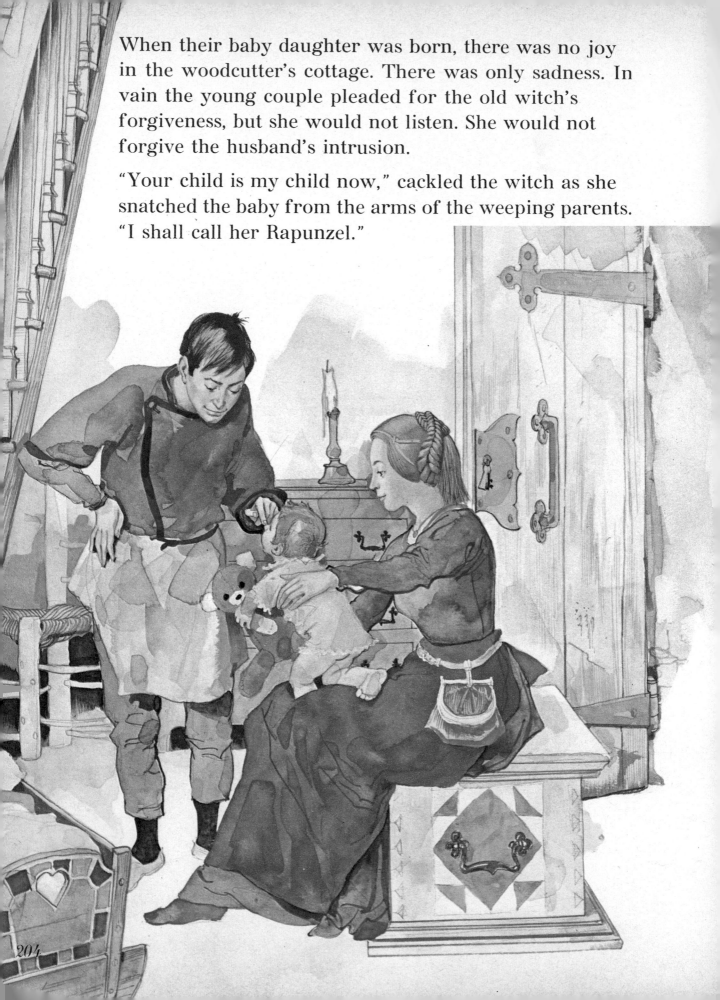

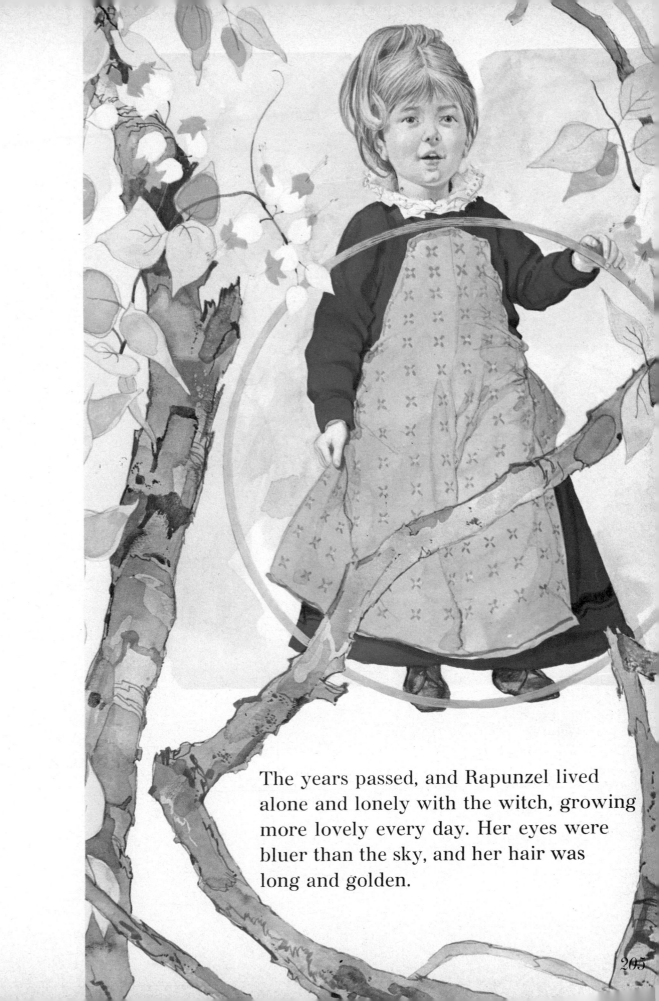

The years passed, and Rapunzel lived
alone and lonely with the witch, growing
more lovely every day. Her eyes were
bluer than the sky, and her hair was
long and golden.

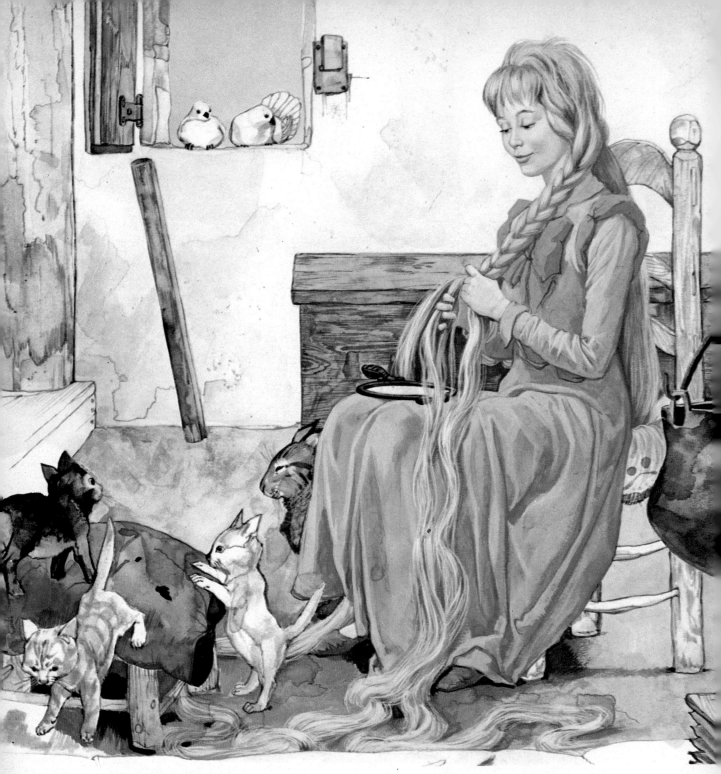

And as Rapunzel grew more beautiful, the witch grew
more jealous.

"I shall lock her away in a distant tower," said the witch
cruelly. "Then I alone shall know her rare beauty."

Rapunzel had been lonely before, but she was even
lonelier in the tower with only her doves and kittens for
company.

The tower had no door and no
stairway, only one small window
high above the ground. Only the old
witch knew the secret of how to enter
it. Every day when she came, she
stood beneath the window and called
out:

"*Rapunzel, Rapunzel!*
Let down your hair."

Whenever she called so, Rapunzel
would drop down her two thick
golden braids, which were long
enough to reach the ground, and
would pull the witch up to the tower
window. The girl's beautiful thick
golden hair became the witch's
ladder.

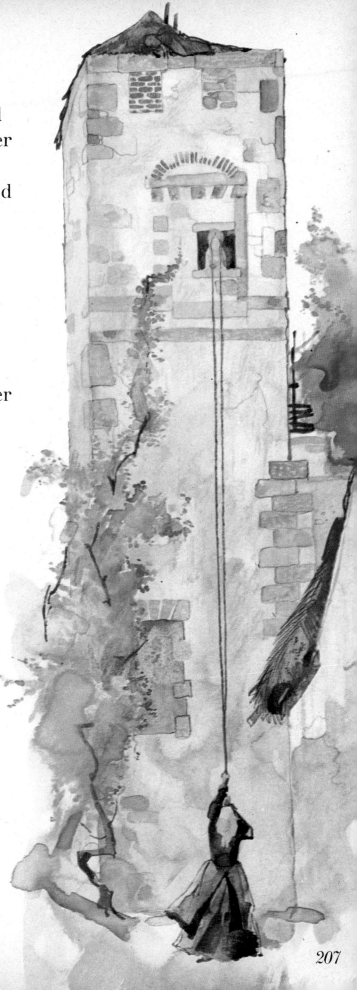

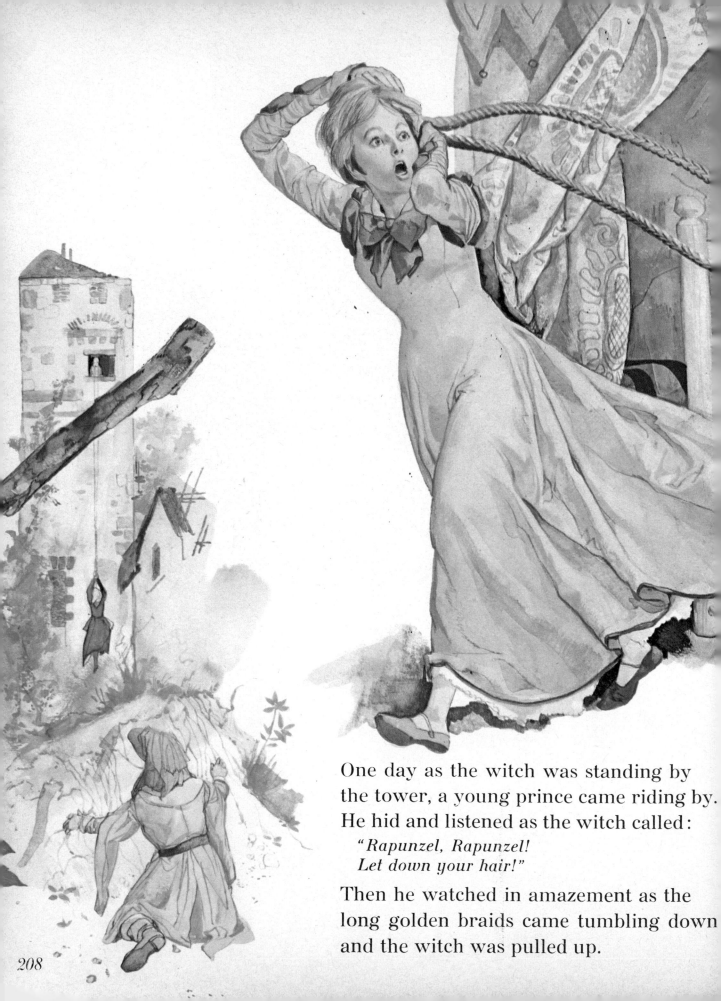

One day as the witch was standing by the tower, a young prince came riding by. He hid and listened as the witch called:

"*Rapunzel, Rapunzel!*
Let down your hair!"

Then he watched in amazement as the long golden braids came tumbling down and the witch was pulled up.

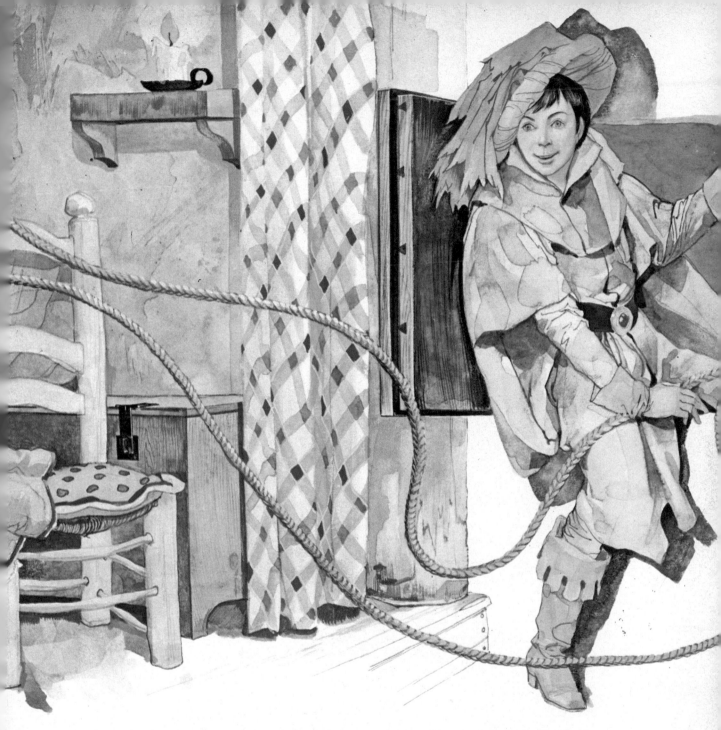

After the witch went away again, the young prince
decided to discover for himself the mystery of the tower.
Standing below the window, he called:

"Rapunzel, Rapunzel!
Let down your hair!"

Instantly, two thick golden braids fell into his hands.
He grasped them tightly and felt himself being pulled up
into the tower window. A moment later he was looking
at the most beautiful maiden he had ever seen.

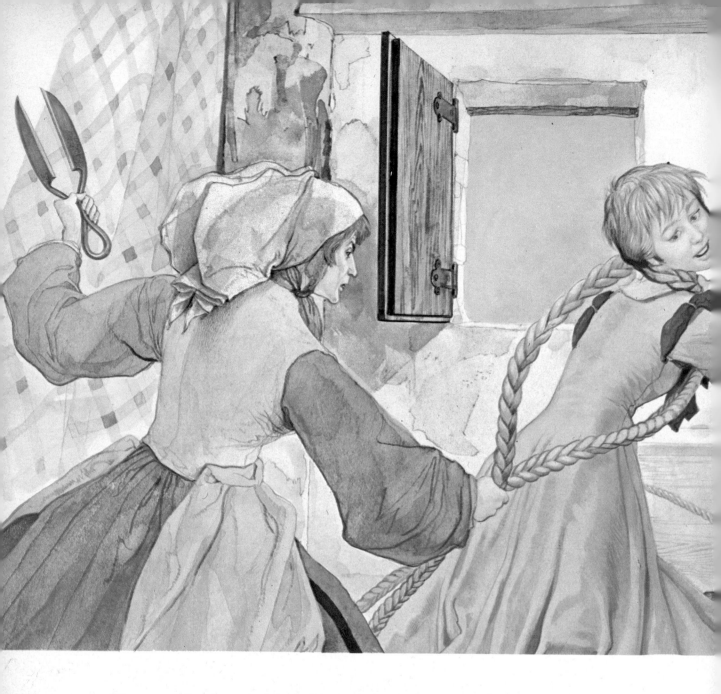

Rapunzel was terrified at first, but not for long. She too
had never seen such a handsome youth before. The
prince was so kind and gentle that within minutes the
two had fallen deeply in love. Although they knew they
risked the witch's fury, every night thereafter the
prince visited the tower. They were very happy, but
their happiness quickly came to an end. One night the
witch returned unexpectedly, just in time to see the
prince at the window.

The witch knew now that she had been deceived, and she took her cruel revenge the very next day. She cut off Rapunzel's beautiful hair and banished her to the wilderness forever. And that night, when the prince climbed up to the tower window, he found the evil witch awaiting him at the top, where she had tied the severed braids to the window frame.

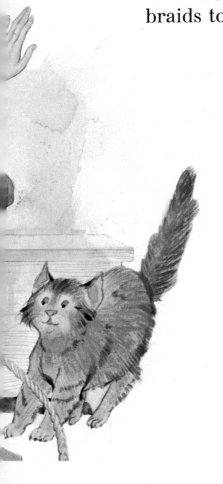

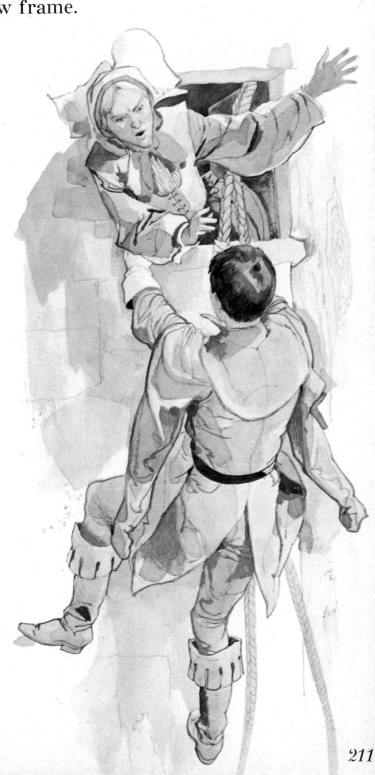

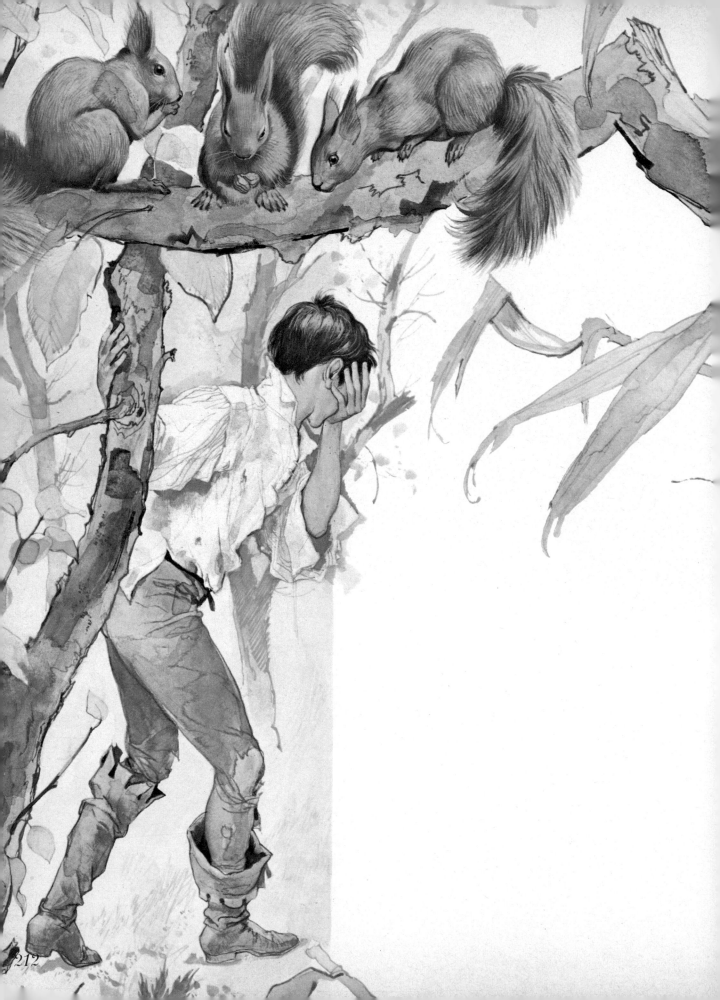

The prince was terribly afraid, but he was no coward.

"What have you done to my Rapunzel, wicked woman?" he shouted bravely, but trying to keep his voice from trembling.

"She is gone forever," cackled the witch. "You will never find her or see her again."

As she spoke, she untied Rapunzel's thick golden braids from the window, and the unlucky prince crashed to the ground below. He was fortunate to fall into a thick bramble bush so that he broke no bones, but its sharp thorns stabbed him cruelly and cut into his eyes and blinded him.

So great was his determination and his love for Rapunzel that, even blind, the prince vowed to continue to search the world over for her. The wild creatures watched him sadly and with sympathy as he stumbled on in his blindness. Through forests and fields, over mountains and down into valleys, he trudged. He seemed a prince no more, but a blind beggar in rags and tatters begging for his food. Wherever he went, he called out pitifully:

"Rapunzel, Rapunzel!
Where can I find you?"

But he was unable to find her. Then, one day he arrived at the edge of the endless wilderness, and could not go on. Sick and weak, he sank to the ground.

"I can't go on," he gasped to himself. "I know I have lost my Rapunzel forever."

The prince lay there delirious, never guessing that at last he had arrived at the place of Rapunzel's banishment. From a distance, Rapunzel saw the ragged figure lying on the ground, and she went toward him to offer help. When she stood over him looking down, she instantly recognized her lost prince. Two hot tears of pity fell from her eyes onto the prince's closed eyelids. Then he opened his eyes slowly—and then wider in wonder, for his blindness had been cured by her tears of genuine love. He saw Rapunzel before him, and with great joy realized his long search was over.

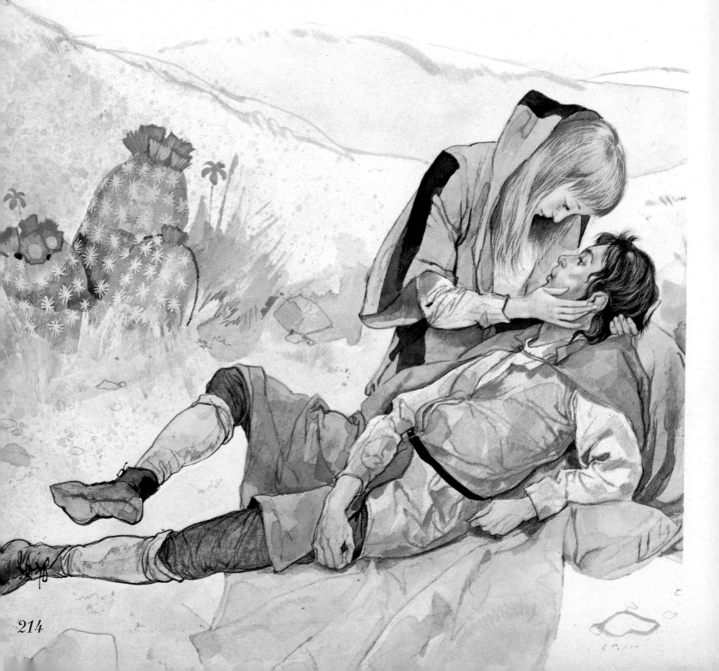

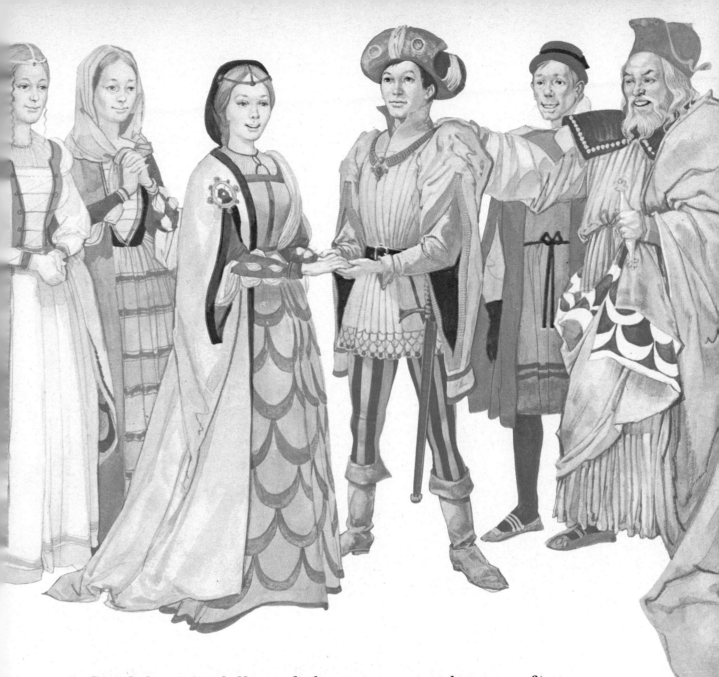

Good fortune followed the young couple ever after.
Together they returned to the prince's palace in the far
country he had left so long ago in his wanderings.
There they were married before the prince's family
and Rapunzel's joyful parents, who had never forgotten
or given up hope of finding their stolen daughter. As
for the envious witch, she flew into a rage and locked
herself in Rapunzel's tower—and never came out again.

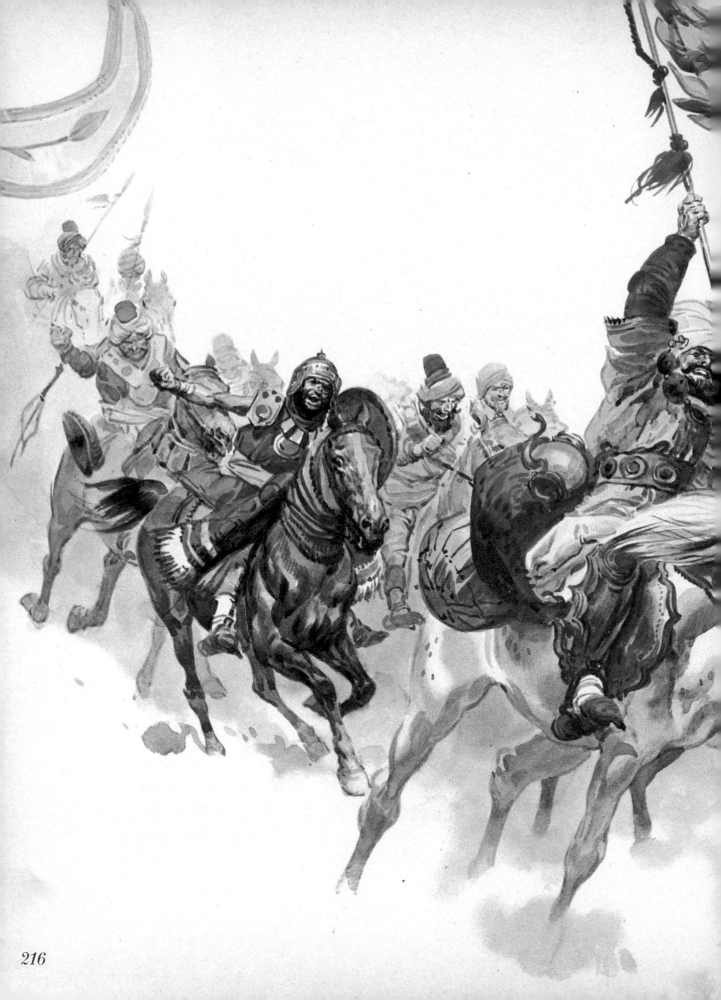

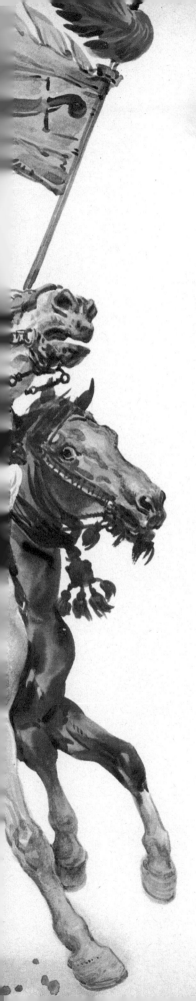

ALI BABA AND THE FORTY THIEVES

Once upon a time, in the country of Persia, there lived two brothers. Cassim, the elder, married a rich wife, but Ali Baba, the younger, married a poor girl and earned their bread chopping wood. One day while Ali was hard at work by a mountainside, he heard the sound of thundering hoof beats coming closer. Just in time he hid behind a tree, because in a moment a band of forty thieves appeared, led by their fierce chieftain Mustafa.

The thieves stopped close by Ali Baba's hiding place, and Mustafa dismounted from his horse. He walked to the mountainside and shouted, "Open, Sesame!"

As if by magic, at these words a door opened, and all forty thieves followed Mustafa into the mountain.

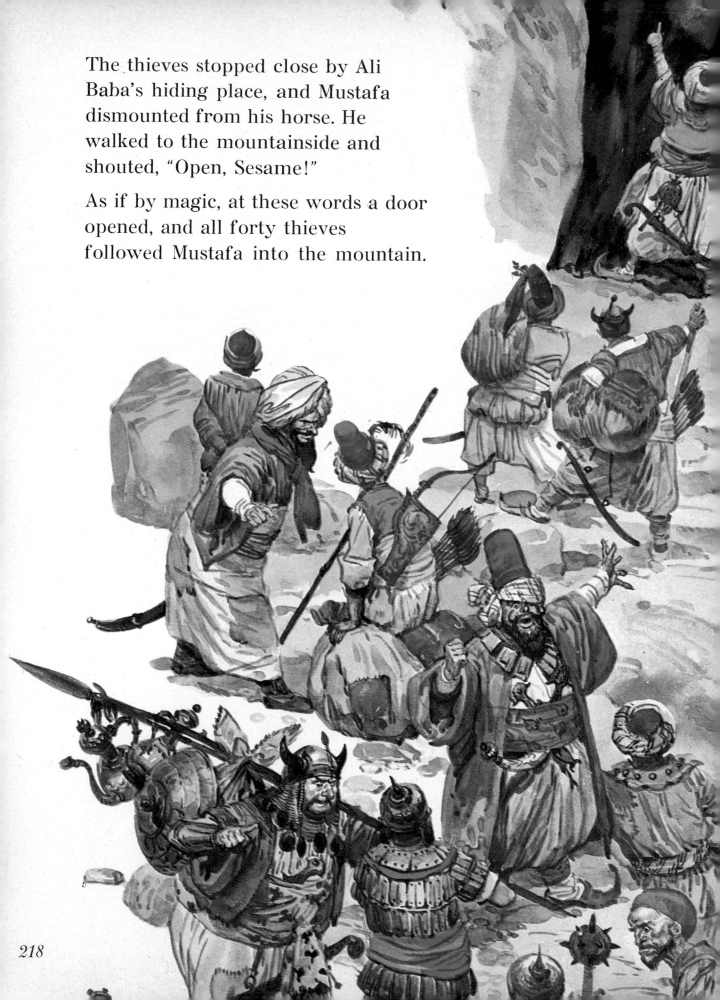

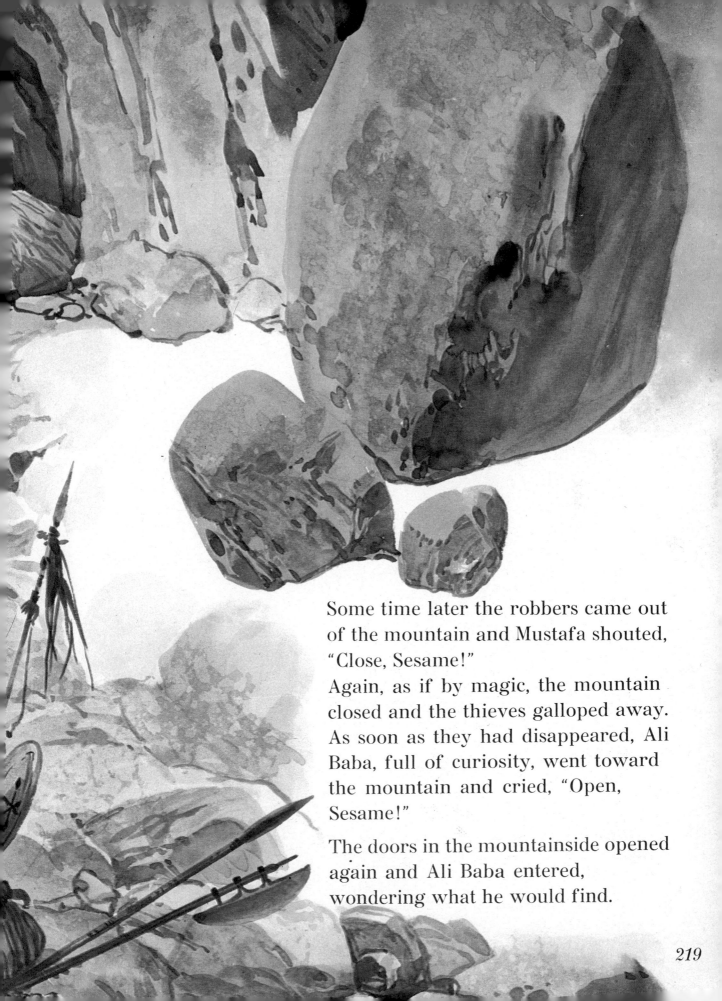

Some time later the robbers came out of the mountain and Mustafa shouted, "Close, Sesame!"

Again, as if by magic, the mountain closed and the thieves galloped away. As soon as they had disappeared, Ali Baba, full of curiosity, went toward the mountain and cried, "Open, Sesame!"

The doors in the mountainside opened again and Ali Baba entered, wondering what he would find.

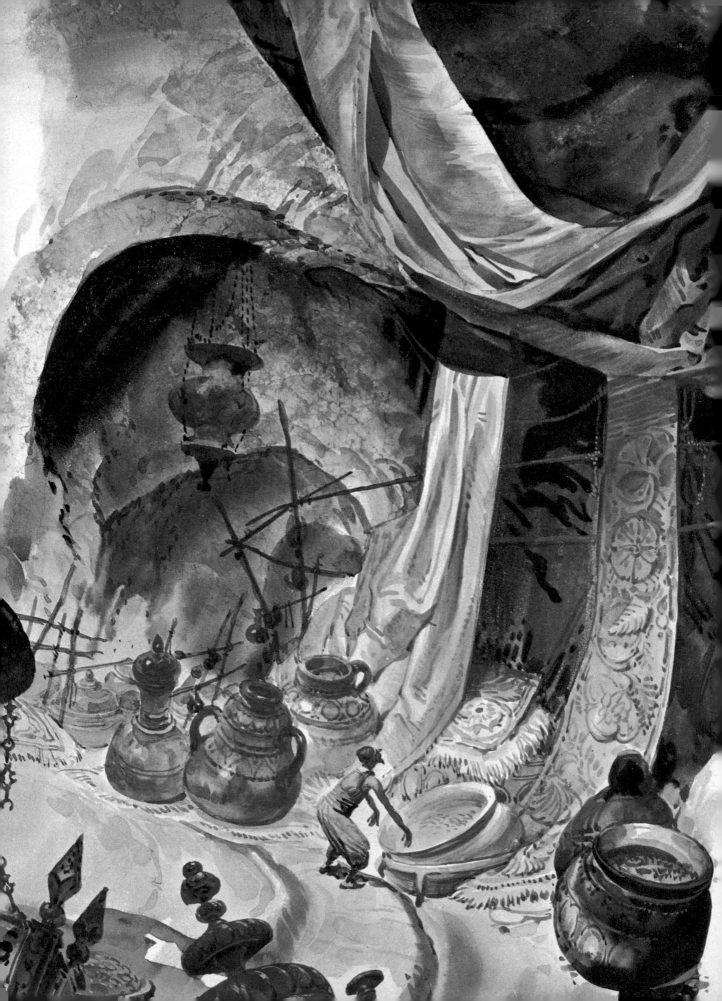

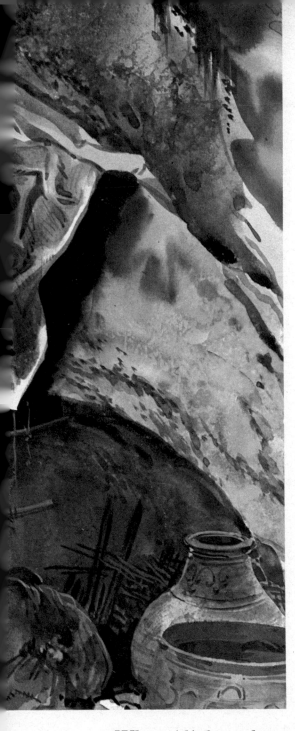

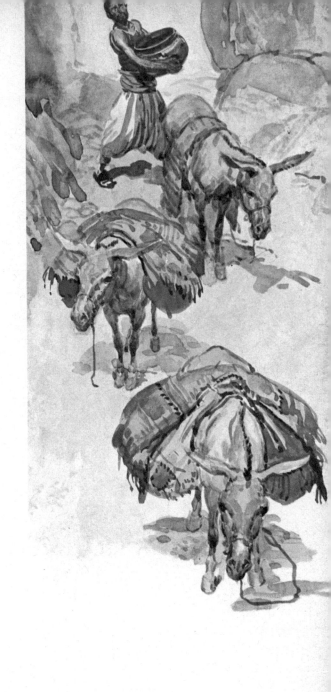

What Ali found made him gasp! Piles of gold coins, precious porcelains, silk tapestries, and sparkling jewels lay all around him.

"What riches!" he cried. "There is so much treasure here, surely no one will notice if I take a little to ease my poverty."

So he loaded his mules with treasure and shouted, "Close, Sesame!"

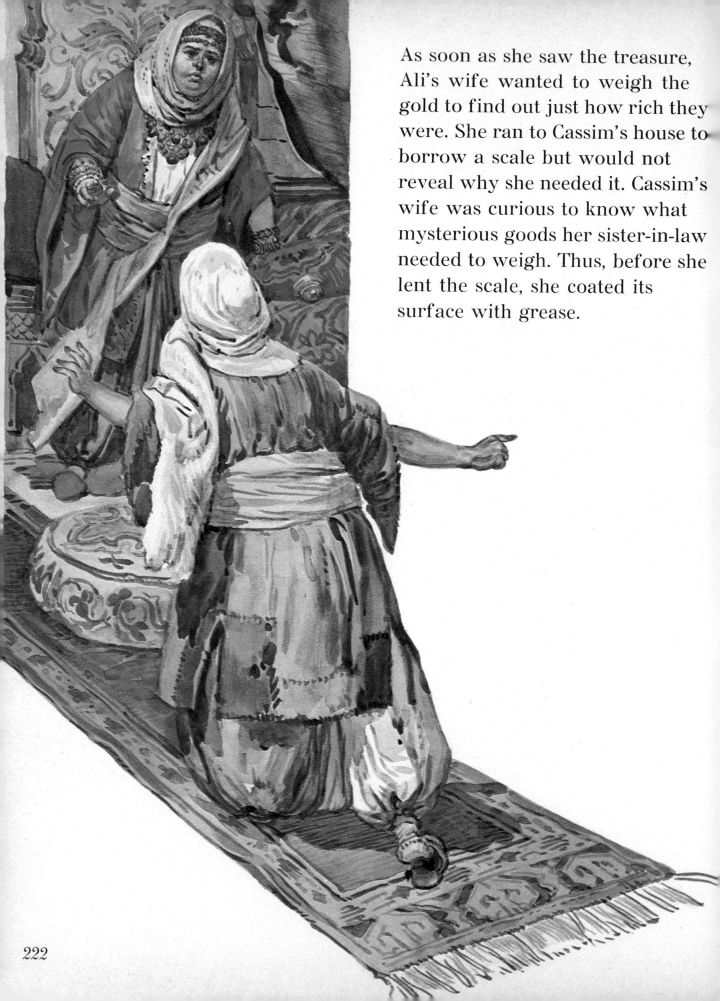

As soon as she saw the treasure, Ali's wife wanted to weigh the gold to find out just how rich they were. She ran to Cassim's house to borrow a scale but would not reveal why she needed it. Cassim's wife was curious to know what mysterious goods her sister-in-law needed to weigh. Thus, before she lent the scale, she coated its surface with grease.

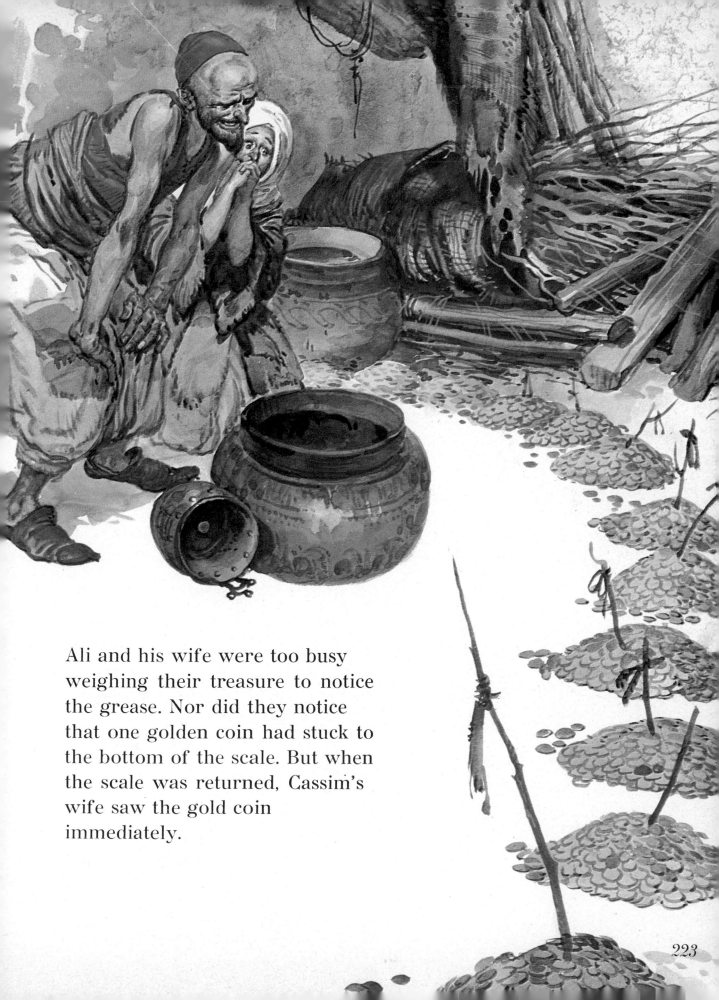

Ali and his wife were too busy
weighing their treasure to notice
the grease. Nor did they notice
that one golden coin had stuck to
the bottom of the scale. But when
the scale was returned, Cassim's
wife saw the gold coin
immediately.

"Look, my husband!" she cried. "Your brother has too much gold to count by hand. He must weigh it instead!"

"How can a miserable woodcutter have such riches?" growled Cassim enviously. "I will find out the truth at once."

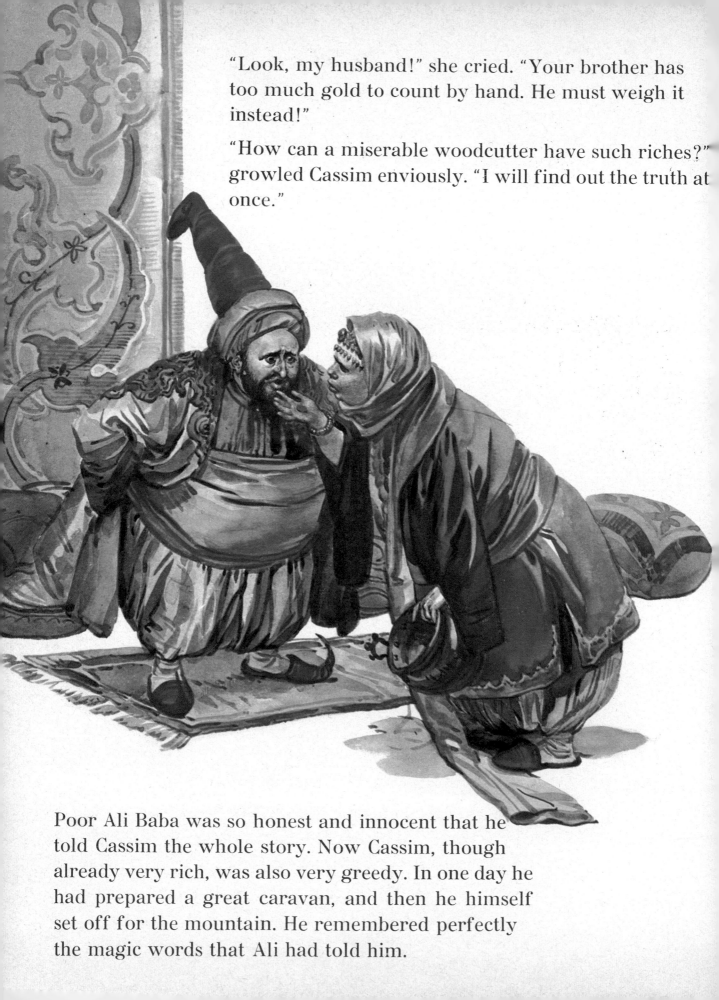

Poor Ali Baba was so honest and innocent that he told Cassim the whole story. Now Cassim, though already very rich, was also very greedy. In one day he had prepared a great caravan, and then he himself set off for the mountain. He remembered perfectly the magic words that Ali had told him.

"Open, Sesame!" Cassim shouted, and once again the doors in the mountainside opened wide. Cassim went in, and the doors shut tight behind him. He stared greedily at the gleaming treasures and quickly began collecting the best. But when he had all he could carry and was ready to leave, he found he had forgotten the magic words to reopen the doors.

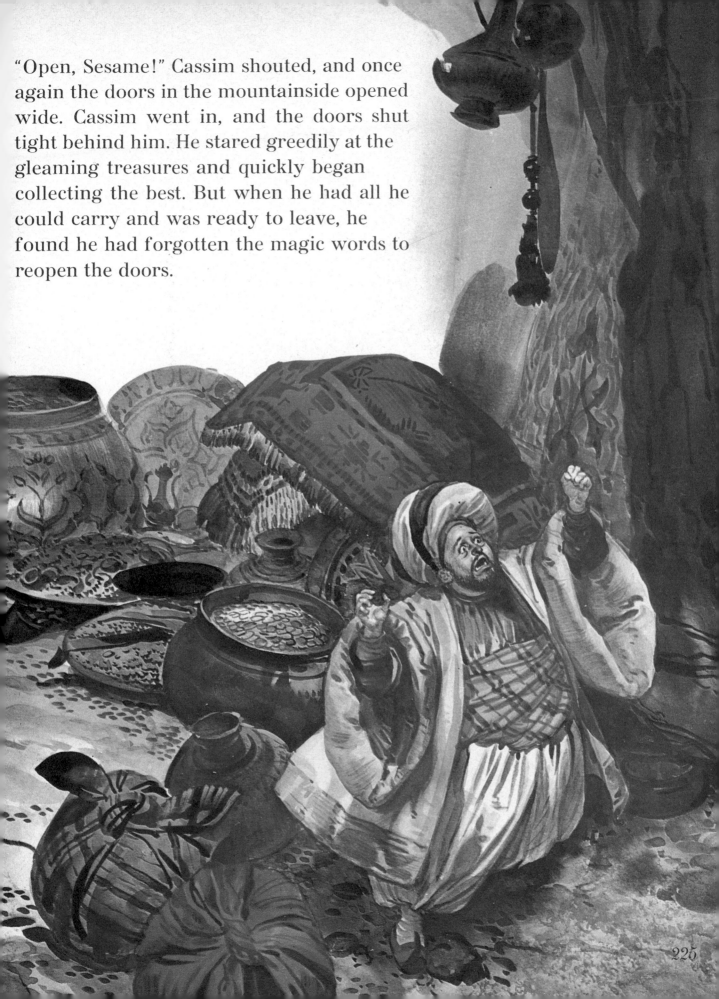

In desperation Cassim tried every name he could think of. "Open, Salvador!" "Open, Sebastian!" "Open, Saxophone!" But the doors stayed shut. The greedy man was fainting with fear when the doors finally opened and all the thieves rushed in and found him there among their treasures.

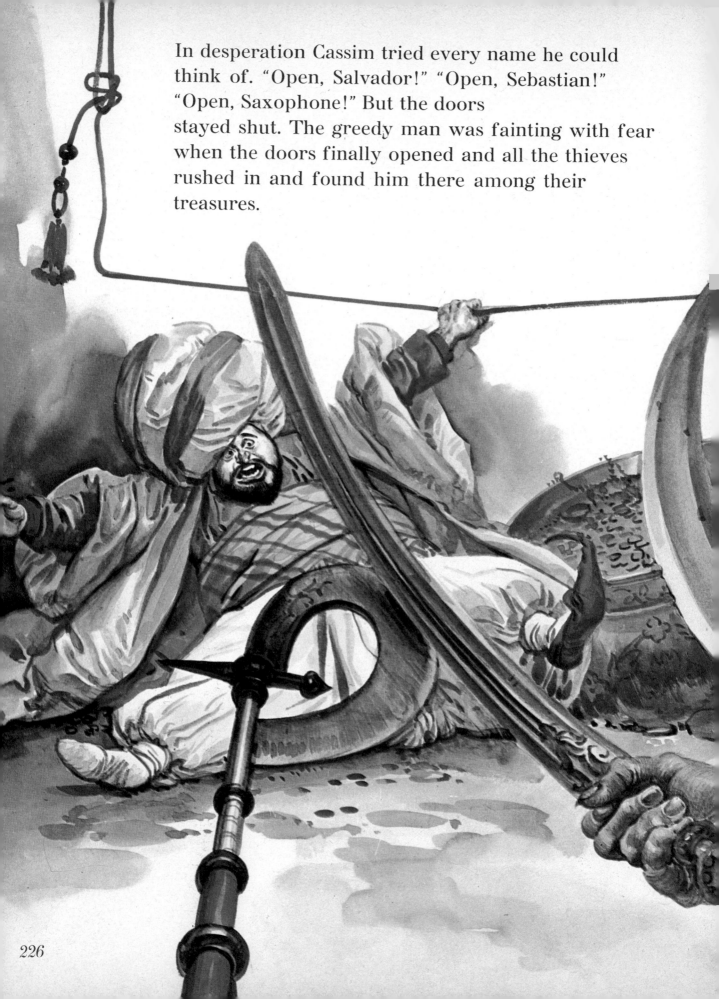

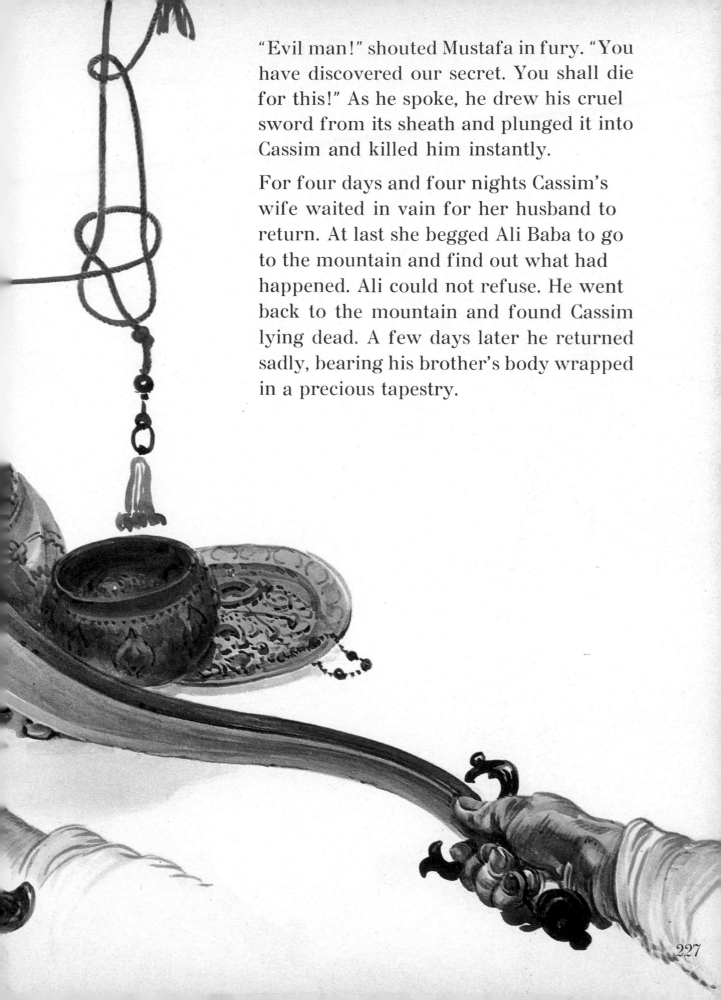

"Evil man!" shouted Mustafa in fury. "You have discovered our secret. You shall die for this!" As he spoke, he drew his cruel sword from its sheath and plunged it into Cassim and killed him instantly.

For four days and four nights Cassim's wife waited in vain for her husband to return. At last she begged Ali Baba to go to the mountain and find out what had happened. Ali could not refuse. He went back to the mountain and found Cassim lying dead. A few days later he returned sadly, bearing his brother's body wrapped in a precious tapestry.

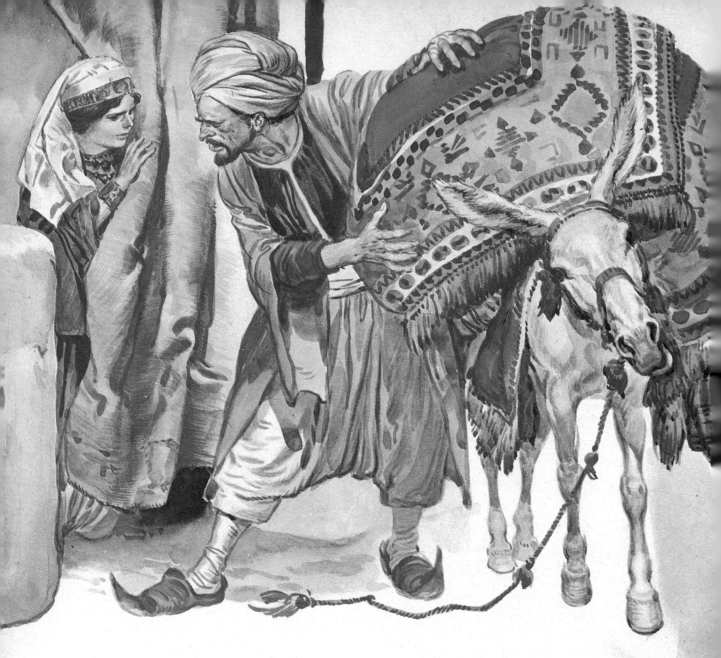

Ali could not comfort the weeping widow, for first he had to warn her of her own immediate danger.

"No one must know how your husband died, my sister-in-law," he said. "If the thieves ever find out his name and where he lived, they may try to kill you too, thinking that you also know their secret."

The grieving widow promised to keep silent, but Ali was still troubled.

He summoned Morgiana, his sister-in-law's quick-witted serving maid, and asked her help.

"I beg you to spread the rumor that your master is sick," Ali asked. "Let the neighbors see you buying medicine and looking heartbroken. After four days, you can tell everyone that your poor master is dead of pneumonia."

Morgiana quickly understood, and luckily she remembered that before he went away Cassim had ordered her to bring a tailor to the house to make him a new suit.

"If the tailor comes, he will surely discover my master's murder," she worried, but then quickly thought of a plan to deceive him.

"I know what I will do. I will bring him here blindfolded and take him home the same way. Then he will never know how to find my master's house again."

"Good girl!" said Ali, much relieved. "I always knew you were clever."

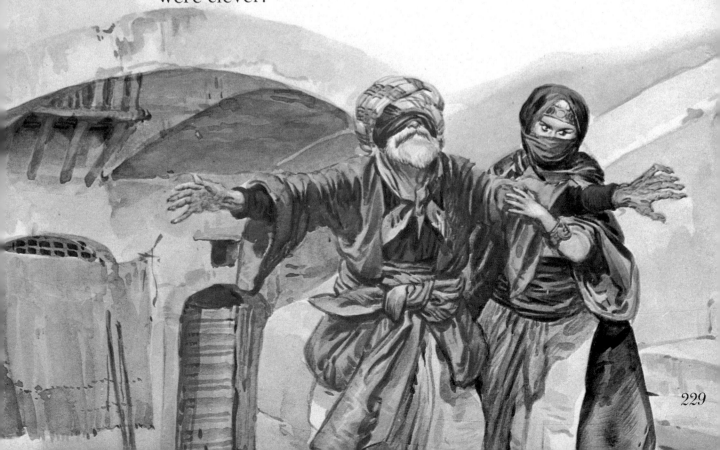

While Ali was making plans, the thieves discovered that Cassim's body was missing. They knew someone must have carried it away and, therefore, that someone else knew their secret. Mustafa was in a rage and ordered his men to find out who this person could be. They searched in the fields, the forest, and the town.

It so happened that one of the thieves, while searching in the town, heard the tailor bragging that he had just made a suit for a murdered man.

"Lead me to this murdered man's house, old one," said the thief eagerly.

"Alas, I cannot, master, for I myself was led there blindfolded," answered the tailor. "But perhaps if you blindfolded me again I could find it once more."

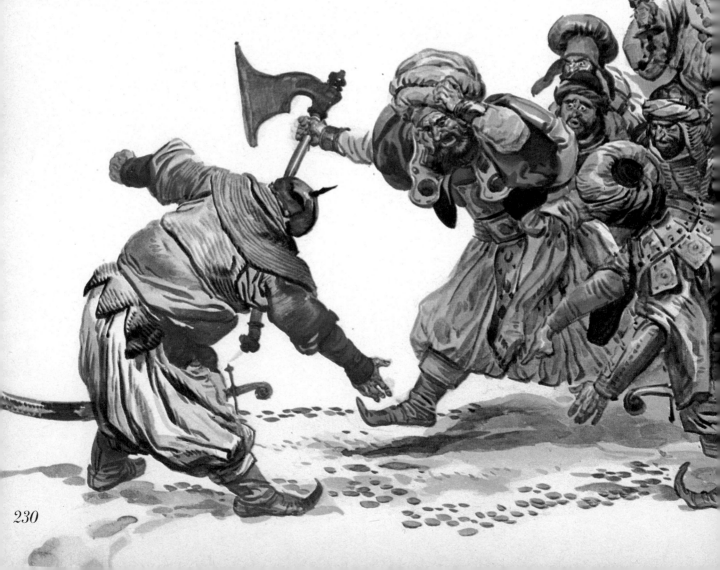

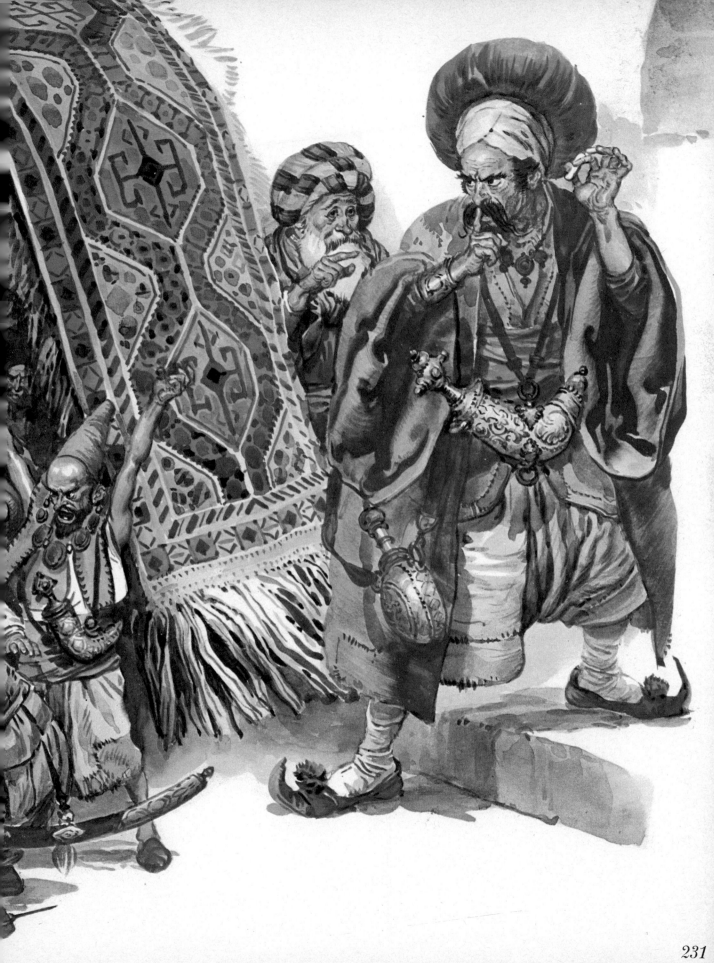

So the thief blindfolded the tailor, and after a few wrong turns they stood before Cassim's house. Quietly the thief drew a cross on the door with chalk and then went back to tell Mustafa of his discovery.

Luckily Morgiana noticed the white cross drawn on her dead master's door and knew it must be the work of the robbers. Quickly she ran through the town making similar chalk crosses on every door, so that when the thieves arrived they did not know which house to attack.

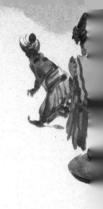

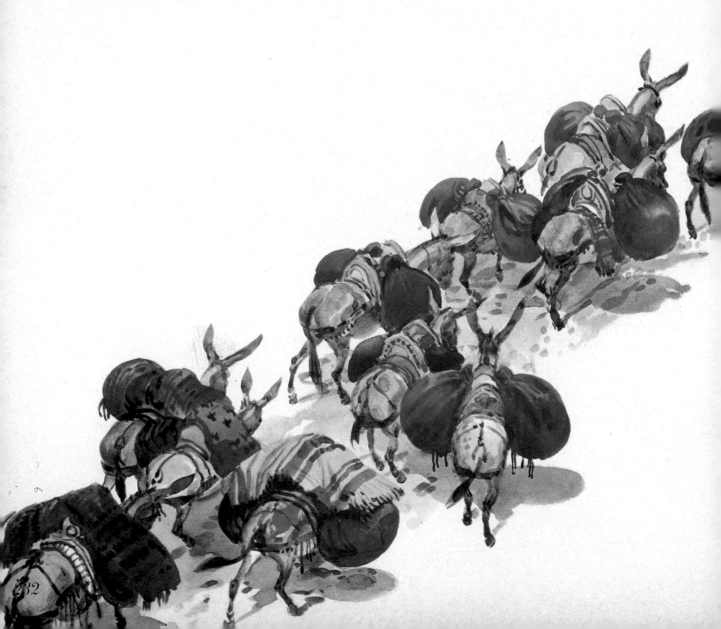

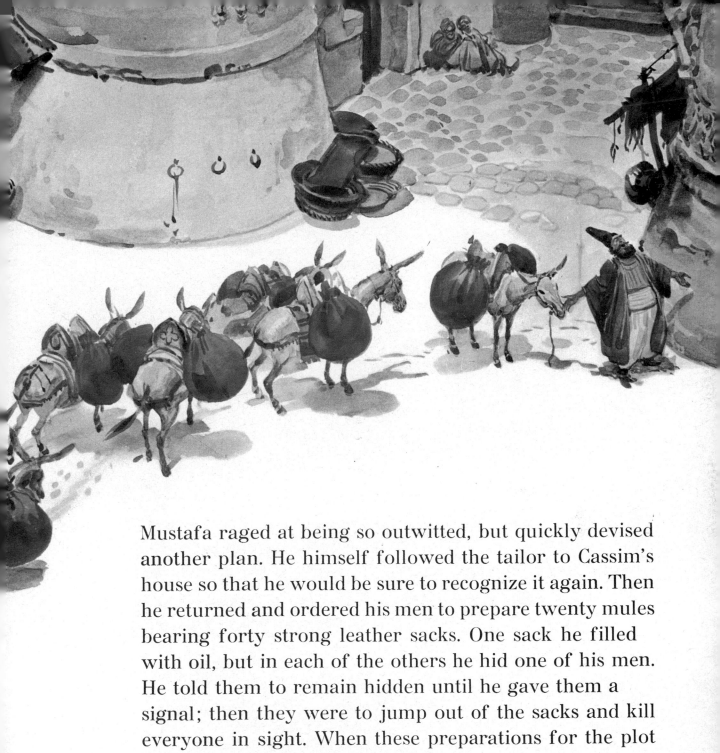

Mustafa raged at being so outwitted, but quickly devised another plan. He himself followed the tailor to Cassim's house so that he would be sure to recognize it again. Then he returned and ordered his men to prepare twenty mules bearing forty strong leather sacks. One sack he filled with oil, but in each of the others he hid one of his men. He told them to remain hidden until he gave them a signal; then they were to jump out of the sacks and kill everyone in sight. When these preparations for the plot were all made, Mustafa led the mule caravan into Cassim's courtyard.

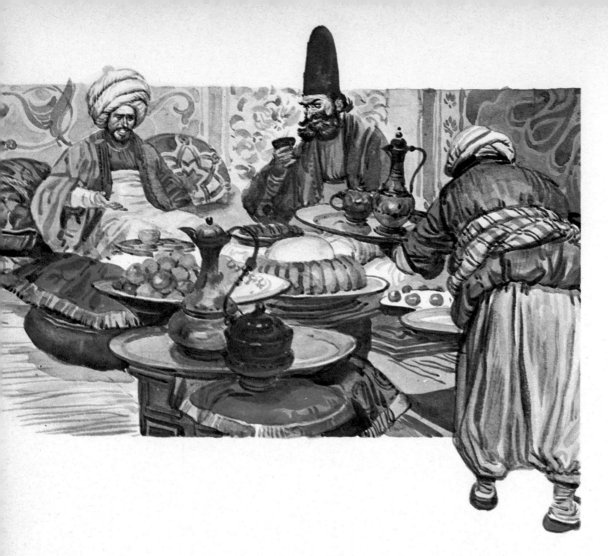

"I am a merchant of fine oil," Mustafa called out.

"Enter, my good merchant," said Ali Baba, who had taken his family to live at his sister-in-law's, "and share our humble meal with us."

Leaving his men hidden in their uncomfortable leather sacks, Mustafa entered the house and accepted food and drink. Soon the maid Morgiana found herself in need of oil and, thinking to borrow a little from the false merchant's sacks, went into the courtyard. As she approached the first mule, she heard a whisper.

"Master," said a voice from the sack, "are you ready yet?"

Morgiana was startled, but she was very clever and a quick thinker.

"Not yet. Later!" she whispered back, imitating the merchant's voice, and then went on to the next mule.

"Now, Master?" whispered another voice.

"Not yet. Later!" Morgiana again replied softly. She suddenly realized that men—not oil—were contained in all the sacks but one. Quickly she took the oil from the fortieth sack, heated it on her stove, and then poured boiling oil into each of the other sacks. And in this way, every one of the thirty-nine thieves was scalded to death.

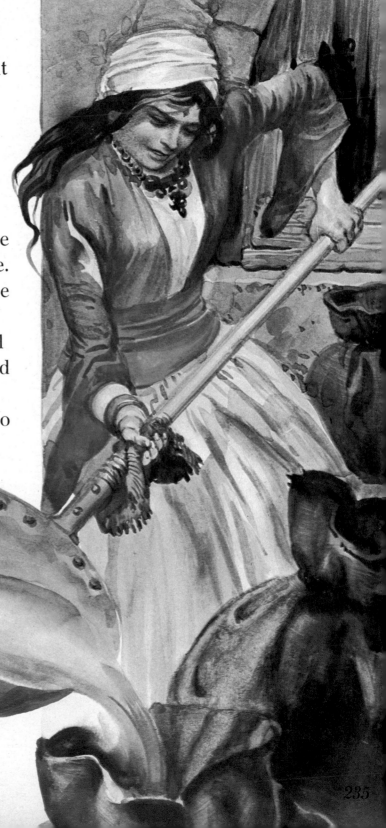

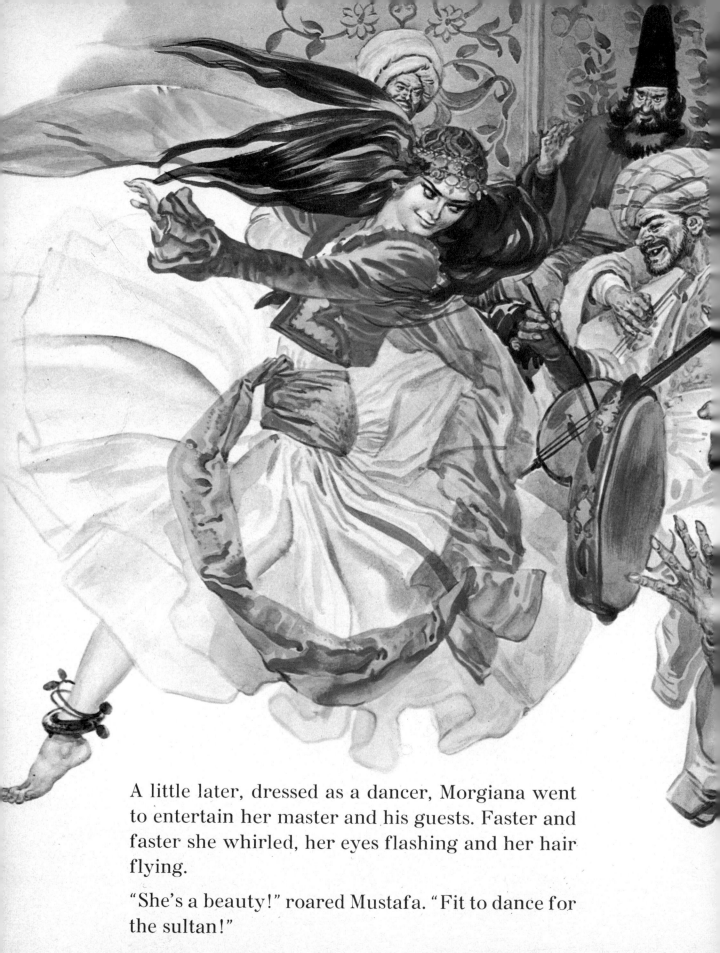

A little later, dressed as a dancer, Morgiana went to entertain her master and his guests. Faster and faster she whirled, her eyes flashing and her hair flying.

"She's a beauty!" roared Mustafa. "Fit to dance for the sultan!"

As Mustafa spoke, Morgiana whirled past him, pulled a dagger from her sash, and plunged it into his heart.

"Morgiana! What have you done?" cried Ali Baba in horror.

"I have saved your life, Master!" answered Morgiana breathlessly. Then she explained what had happened.

In gratitude for her devotion Ali Baba rewarded her richly and married her to his only son. They all lived together in luxury and contentment ever after.

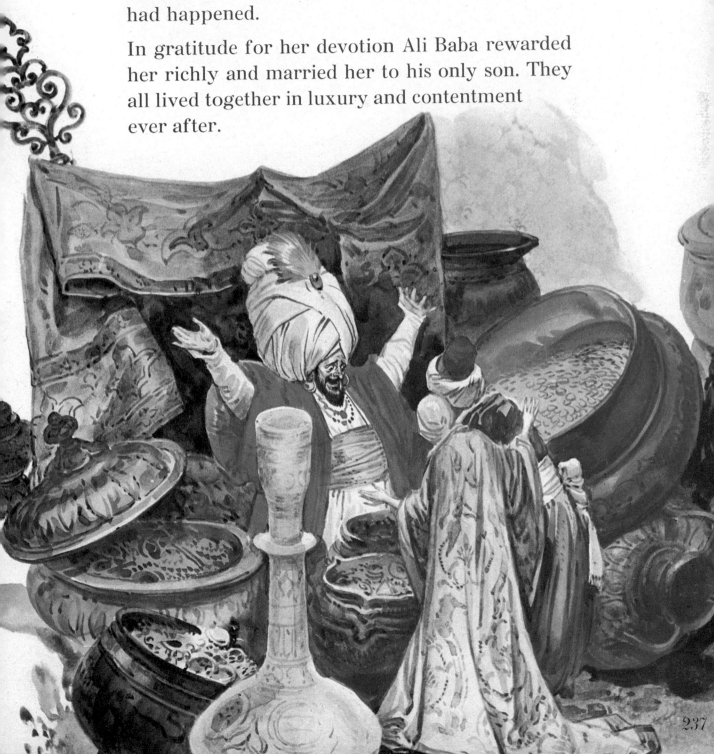

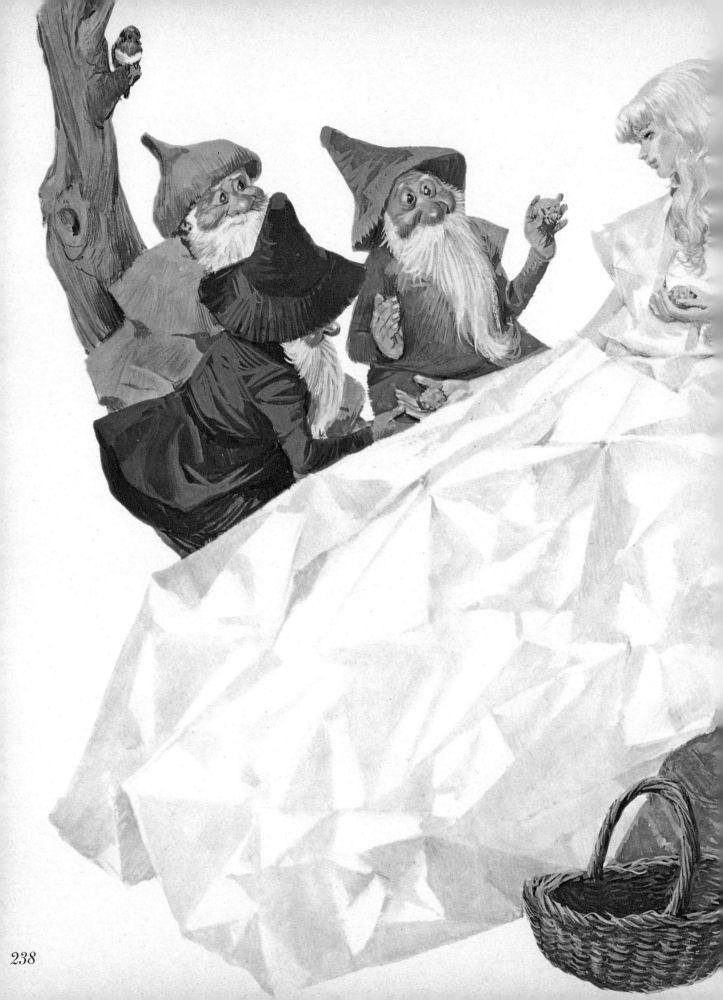

THE THREE DWARFS IN THE WOOD

Once upon a time the young wife of a rich merchant died suddenly, and her heartbroken husband tried to care for their only daughter by himself. After several years, he met a young widow who also was trying to care for her only daughter and, considering himself fortunate, married her immediately. His new wife pretended to be sweet and gentle, so the poor man did not realize she was hard-hearted and jealous of his beautiful daughter. He died soon after their wedding. The poor girl was then left alone with her evil stepmother and ugly stepsister.

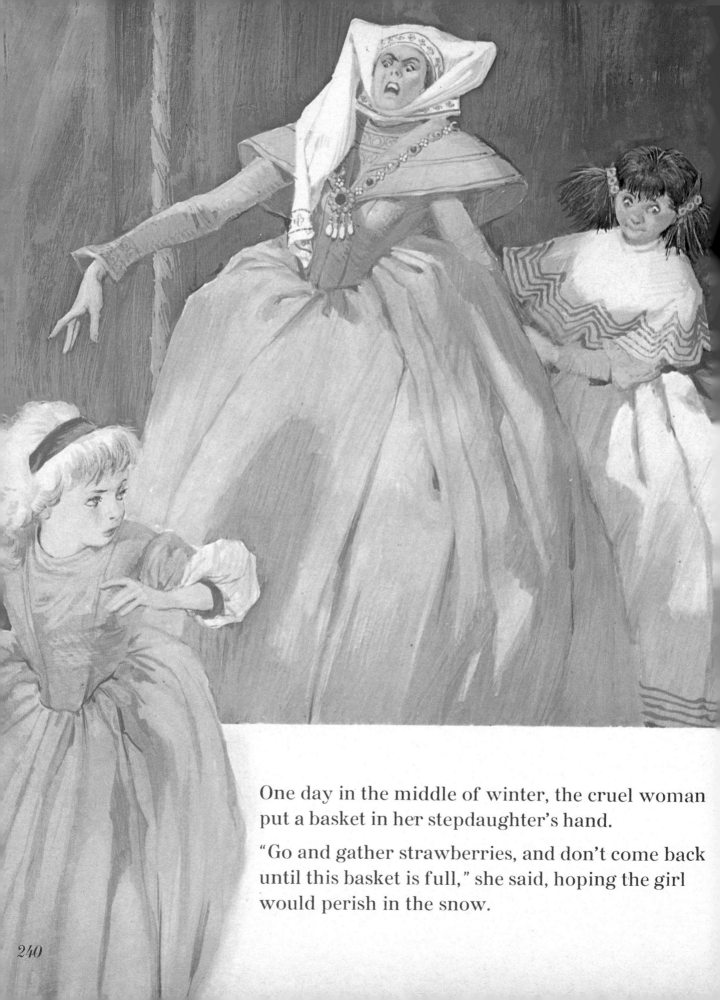

One day in the middle of winter, the cruel woman put a basket in her stepdaughter's hand.

"Go and gather strawberries, and don't come back until this basket is full," she said, hoping the girl would perish in the snow.

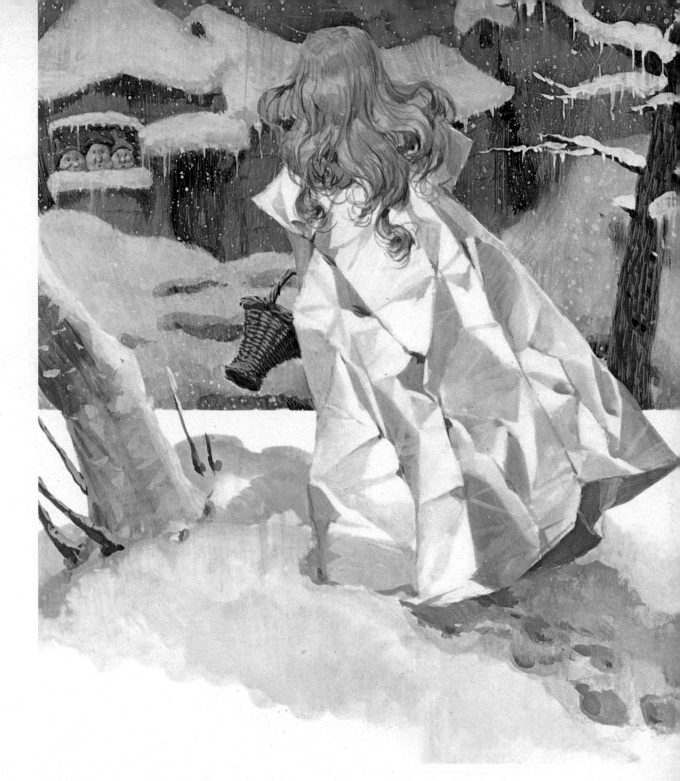

After she had given the child a paper dress to wear and a crust of dry bread to eat, the wicked woman sent her out into the howling storm.

"Ungrateful wretch!" she shouted after her. "I give you clothes to wear and food to eat and don't even get a word of thanks!"

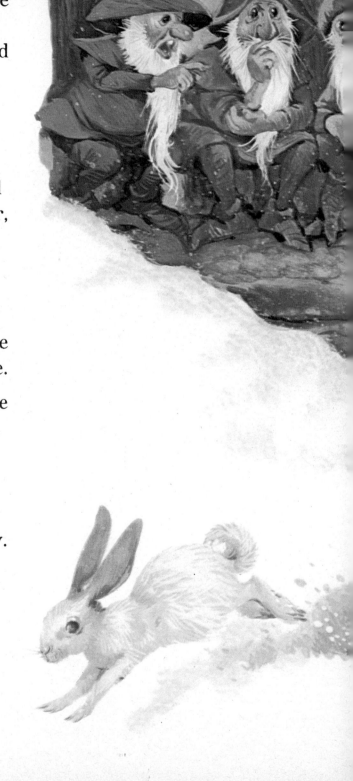

The shivering girl walked barefoot through the snow and after a time came upon a tiny cottage where three dwarfs greeted her and invited her in. They led her to a warm place by the fire, and when she began to eat her dry bread, they begged her to share it with them.

"Gladly," she said and then divided the little crust. As they ate together, she told them about her evil stepmother. The dwarfs were outraged that so gentle a child should be so cruelly treated, and they decided to help her. But before they did, they needed to test her more.

"Please, child, would you sweep the snow off our steps?" they asked.

"I would gladly do anything to repay your kindness," the girl answered. She took a broom and walked barefoot out into the snow.

The dwarfs looked at one another and nodded in satisfaction.

"Good deeds should be richly rewarded," they agreed, so they immediately gave the sweet girl three magic gifts.

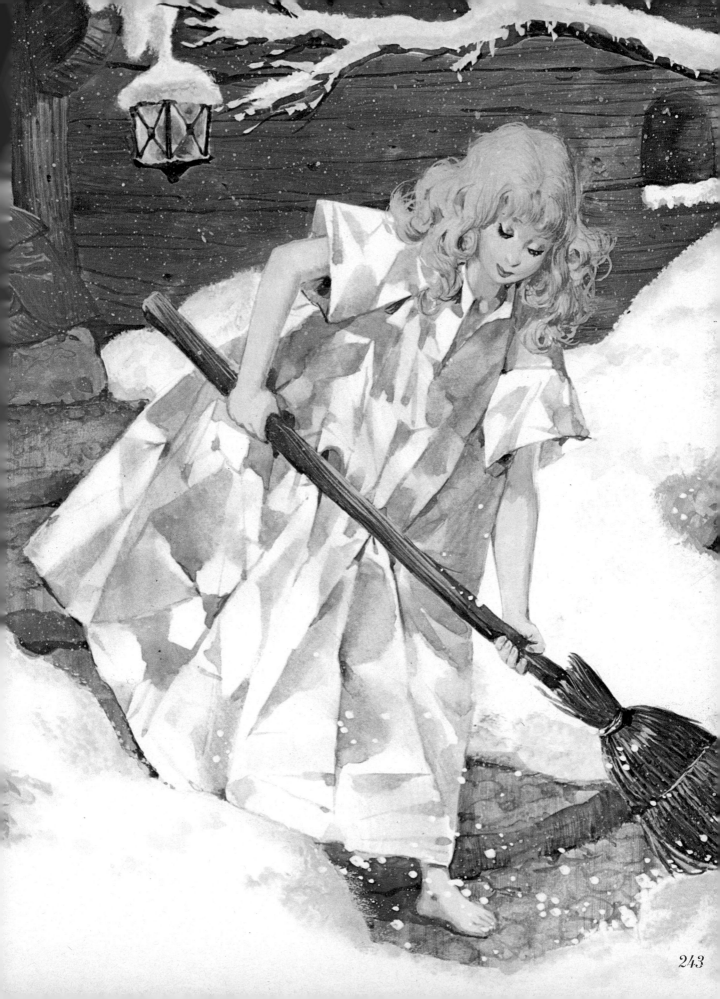

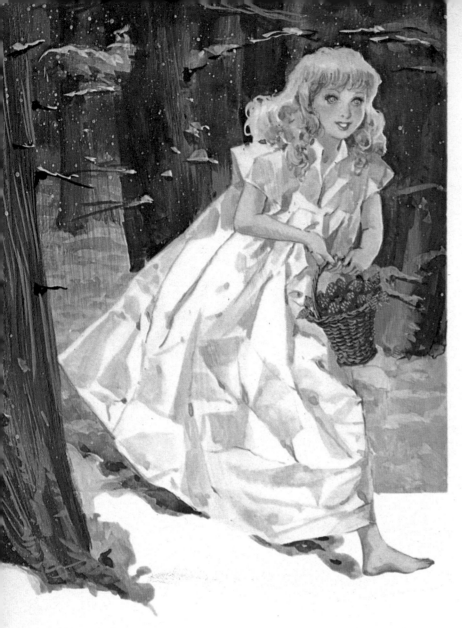

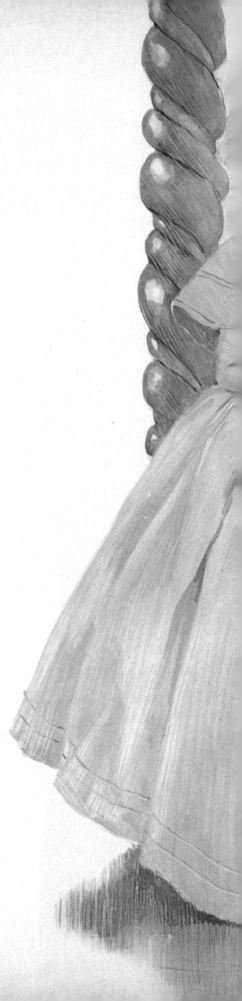

The dwarfs promised that every day she would grow more beautiful, that gold coins would drop from her mouth whenever she spoke, and that a handsome king would marry her.

Meanwhile, as the girl was sweeping the steps she suddenly gasped in astonishment for beneath the snow she found the biggest strawberries she had ever seen. She filled her basket to overflowing and, after calling a hasty farewell to the dwarfs, ran home.

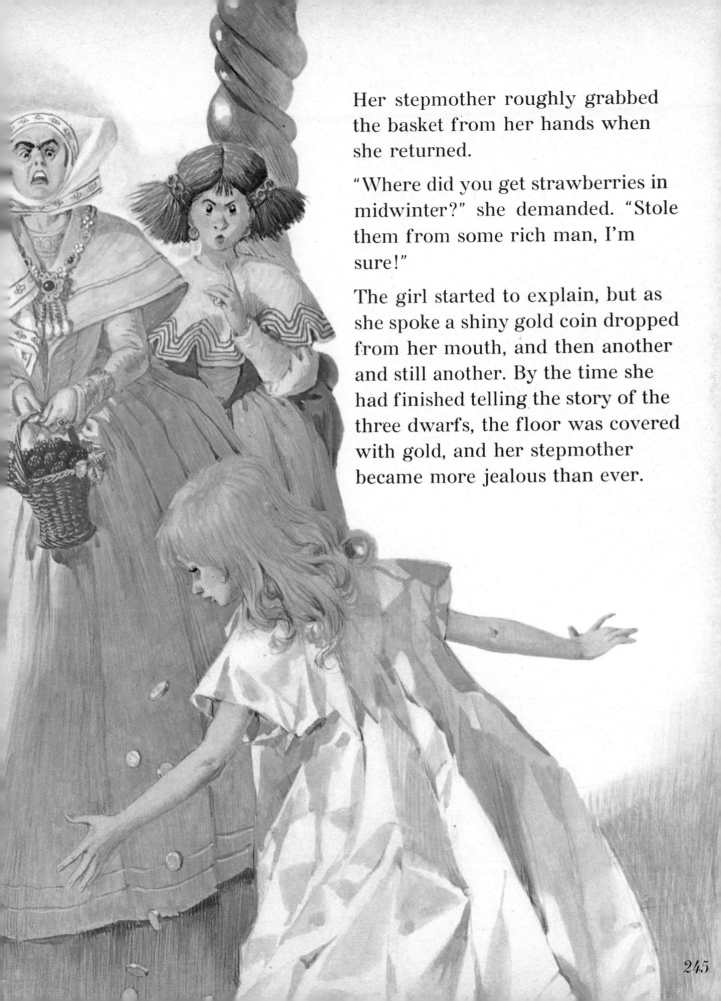

Her stepmother roughly grabbed the basket from her hands when she returned.

"Where did you get strawberries in midwinter?" she demanded. "Stole them from some rich man, I'm sure!"

The girl started to explain, but as she spoke a shiny gold coin dropped from her mouth, and then another and still another. By the time she had finished telling the story of the three dwarfs, the floor was covered with gold, and her stepmother became more jealous than ever.

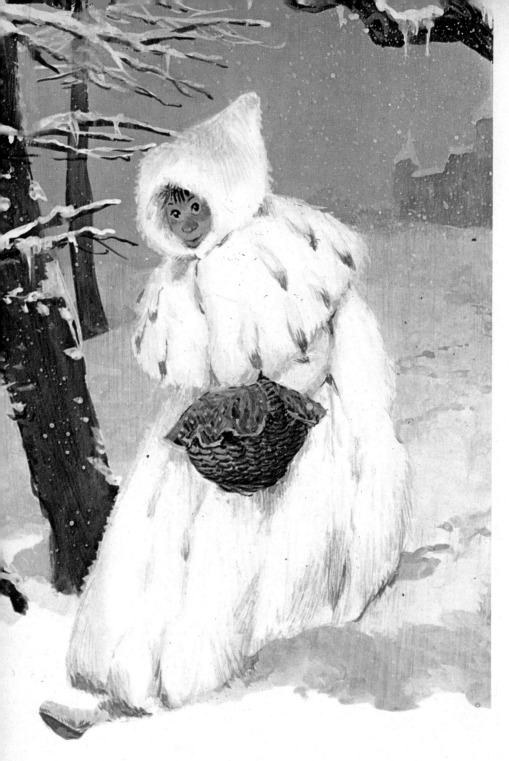

The woman desired the same good fortune for her own ugly daughter, and so decided that she too must visit the three dwarfs in the wood. But before she sent the dreary girl out into the snow, she gave her a warm coat of heavy white fur to wear and a large basket of goodies.

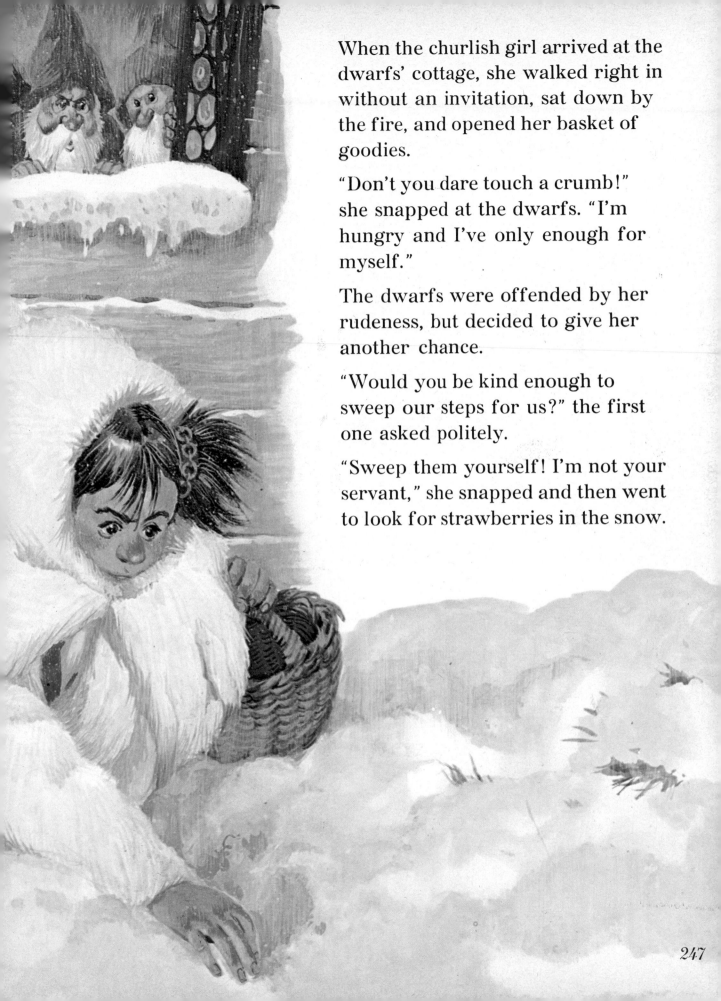

When the churlish girl arrived at the dwarfs' cottage, she walked right in without an invitation, sat down by the fire, and opened her basket of goodies.

"Don't you dare touch a crumb!" she snapped at the dwarfs. "I'm hungry and I've only enough for myself."

The dwarfs were offended by her rudeness, but decided to give her another chance.

"Would you be kind enough to sweep our steps for us?" the first one asked politely.

"Sweep them yourself! I'm not your servant," she snapped and then went to look for strawberries in the snow.

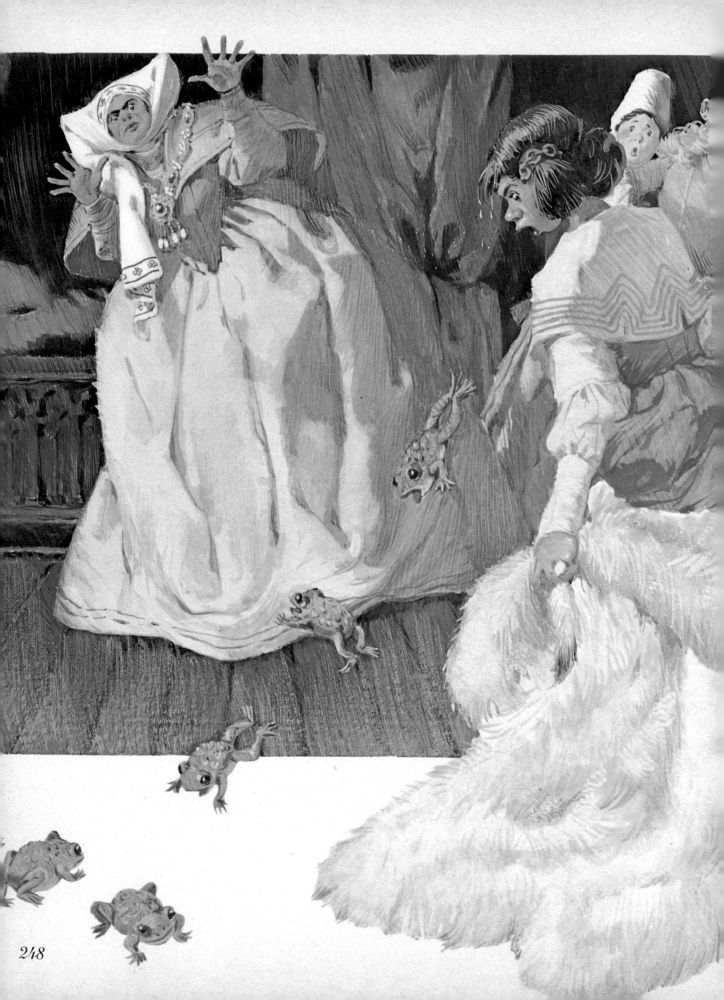

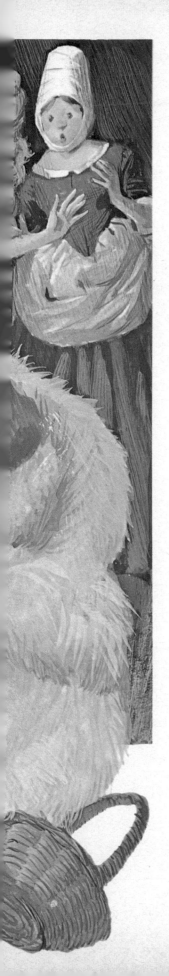

"Unkind deeds must be rewarded, too," the dwarfs said to each other as she left.

"I promise that she shall grow uglier every day," said the first dwarf.

"And I promise that, every time she speaks, toads shall jump from her mouth," said the second.

"And I promise that she shall die a miserable death," said the third.

Outside in the snow the rude girl was in a terrible temper because she could find no strawberries. Finally she gave up and ran home. She began complaining the moment she entered the house, but everyone jumped back in horror when an ugly speckled toad hopped from her mouth, and then another and still another, until the floor was covered with the slimy creatures.

"Shut your mouth and go to your room!" screamed her mother frantically. "Or you'll fill the whole house with these hateful things."

From that day on, the evil woman was more enraged than ever. Jealously she noticed that her stepdaughter grew more beautiful every day, and richer too.

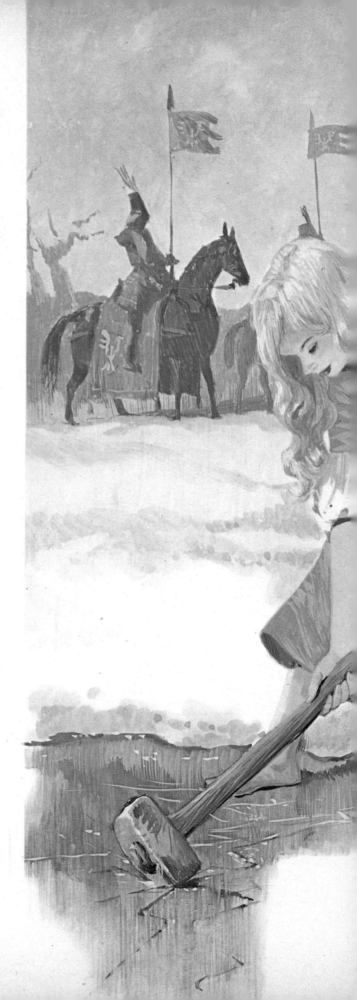

"It's all your fault!" she screamed at the girl one day. "You with your false stories of dwarfs and strawberries in the snow. Take this blanket and wash it in the river, and don't come back until it's clean."

The beautiful girl asked forgiveness and begged for pity.

"The river is frozen solid," she cried.

"Then take a hammer and break the ice!" shouted her stepmother.

"But the blanket is badly stained, and I'll surely freeze to death before it's clean," sobbed the girl.

"Then you'll freeze, and good riddance to you!" said the terrible woman.

Once again the unfortunate girl went out into the cold winter and walked shivering to the riverbank. But as she was trying to break the thick ice, the royal coach happened to pass. The young king riding inside saw the beautiful girl struggling with the heavy hammer. He ordered his coachman to halt, then jumped down, ran swiftly to the frozen river, and gently took the hammer from the poor girl's icy hands.

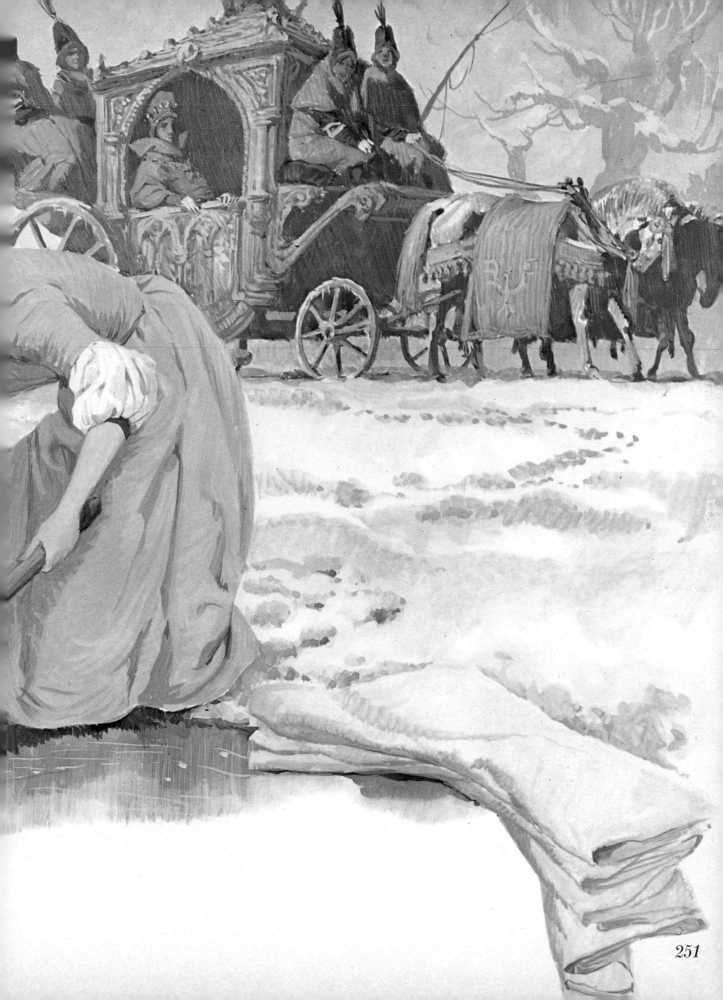

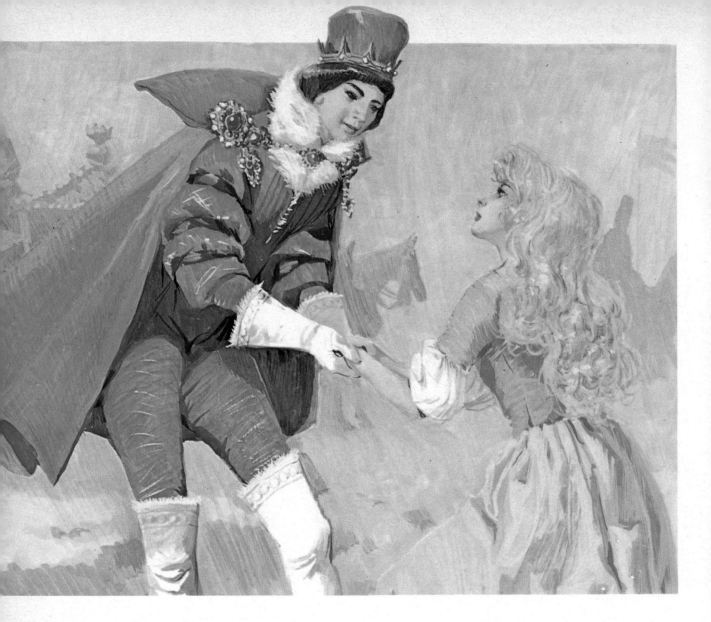

"I am here to help you," he said, looking down as she knelt before him.

"Alas, no one can help me!" she cried desperately.

Their eyes met, and in an instant they were in love.

"Will you ride with me to my castle?" asked the king.

"Willingly," whispered the girl.

"And will you be my queen?" he added.

"Gladly! Gratefully!" she sighed.

The very next day they were married in great splendor.

Within the year a beautiful son was born to them, and their happiness was complete. The cruel stepmother and her ugly daughter, still full of envy, came to the royal bedchamber pretending to admire the baby and to beg the queen's forgiveness. The gentle queen willingly forgave them, but when the king left her side for a minute, the evil women seized her and threw her out the window into the lake below. There she was magically transformed into a beautiful white duck with a tiny golden crown on her head.

Swiftly the woman pushed her ugly daughter into the royal bed and drew the curtains round her. When the king returned, the stepmother told him his wife was sleeping and must not be disturbed.

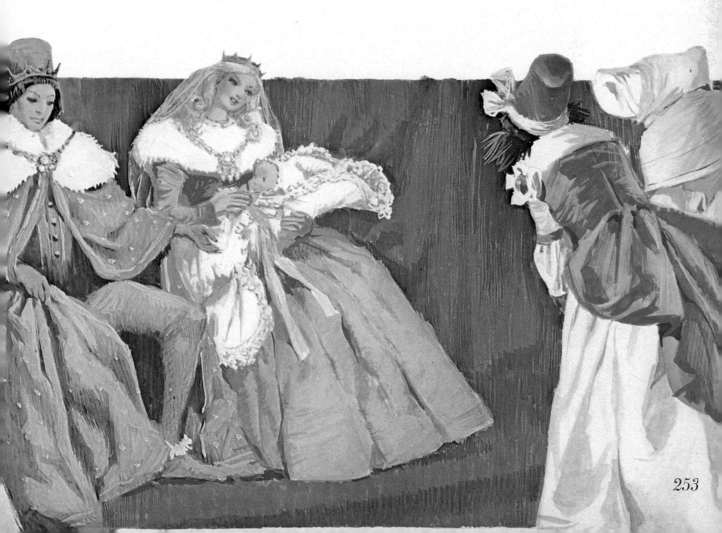

The next day a young page noticed the crowned duck swimming in the lake of the castle. As he reached down to pet it, he was amazed to hear it speak.

"I am your queen, master page, and I command you to take me to my baby," the bird said.

The page dared not refuse and carried the duck to the threshold of the royal nursery, where it was transformed instantly into the lovely queen. She ran to her baby's side, tucked him into his cradle gently, and kissed him tenderly.

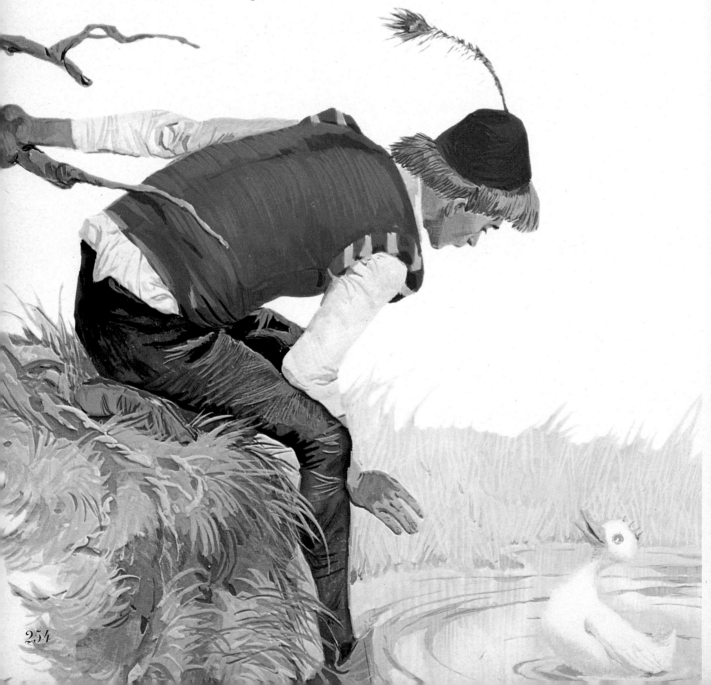

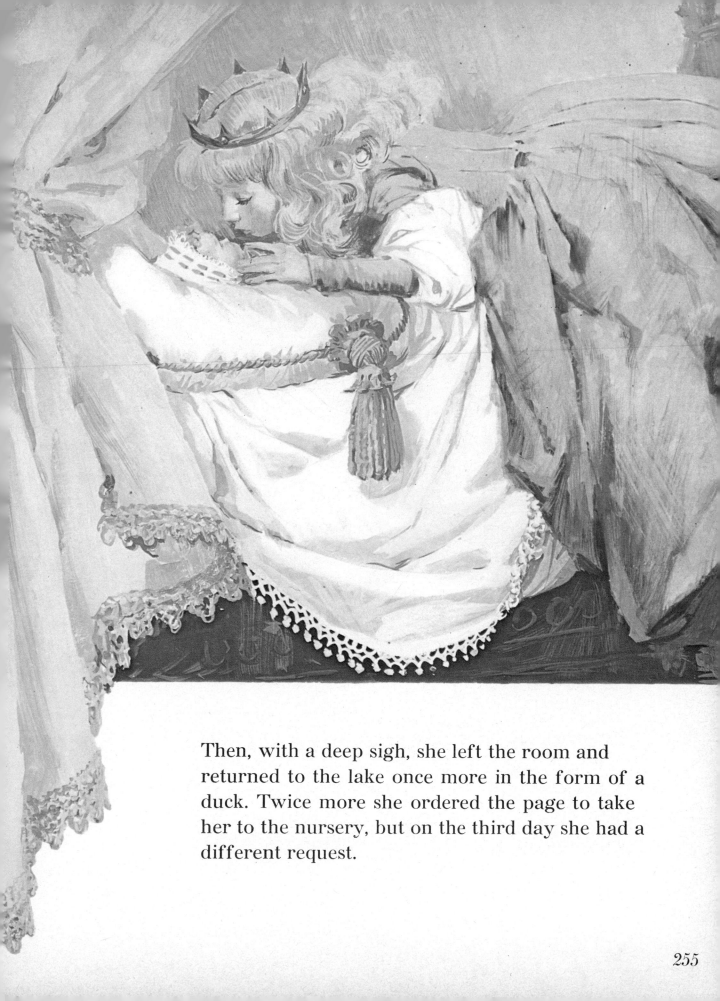

Then, with a deep sigh, she left the room and returned to the lake once more in the form of a duck. Twice more she ordered the page to take her to the nursery, but on the third day she had a different request.

"Go to His Majesty," she said, "and beg him to come here and swing his sword over my head in three wide circles."

The king came directly to the lake and swung his sword in three wide circles over the duck's head, just as commanded. As he finished the third circle, the duck vanished and in its place stood his beautiful queen.

When the king learned the story of the evil stepmother's treachery, he vowed that she and her ugly daughter should be justly punished.

"Tell me a suitable punishment for evildoers who have tried to drown an innocent person," he demanded when he found the wicked women.

"They should be shut up in a barrelful of spikes and rolled into the water to drown," they answered.

"You have just pronounced your own fate," shouted His Majesty.

The king ordered this punishment to be carried out at once. Ever after, he and his queen could live in peace and happiness, just as the three dwarfs in the wood had promised the gentle maiden.

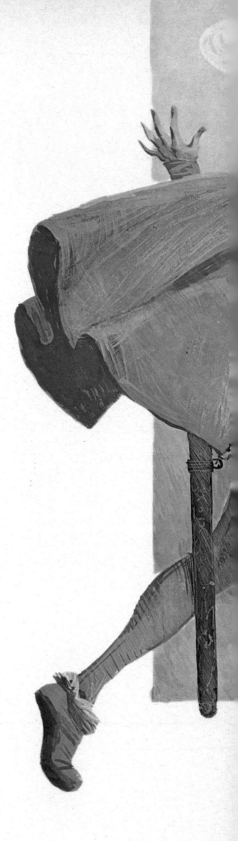

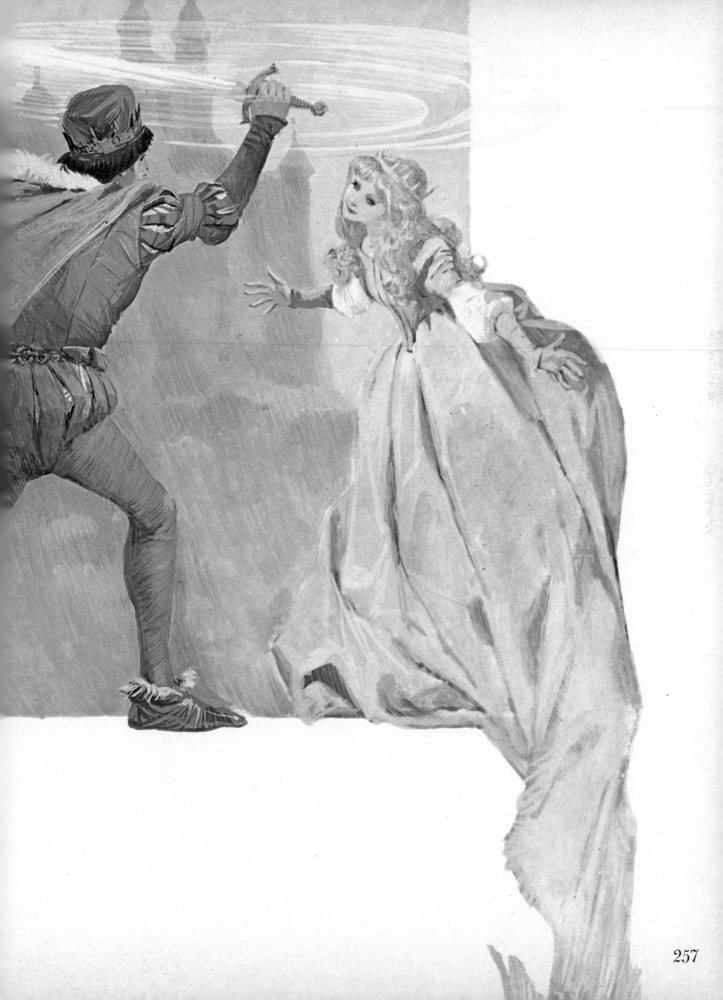

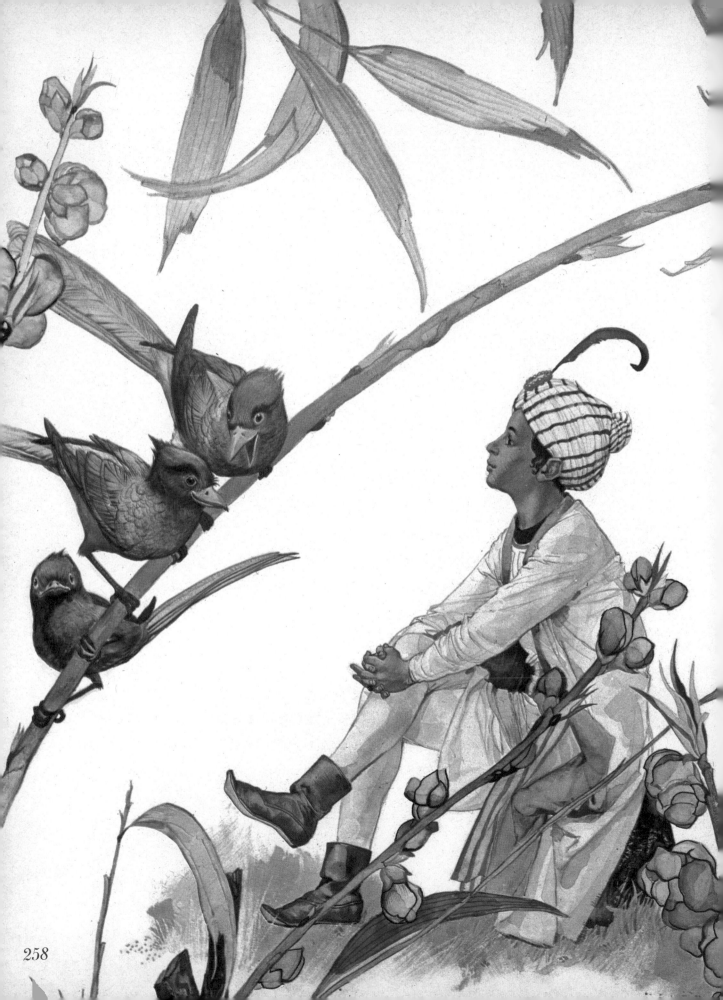

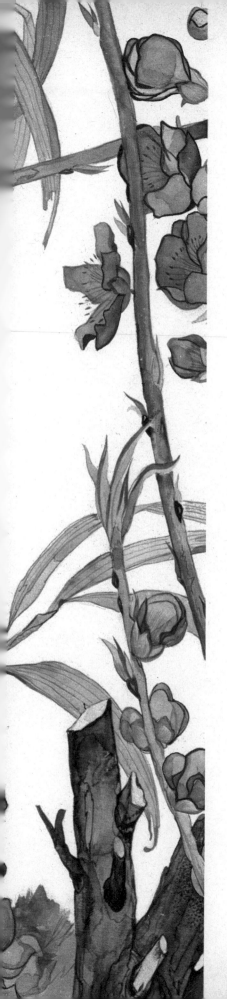

PRINCE KAMAR AND PRINCESS BUDUR

Once upon a time, on a faraway island in the middle of the vast China Sea lived a rich sultan whose greatest joy in life was his only son, Prince Kamar. The young prince was beloved also by the sultan's loyal subjects, who all claimed he was the most handsome youth in the realm. The sultan cherished his son more than he valued his riches and his palaces. But the ruler was getting older, and one day, when he and the prince were sitting in the royal gardens, he felt it was time for some fatherly advice.

"My dear son," he said, "it would be good for you to choose a wife."

"Not yet, Father," answered the handsome prince. "I'm happy as I am."

"I would dearly love to hold my own grandchildren on my knees before I die," argued the sultan.

"Beloved father, may you live forever!" laughed the prince. "I have plenty of time yet for raising children."

But his reply threw the sultan into a rage. "Since you will not take your father's advice," he shouted angrily, "you must now obey your sultan's command. Marry within the coming year, or you shall face imprisonment!"

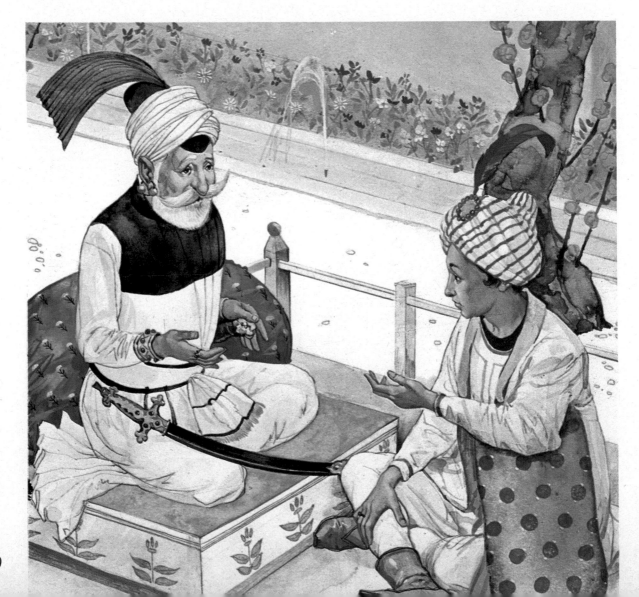

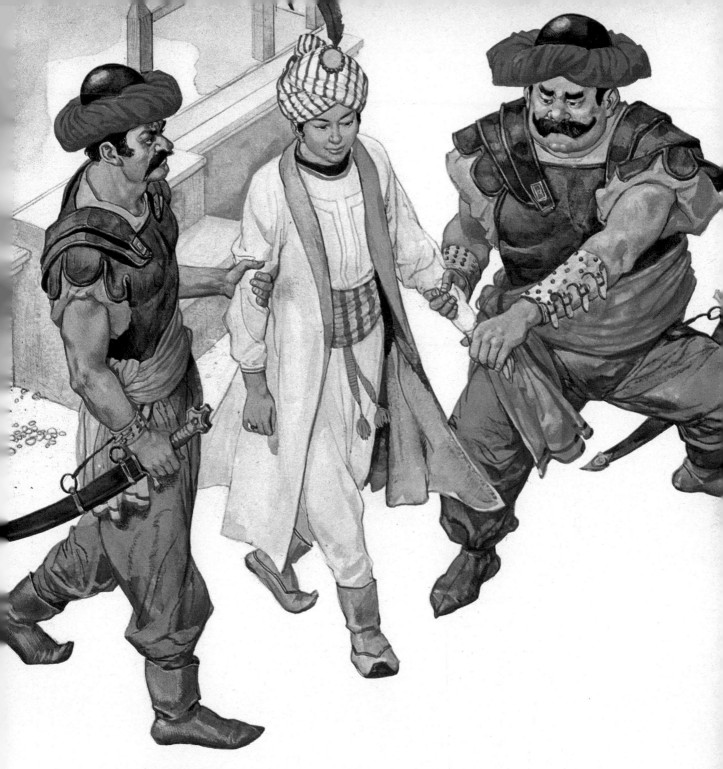

And so Prince Kamar obediently devoted himself to
serious study of the kingdom's beautiful maidens. It was
hard for him to concentrate on his task, and at the end
of the year when he had not yet found the princess
of his dreams, the sultan threw his son in prison.

At the very same time, in faraway China, the emperor gave the same fatherly advice to his beautiful daughter, Princess Budur.

"Marry within the year, or I shall lock you in your room!" he thundered.

The princess obediently studied every handsome youth in China, but at the end of the year when she had not yet found the prince of her dreams, her father locked her in her room.

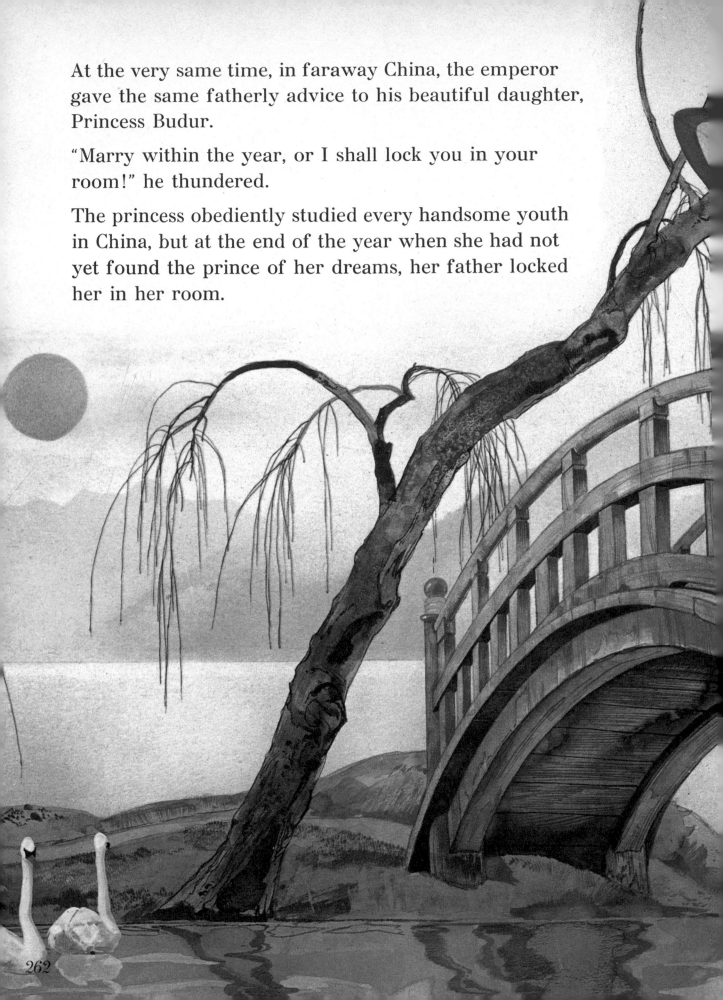

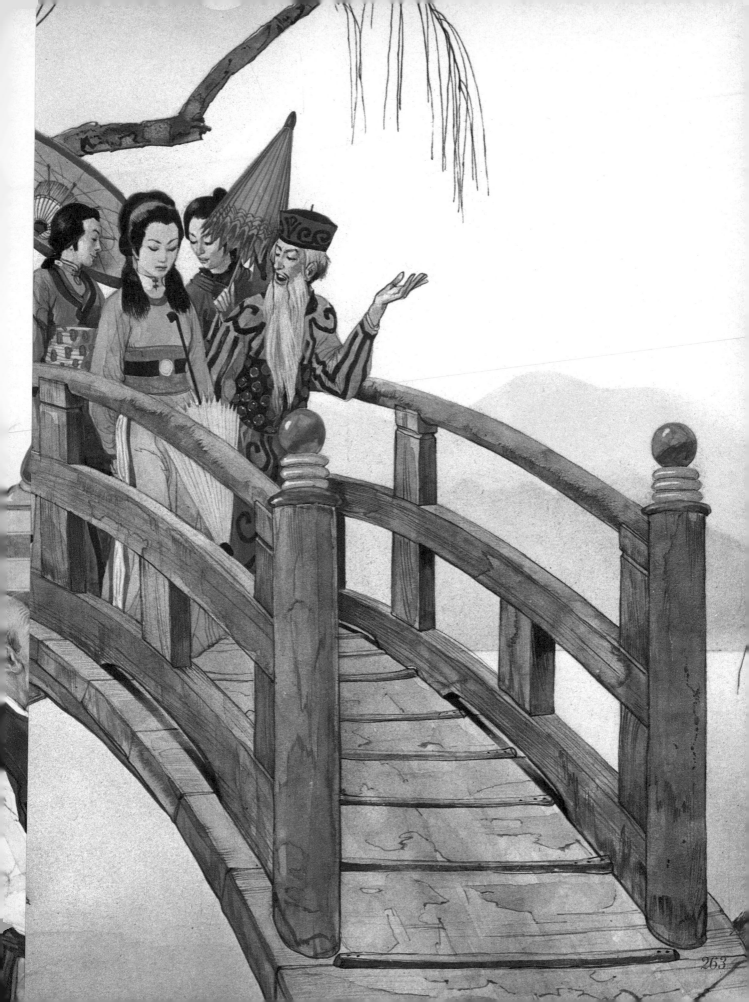

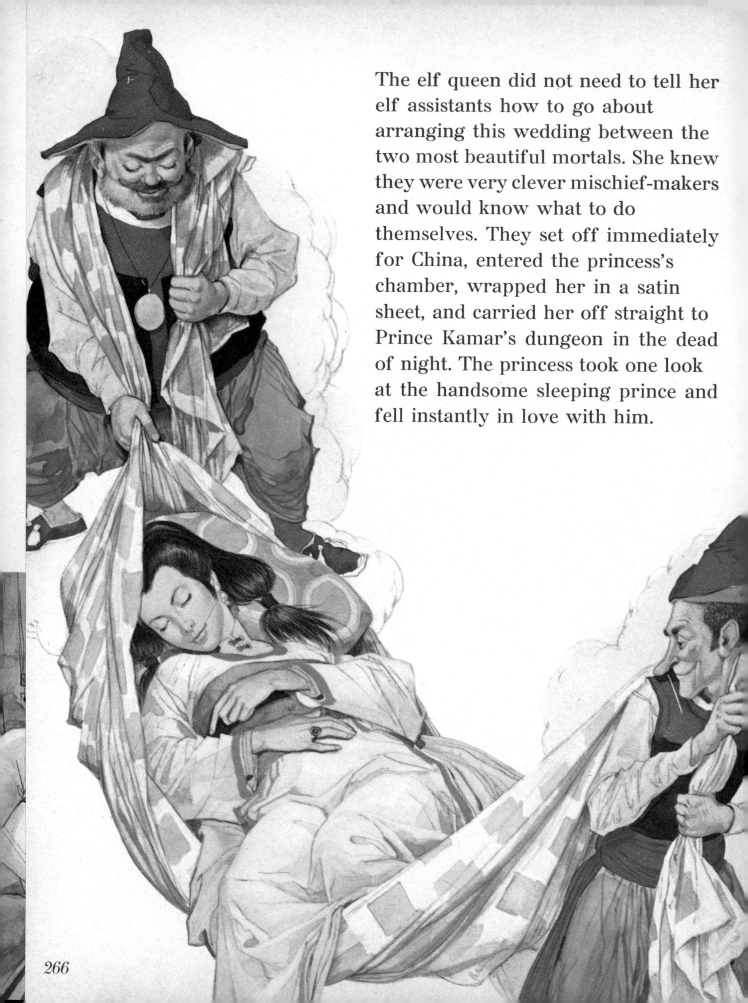

The elf queen did not need to tell her
elf assistants how to go about
arranging this wedding between the
two most beautiful mortals. She knew
they were very clever mischief-makers
and would know what to do
themselves. They set off immediately
for China, entered the princess's
chamber, wrapped her in a satin
sheet, and carried her off straight to
Prince Kamar's dungeon in the dead
of night. The princess took one look
at the handsome sleeping prince and
fell instantly in love with him.

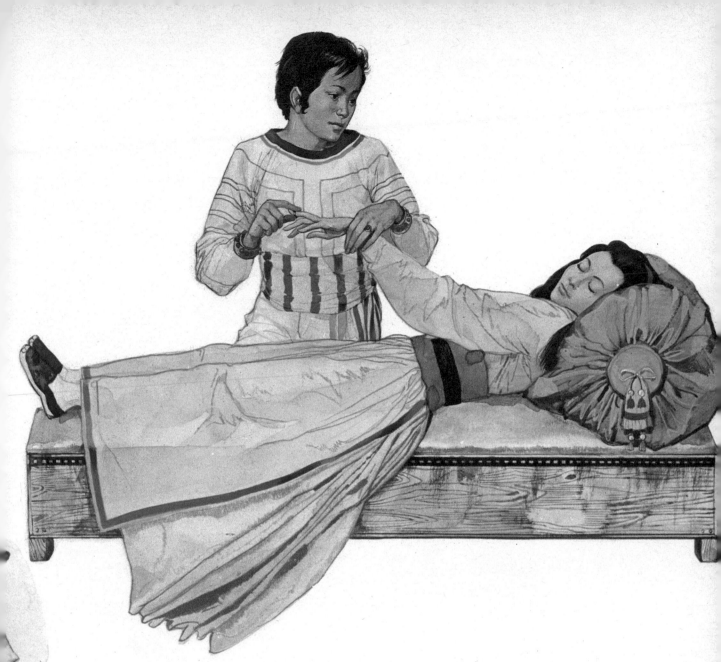

As proof of her undying love and devotion, Princess Budur put a great emerald ring on his finger. Then she fell asleep to dream of her love.

When the prince awoke and took one look at the sleeping princess, he too fell instantly in love. As proof of his love and devotion, he put a great pearl ring on her finger and then fell off to sleep again to dream of his beloved.

The elves watched happily as the beautiful lovers slept, but then one elf thought up even more mischief.

"Let's take the princess back to China!" he cried.

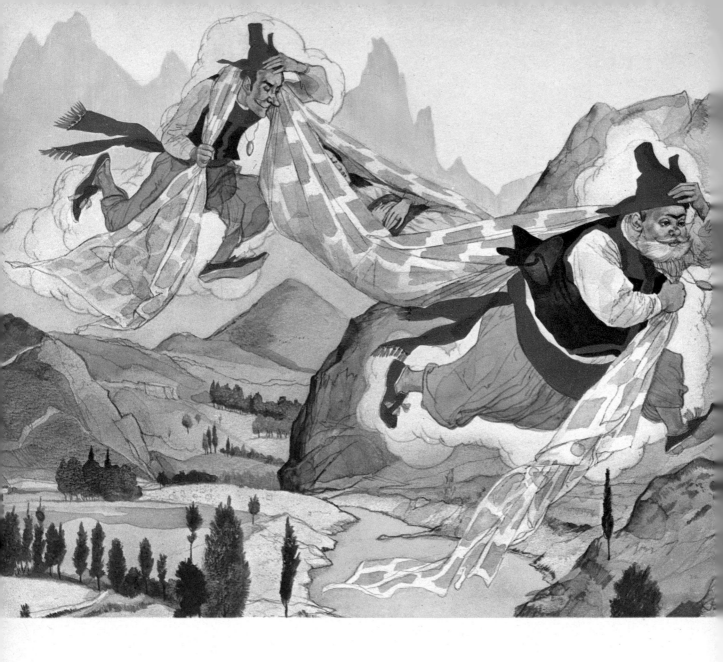

"Why?" asked his brother. "She and the prince have just fallen in love. Why separate them now?"

"To test their love, of course, silly!" shouted the first elf. "If they are truly in love, they will not rest till they find each other again."

Delighted with their latest mischief, the two elves quickly returned the princess to her prison bed in China. When the prince awoke and found himself alone in his cell, he became desperate.

"I will have no other bride!" he shouted when his father arrived.

"Your lovely princess exists only in your dreams," the sultan answered.

But the prince looked at the emerald ring on his finger and knew he had not been dreaming. He lay on his bed with his heart breaking, while the royal physicians tried in vain to cure him.

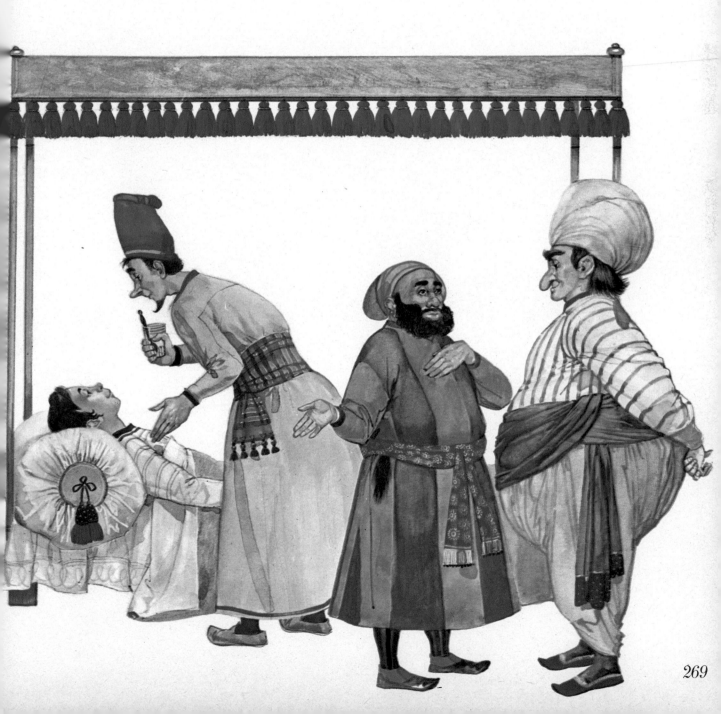

When Princess Budur awoke and found herself alone, she too became desperate.

"I will have no other bridegroom," she sobbed when visited by her anxious father.

"Your handsome young prince exists only in your dreams, my child," the emperor insisted.

But the princess looked at the pearl ring on her finger and knew that she had not been dreaming. She sat in her garden with her heart breaking, growing paler and thinner every day, while the imperial physicians tried without success to cure her. She grew so weak that one day she could not rise from her bed, and the old emperor was in despair.

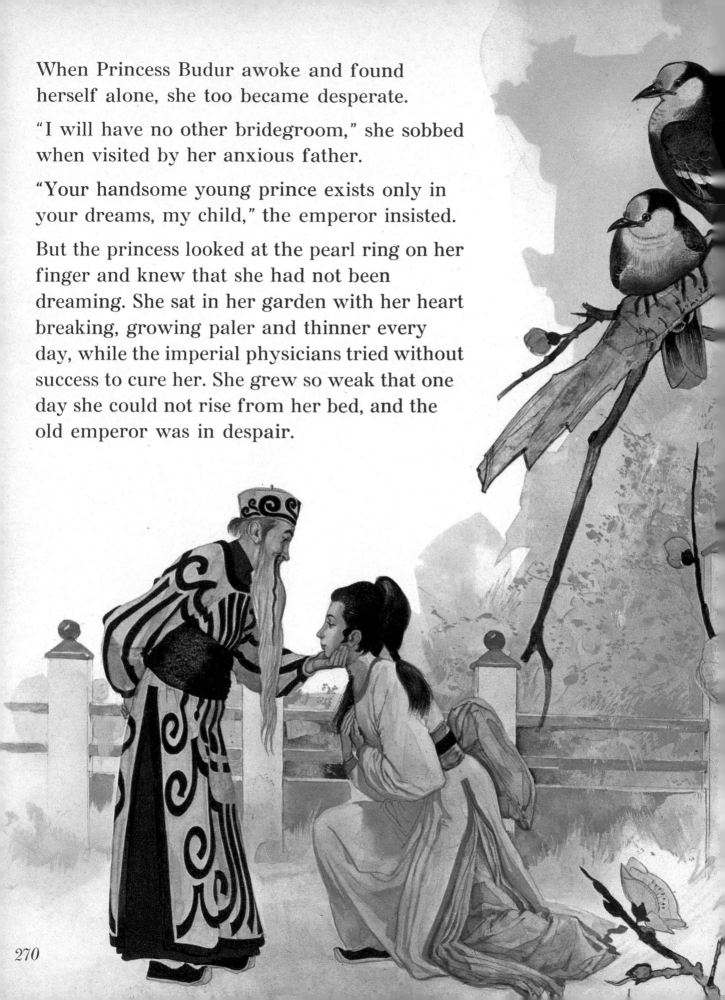

Finally, her handsome young brother, Prince Chang, came to comfort her. "I see the ring on your finger, my sister, and I do believe your prince exists," he said kindly, taking her hand in his.

"Thank you, dear brother," the princess whispered weakly. "But if you do believe me, I beg you to find him for me."

"If he lives across the wide ocean, or in the burning desert, or on the highest mountain, I will find him, never fear," vowed her brother as he left her bedchamber.

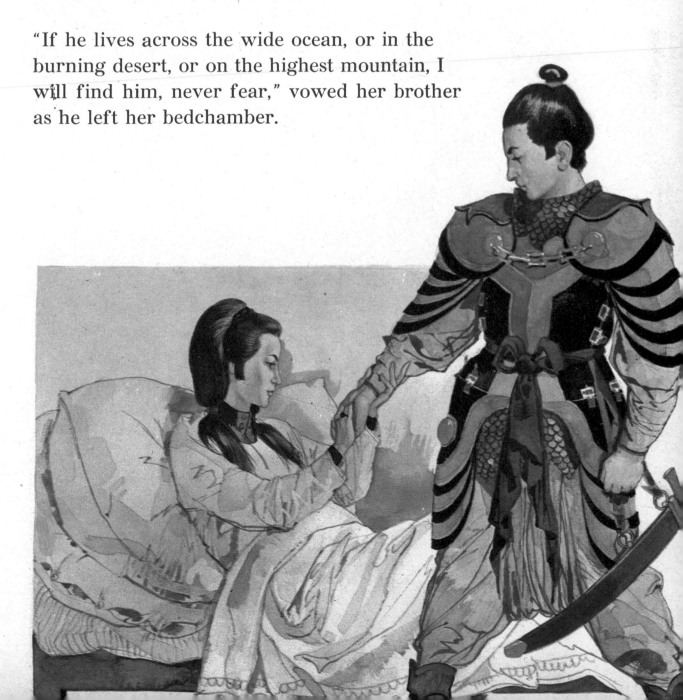

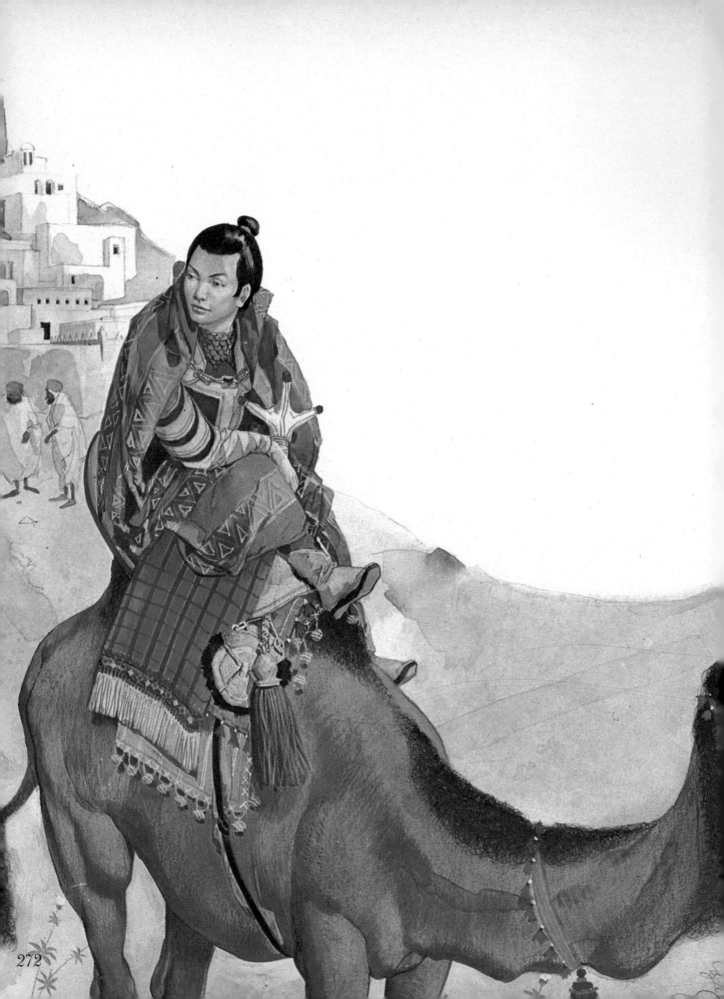

The very next day Prince Chang set forth on his long and perilous search for his sister's lost prince. He traveled across deep rivers, scaled high mountains, and rode a camel across a burning desert, but nowhere did he find Prince Kamar. Then, one day he heard a traveler speak of a distant land where the sultan's handsome son lay dying of an unknown illness.

"Does this prince wear a priceless emerald ring on his finger?" cried Chang eagerly.

"He wears such an emerald," answered the traveler. "They say it is as big as a swallow's egg."

"At last I have found my sister's dream prince!"

Quickly Prince Chang bought a sturdy boat and started off on a dangerous voyage across the China Sea. But before long a terrible storm came up, and his ship sank in the churning waters.

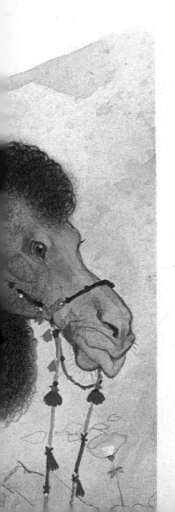

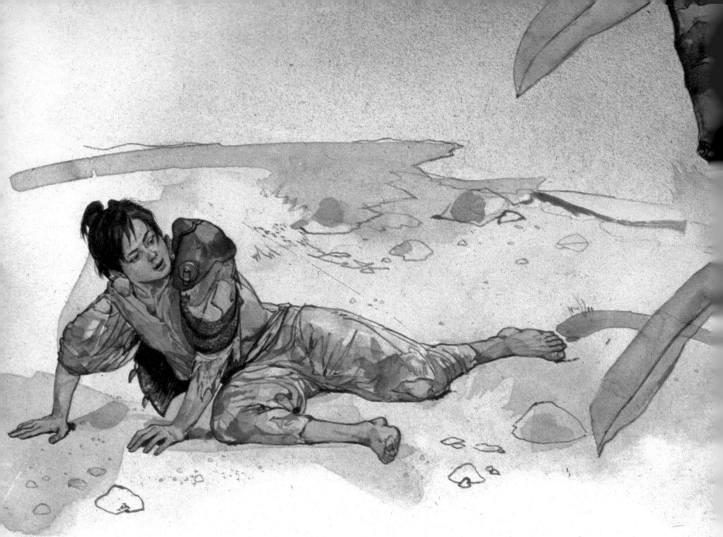

Fortunately, Prince Chang managed to cling to some timber which floated away toward land, and several days later he was washed up, half-drowned and exhausted, on the white sands of a distant shore.

Still dazed by his terrible ordeal, he had no idea where he was, but soon a horseman came riding by.

"What land is this?" Chang called weakly.

"This land belongs to our unhappy sultan," answered the horseman, who was a palace guard. "Our ruler's poor son lies dying of an unknown malady, and perhaps may already be dead."

"Take me to your sultan! Quickly, I beg you, before it is too late," Prince Chang gasped.

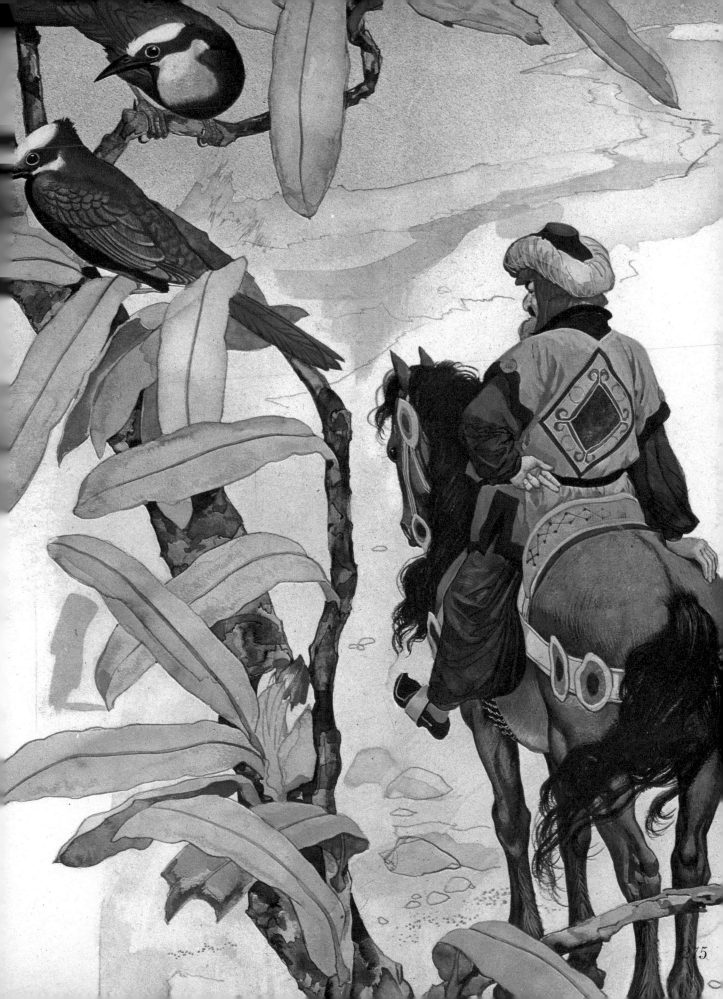

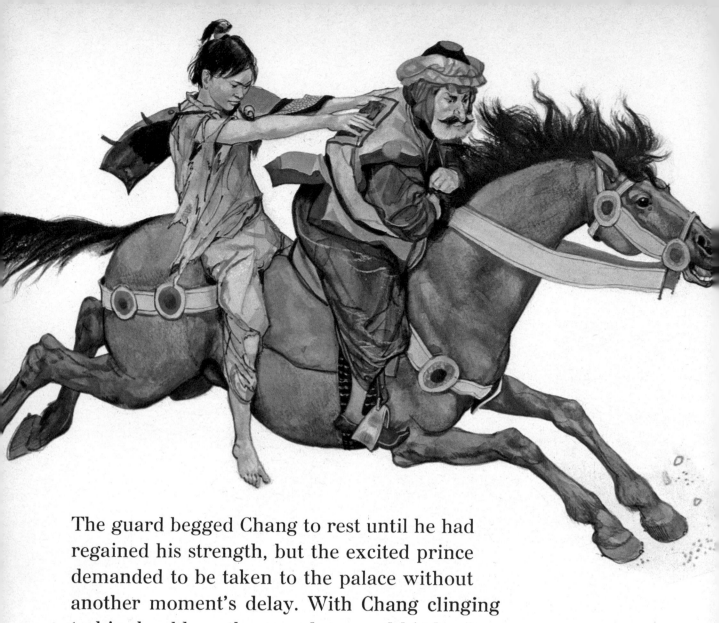

The guard begged Chang to rest until he had
regained his strength, but the excited prince
demanded to be taken to the palace without
another moment's delay. With Chang clinging
to his shoulders, the guard spurred his horse
on and together they galloped to the palace at
breakneck speed.

Chang was immediately taken to the royal
bedchamber, where the young prince lay pale
and nearly lifeless on satin pillows. His eyes
were closed, and his breathing was very faint.
The royal physicians hovered around his bed
trying desperate remedies, since the sultan had
sworn to kill them if they failed to cure his son.

As Chang looked down at the pale face on the pillows, the young prince opened his eyes.

"No one believes I ever saw my beautiful princess," Prince Kamar whispered softly.

"I believe you," replied Prince Chang. "Your princess does exist, and she has sent me to find you. From the moment you gave her your pearl ring she has thought of no one but you. I know this well because the lovely Princess Budur is my sister."

The mischievous elves watched delightedly as the prince sat up in bed. The color returned to his face, and his eyes opened wide with joy. Within seconds he was healthy and handsome as ever.

"At last!" he cried. "I have found my princess!"

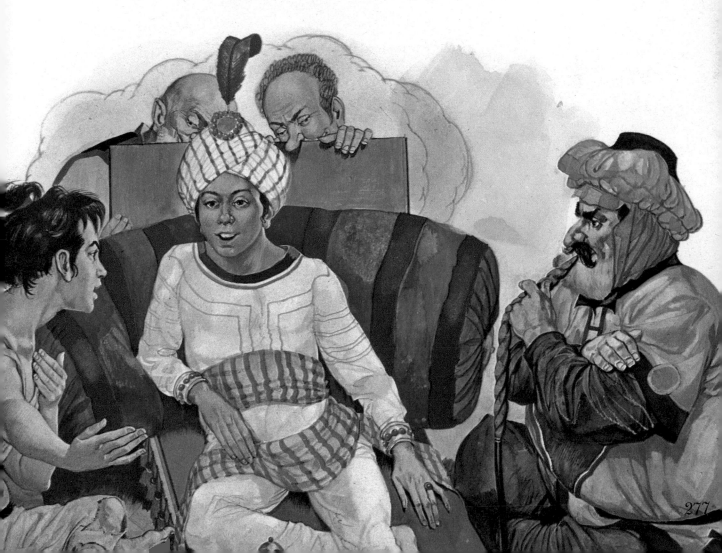

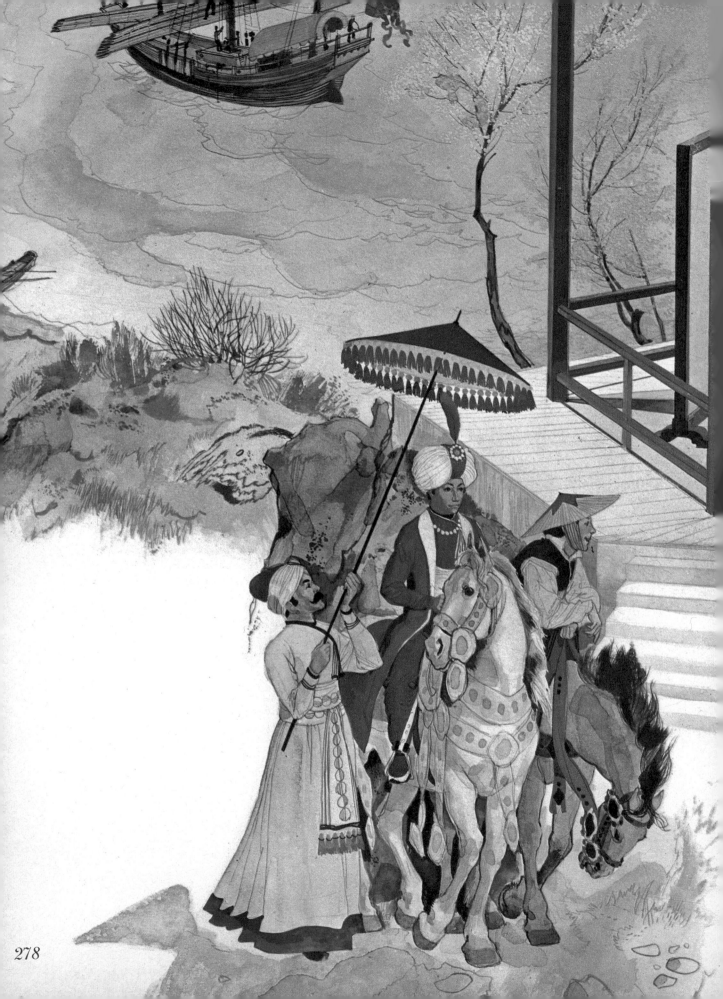

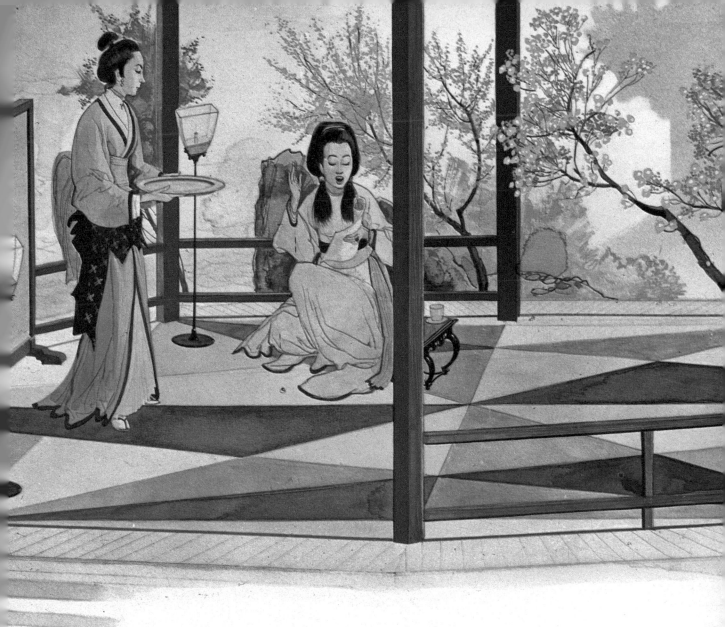

Prince Kamar ordered a messenger to rush ahead and bear the emerald ring as a sign to Princess Budur, and as soon as he could he sailed across the China Sea with Prince Chang to find his beloved once again.

When Princess Budur saw her ring and knew that her prince was coming to claim her, she too became strong and beautiful once more. And when the prince arrived, the two most beautiful of mortals were married. They never knew unhappiness again, because the mischievous elves had flown away to play their tricks in other distant lands.

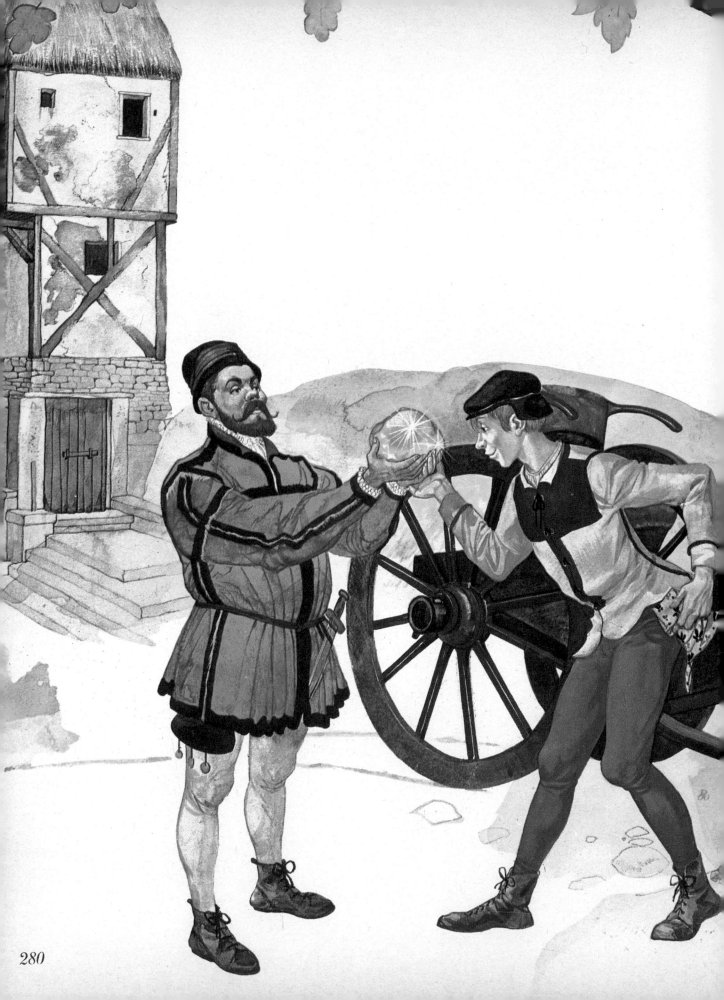

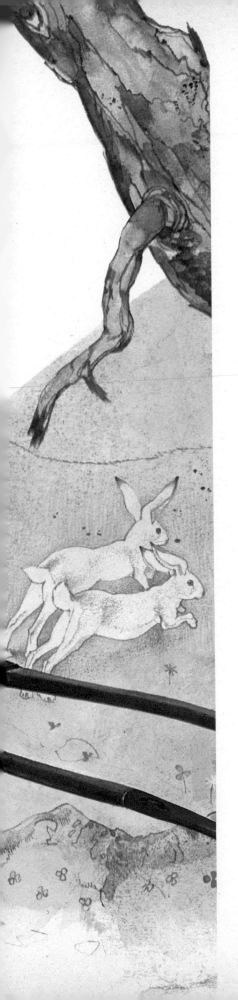

HANS IN LUCK

Once upon a time there was a cheerful young man named Hans who had worked hard for seven years as a baker's apprentice.

One spring day Hans decided it was time to go home, so he politely asked for his wages.

"You have been a good worker, so your pay shall be handsome," said his master, and he rewarded Hans with a lump of gold as big as his head.

"How lucky I am," cried Hans. "I shall come home a rich man."

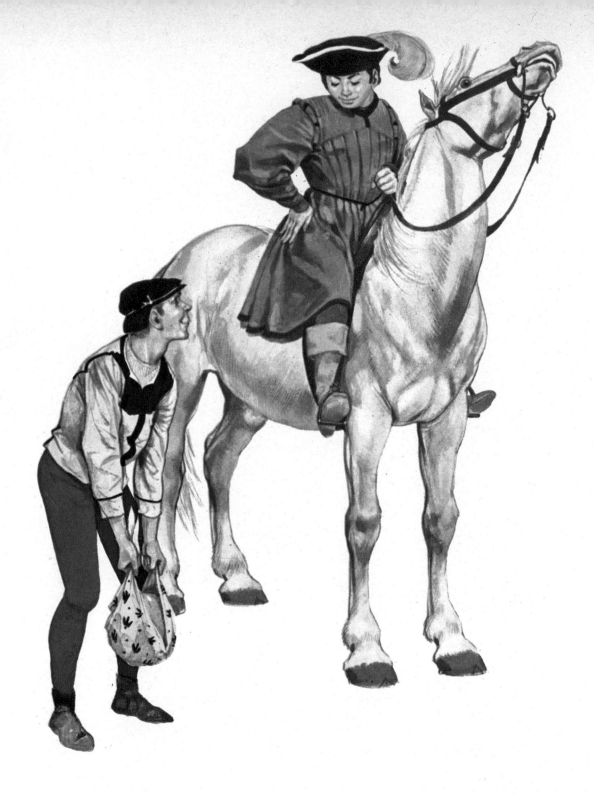

He carefully wrapped the gold in a handkerchief, bade farewell to his master and started home with a light heart. But such a great lump of gold is heavy, and soon Hans became hot and tired.

As he walked wearily along, a young man came trotting by, sitting comfortably on a handsome horse.

"Ah!" said Hans admiringly. "What a fine thing it is to ride on horseback!"

"Then why do you walk?" asked the rider.

"I have no horse, sir," Hans replied. "And this great lump of gold is a heavy burden."

"Then let's make an exchange," suggested the clever rider. "Your burden for my horse."

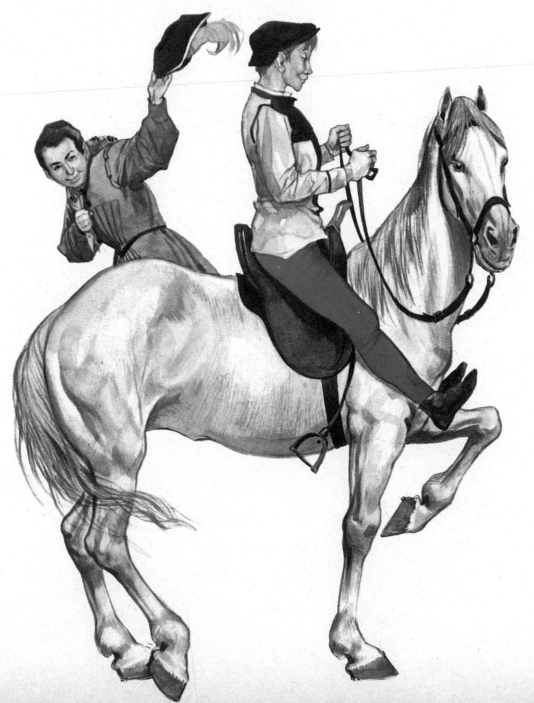

"How lucky I am to ride so comfortably on this handsome horse," Hans said to himself. "And how silly of that man to change."

He rode merrily along, whistling a cheerful tune. After a time he wondered whether his horse would not go a little faster. So he cracked his whip sharply.

Away galloped his handsome horse at full speed, and before Hans knew what was happening, he flew through the air and landed on his back by the roadside.

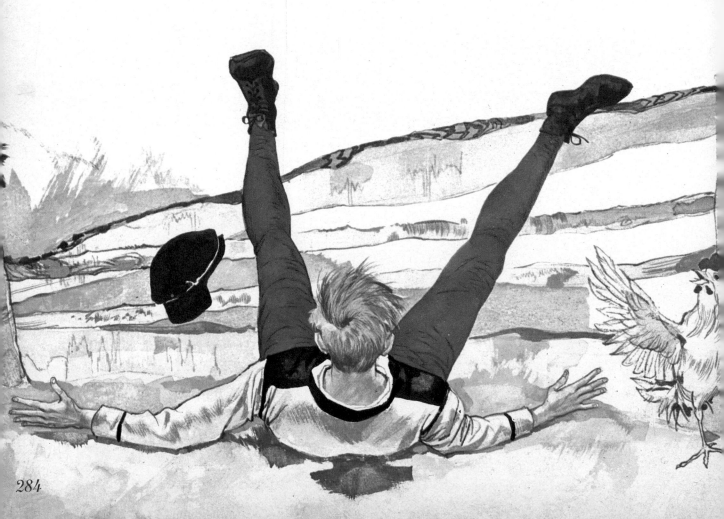

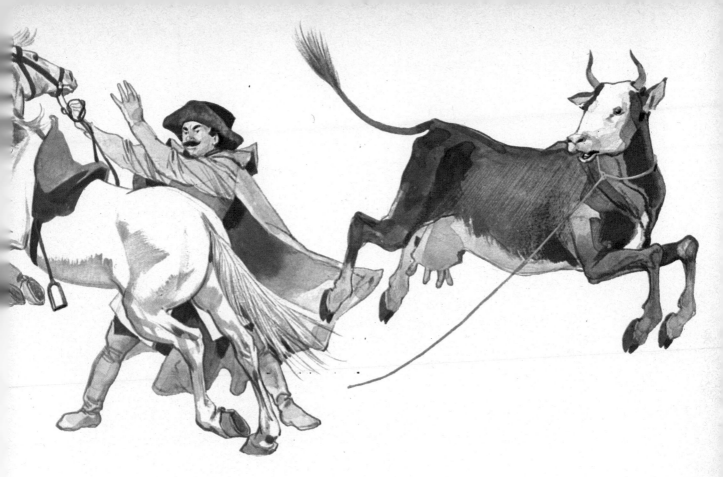

A farmer passing by with his cow caught the runaway horse. Hans thanked him politely and looked at the cow with great admiration.

"What a fine animal you have," he said to the farmer. "And far less dangerous than this wild horse of mine. If I had such a cow I could walk along leisurely with her and have milk and butter and cheese free of charge."

"Then let's make an exchange," said the farmer, looking at the beautiful horse with greedy eyes.

"I'll take this dangerous horse off your hands and you can have my gentle cow."

"How kind you are!" cried Hans, and the exchange was speedily arranged.

The farmer galloped away on the horse, happy with his clever bargain, but Hans was just as proud.

"How lucky I am," he said to himself. "All I need to buy is a piece of bread, which is certainly cheap enough, and then, whenever I'm hungry I can eat it with good rich butter and cheese and wash it down with the freshest milk."

He was already so fond of his cow that he stopped by a pasture fence just to let it rest while he petted it.

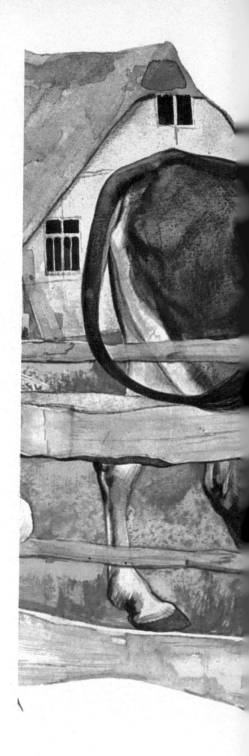

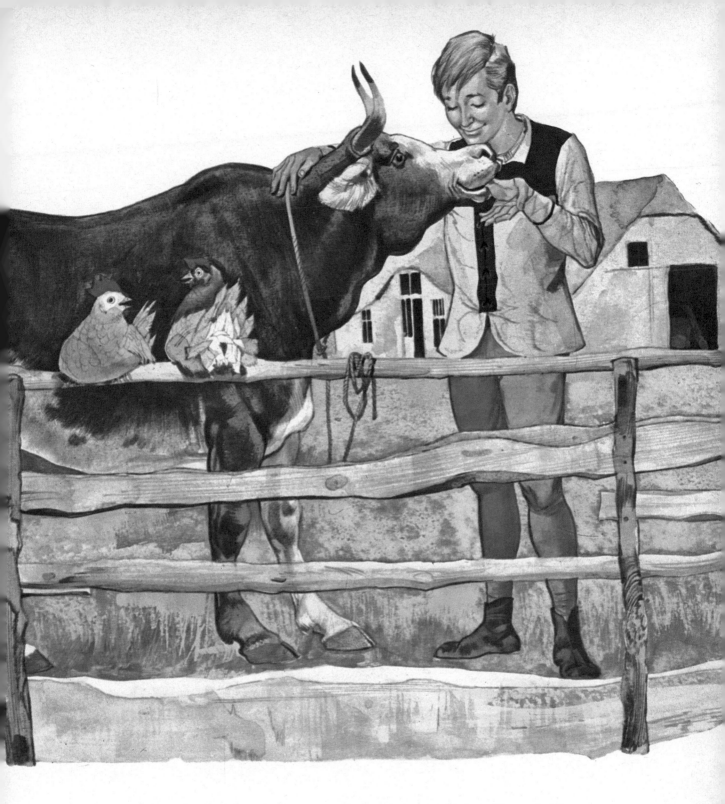

But before long he felt very hungry and, leading his patient cow by her halter rope, he hurried straight to the nearest village to find an inn.

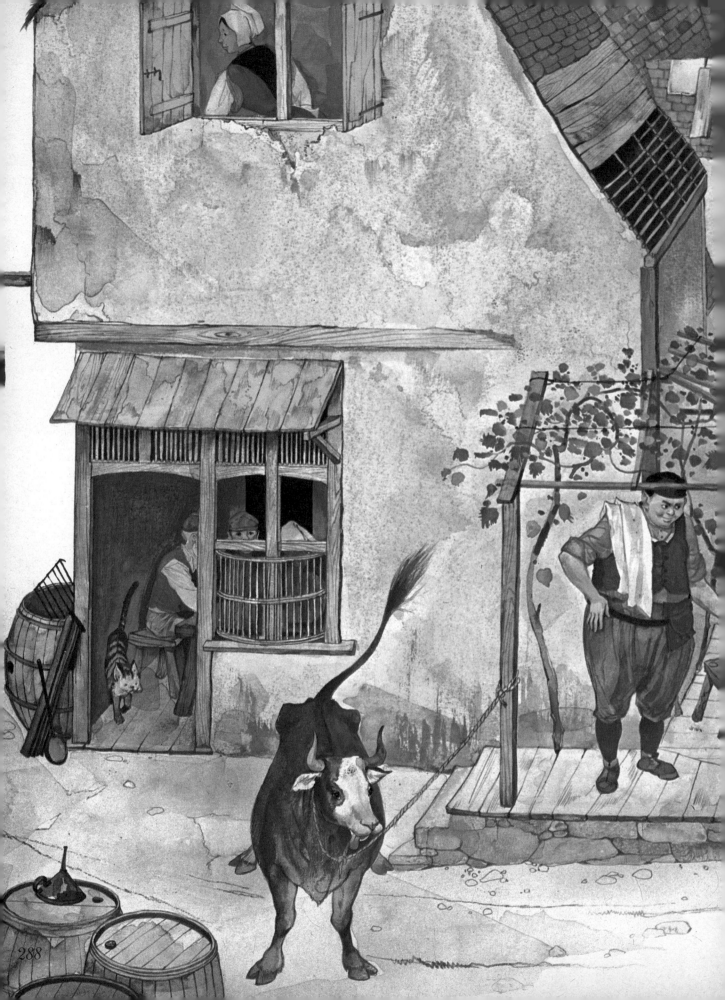

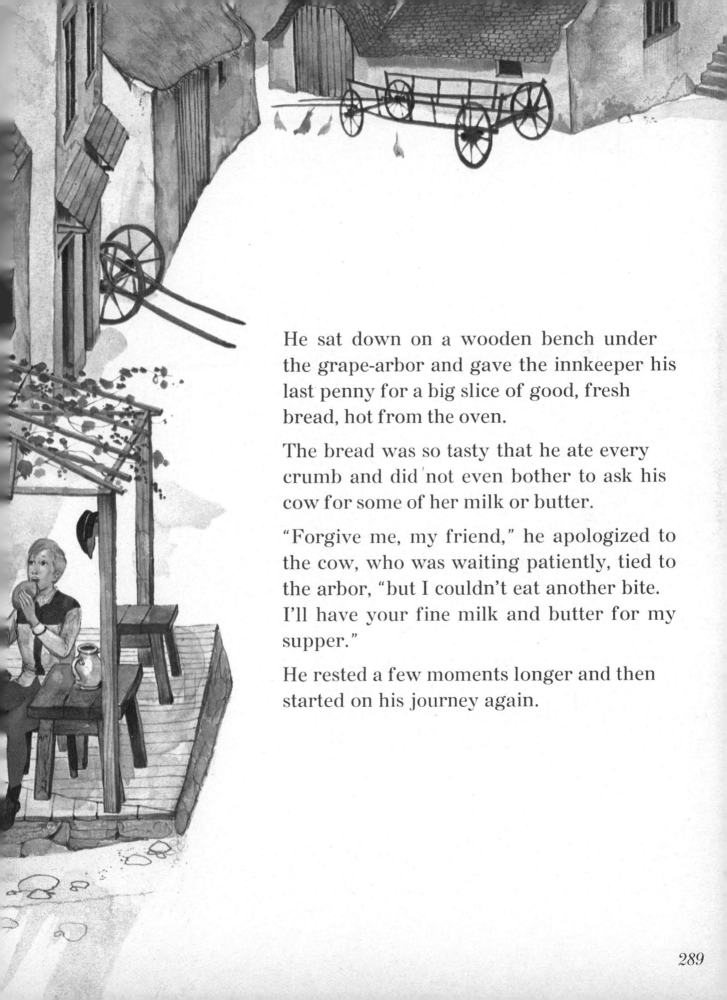

He sat down on a wooden bench under the grape-arbor and gave the innkeeper his last penny for a big slice of good, fresh bread, hot from the oven.

The bread was so tasty that he ate every crumb and did not even bother to ask his cow for some of her milk or butter.

"Forgive me, my friend," he apologized to the cow, who was waiting patiently, tied to the arbor, "but I couldn't eat another bite. I'll have your fine milk and butter for my supper."

He rested a few moments longer and then started on his journey again.

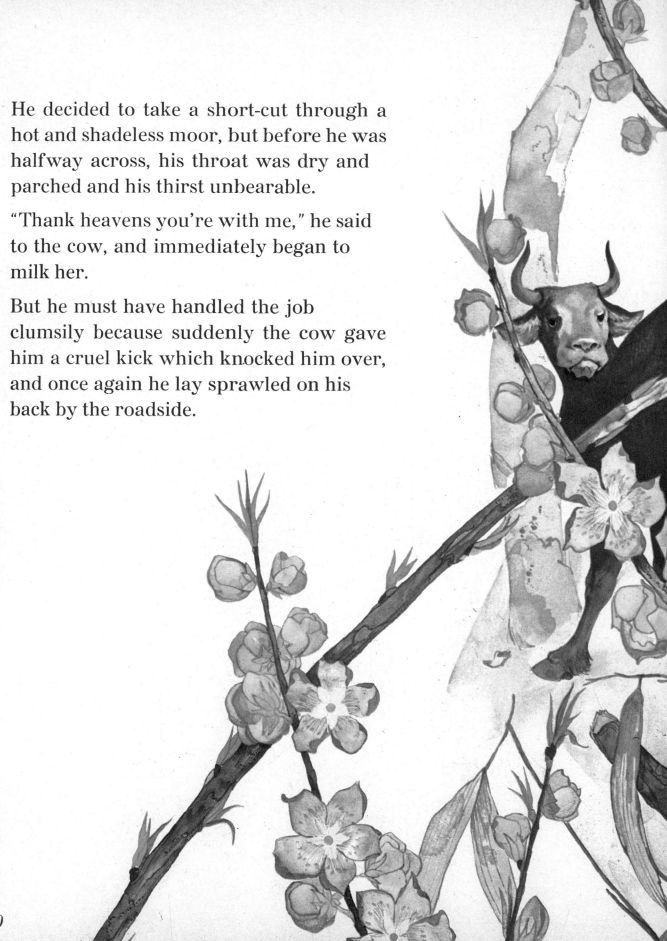

He decided to take a short-cut through a hot and shadeless moor, but before he was halfway across, his throat was dry and parched and his thirst unbearable.

"Thank heavens you're with me," he said to the cow, and immediately began to milk her.

But he must have handled the job clumsily because suddenly the cow gave him a cruel kick which knocked him over, and once again he lay sprawled on his back by the roadside.

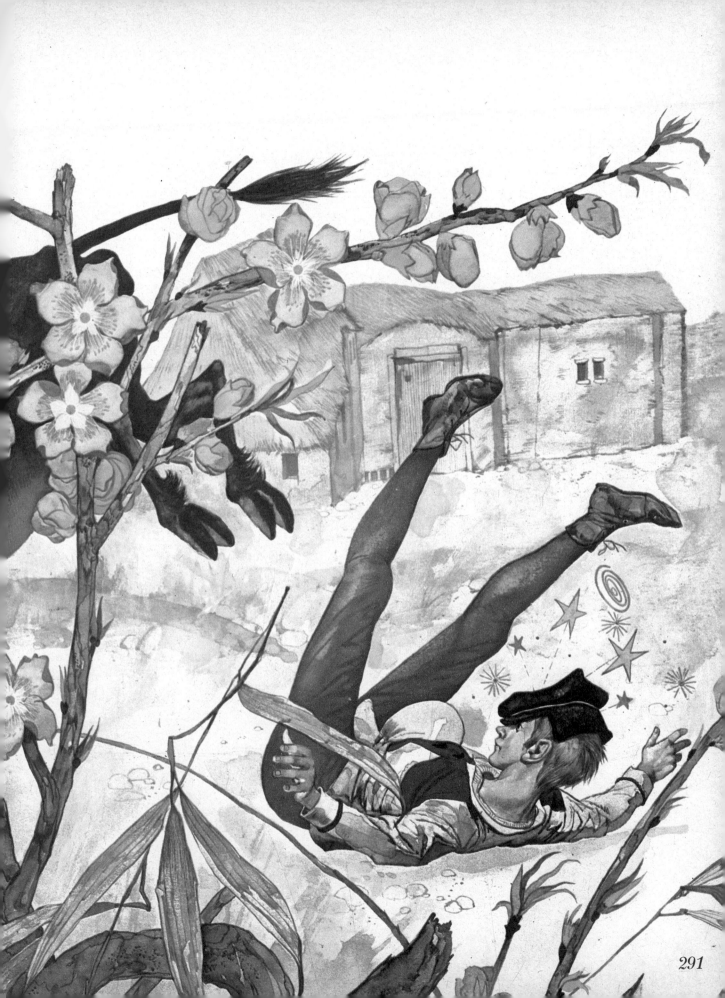

291

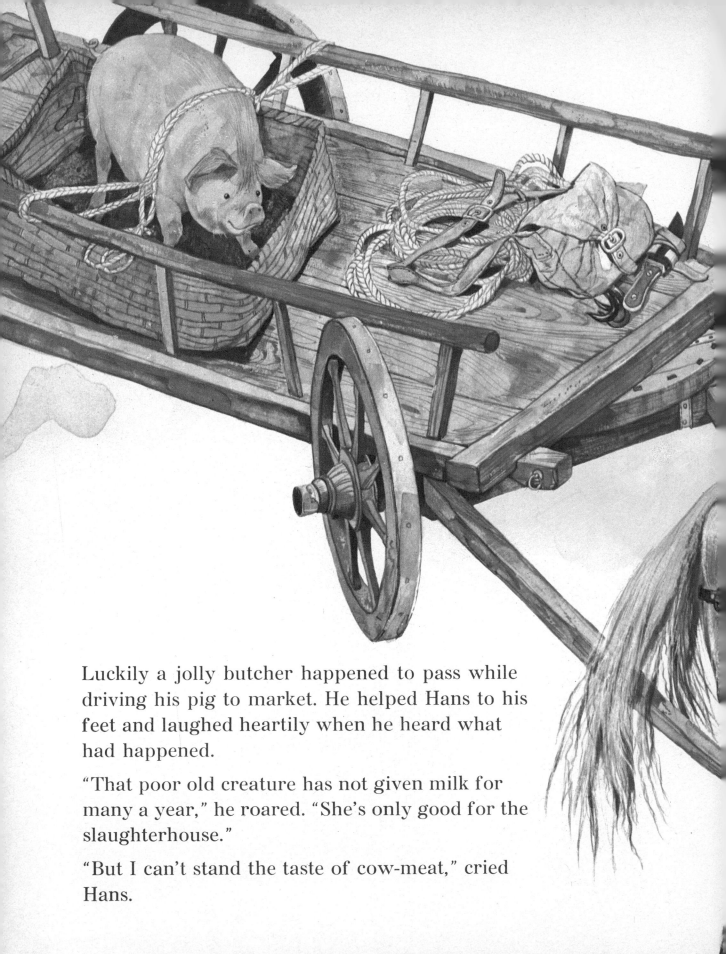

Luckily a jolly butcher happened to pass while driving his pig to market. He helped Hans to his feet and laughed heartily when he heard what had happened.

"That poor old creature has not given milk for many a year," he roared. "She's only good for the slaughterhouse."

"But I can't stand the taste of cow-meat," cried Hans.

"Now, if only I had a good fat pig, I would have all the bacon and sausage I could eat."

"Then let's make an exchange," suggested the butcher, who already had decided that the cow would fetch a good price at the market. "I'll take this scrawny beast and give you my pig in return."

"How kind you are," cried Hans, and the trade was quickly made.

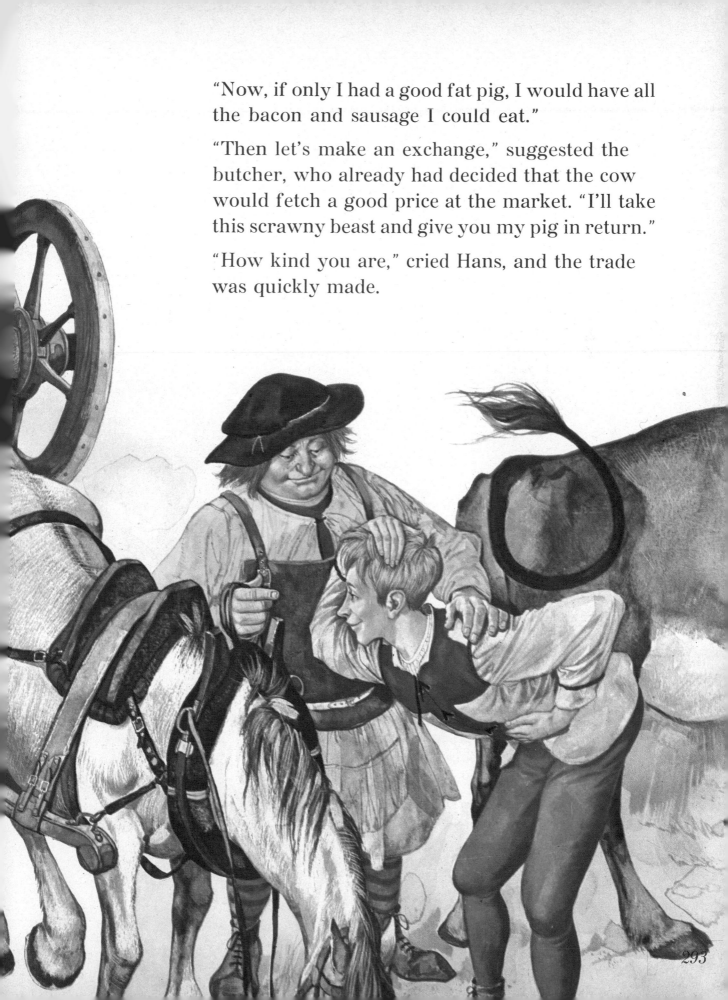

"How lucky I am," Hans chuckled to himself, admiring his prize pig as he dragged her along the dusty road. They had to walk so slowly that soon they were overtaken by a farmer's boy carrying a great white goose.

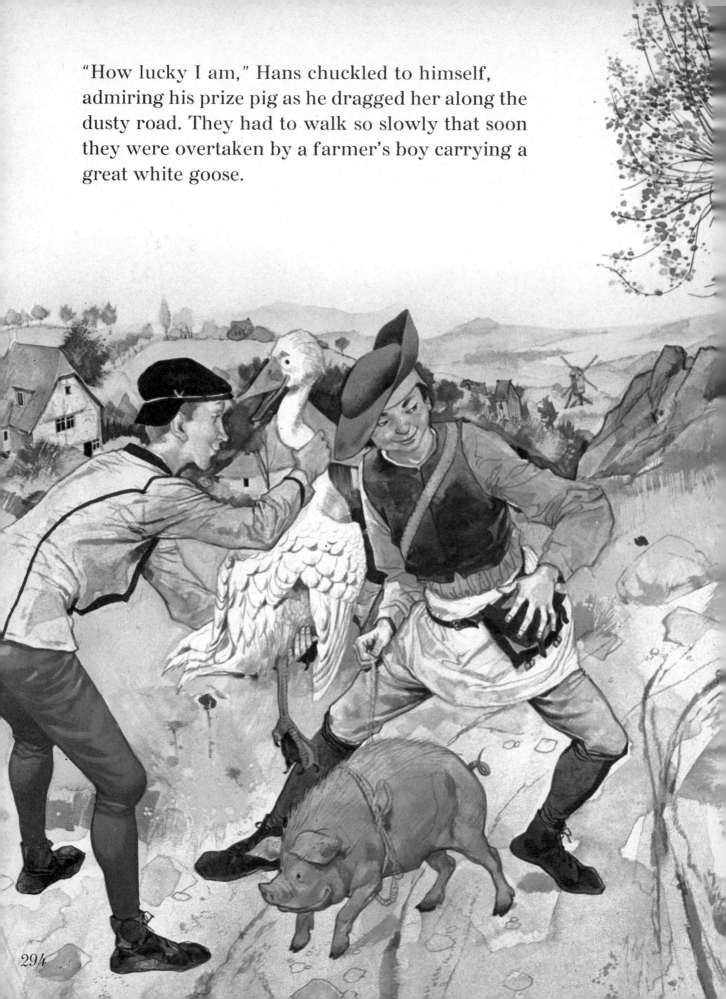

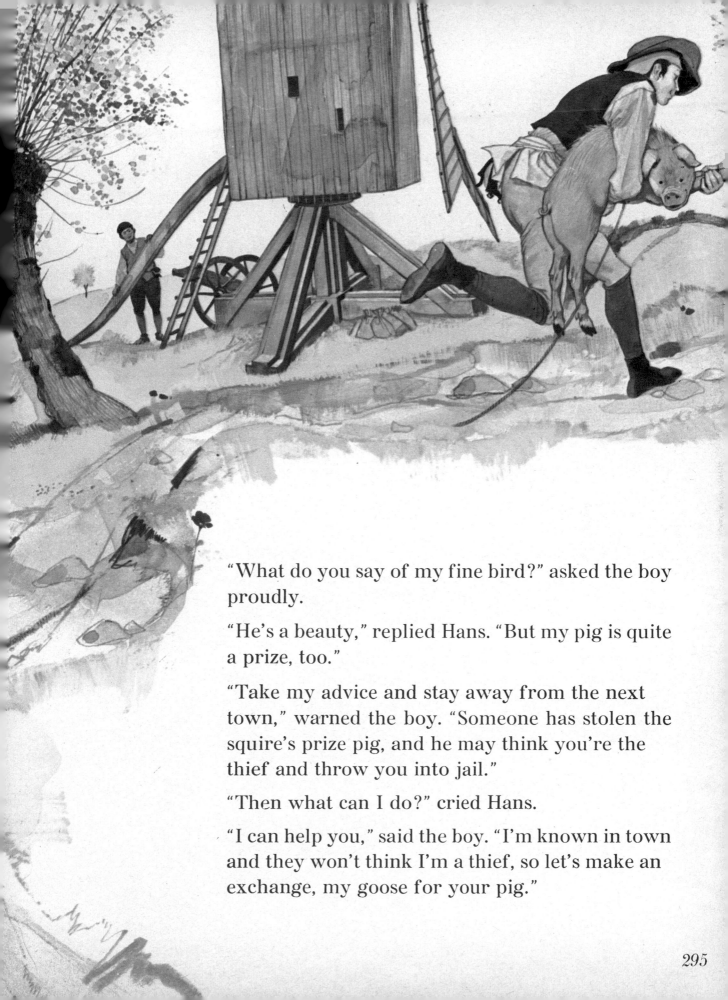

"What do you say of my fine bird?" asked the boy proudly.

"He's a beauty," replied Hans. "But my pig is quite a prize, too."

"Take my advice and stay away from the next town," warned the boy. "Someone has stolen the squire's prize pig, and he may think you're the thief and throw you into jail."

"Then what can I do?" cried Hans.

"I can help you," said the boy. "I'm known in town and they won't think I'm a thief, so let's make an exchange, my goose for your pig."

Hans was delighted with the exchange.

"I'm lucky as always," he thought happily to himself as he strolled down the road. "First, my mother will cook an excellent roast from my fine goose. Then the fat will keep us in goose-grease for six months, and there will be so many beautiful feathers that we shall make soft pillows for each of us. Yes, it's true, good luck seems to follow me wherever I go."

Finally he came to the last village before his own and passed a knife-grinder working at his grindstone and singing cheerfully.

"You seem happy at your trade," Hans remarked pleasantly.

"It's a good one, indeed," said the grinder. "Knives always get dull and need sharpening, so a knife-grinder always has money in his pocket. Now tell me, where did you get that fine goose?"

"I traded it for my pig," answered Hans.

"And where did you get your pig?" the grinder went on.

"In exchange for the cow I had traded for the horse which I bought with the gold I earned in seven years of hard work," replied Hans.

"And now what you need is money in your pocket," said the grinder. "A grindstone is your answer. Let's make an exchange—your goose for one of my stones."

"Done!" cried Hans gratefully and quickly made the exchange.

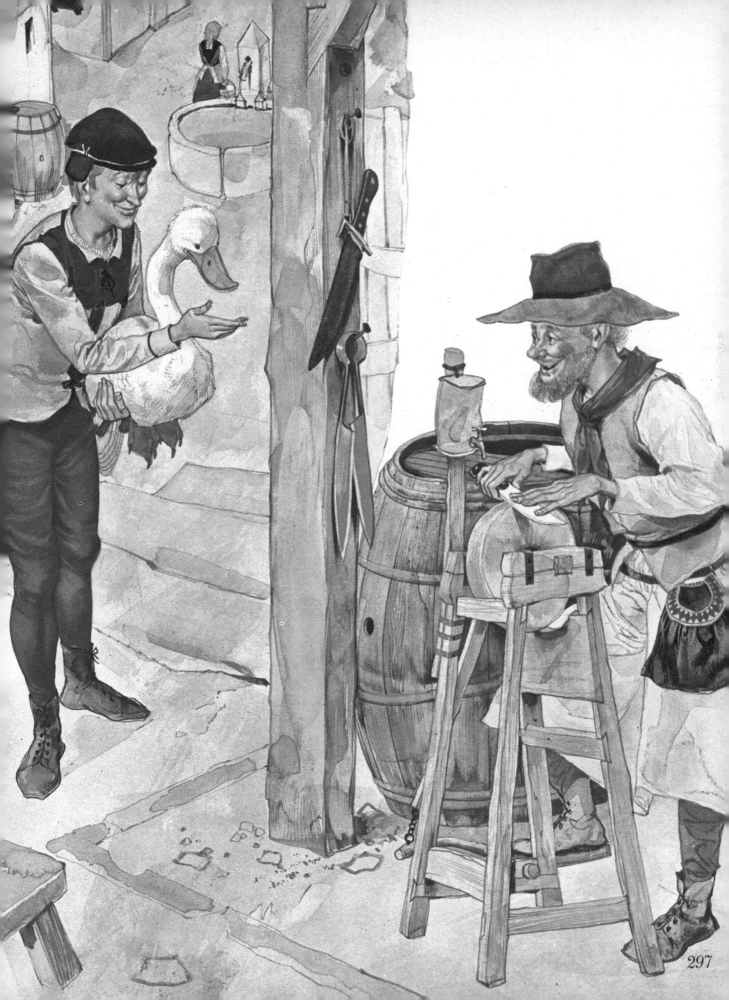

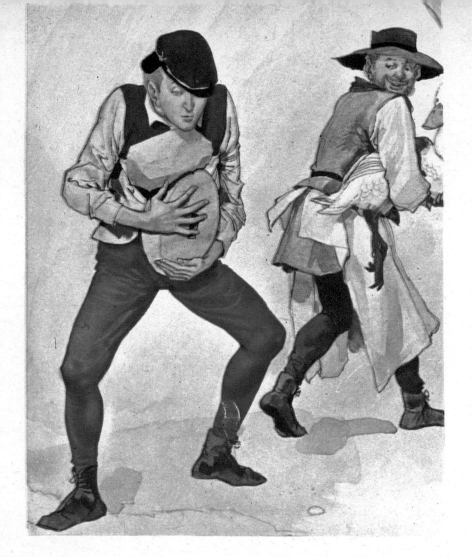

Hans took the heavy stone, already counting the coins that would soon jingle in his pocket.

"I must have been born under a lucky star," he said once again. "I seem to get everything I need without even trying."

But the grindstone was heavy, and soon Hans was weary and thirsty. By the time he reached his village he could barely drag himself to the well.

As he reached over to drink, he knocked the grindstone over the side of the well, and down it sank, down to the very bottom.

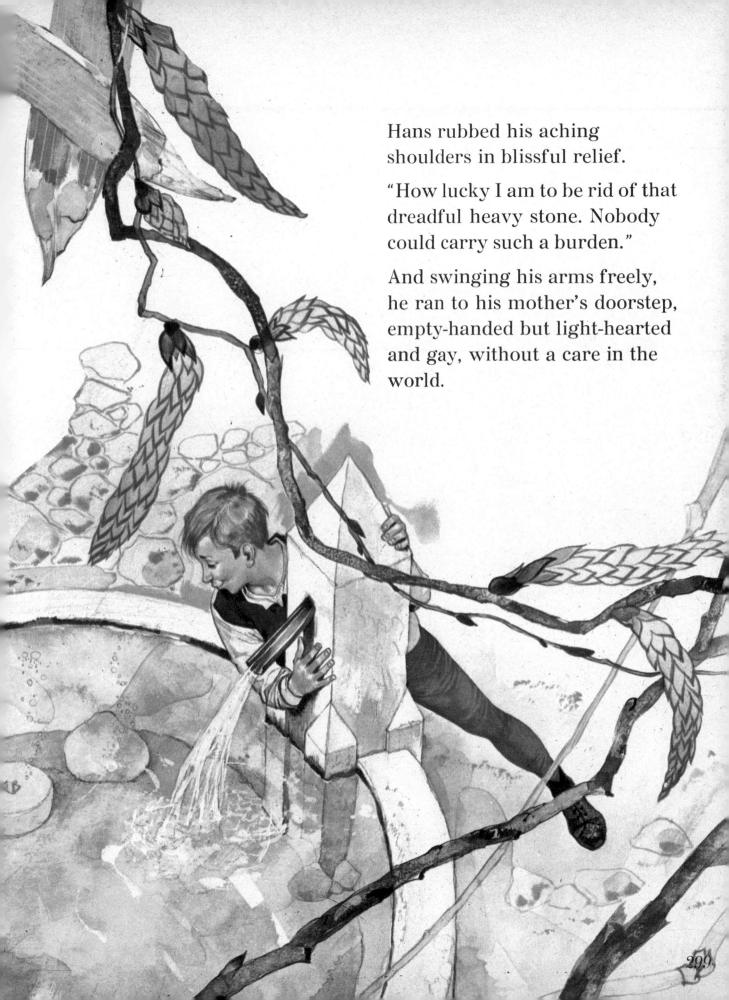

Hans rubbed his aching shoulders in blissful relief.

"How lucky I am to be rid of that dreadful heavy stone. Nobody could carry such a burden."

And swinging his arms freely, he ran to his mother's doorstep, empty-handed but light-hearted and gay, without a care in the world.

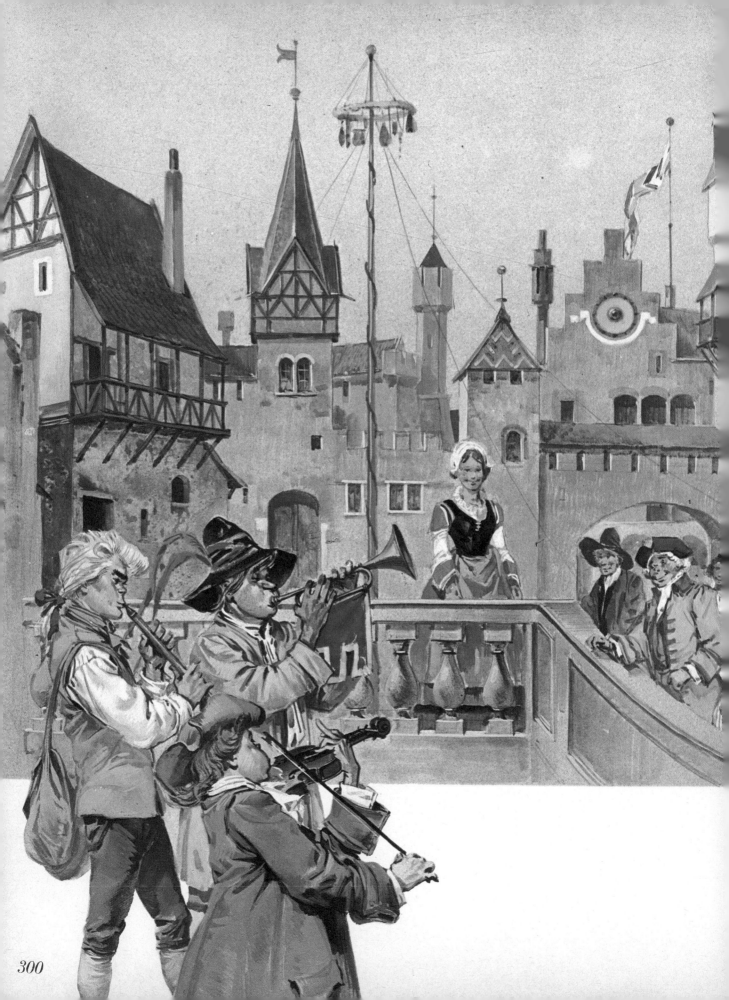

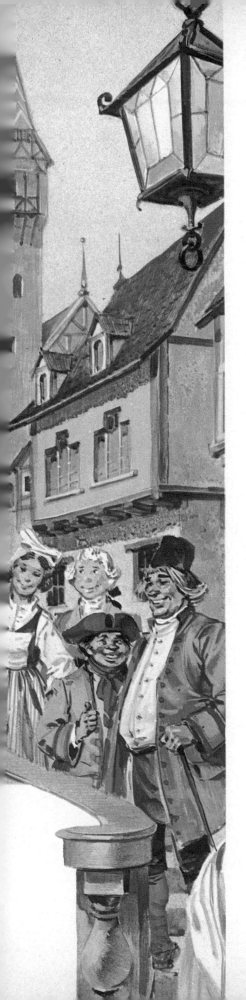

THE THREE MUSICIANS

Once upon a time there were three brothers who earned their living as traveling musicians, going from place to place and entertaining the populace with their lively tunes at banquets and village fairs. And when they were done with their playing, they would often join the local folk in feasting and drinking and storytelling.

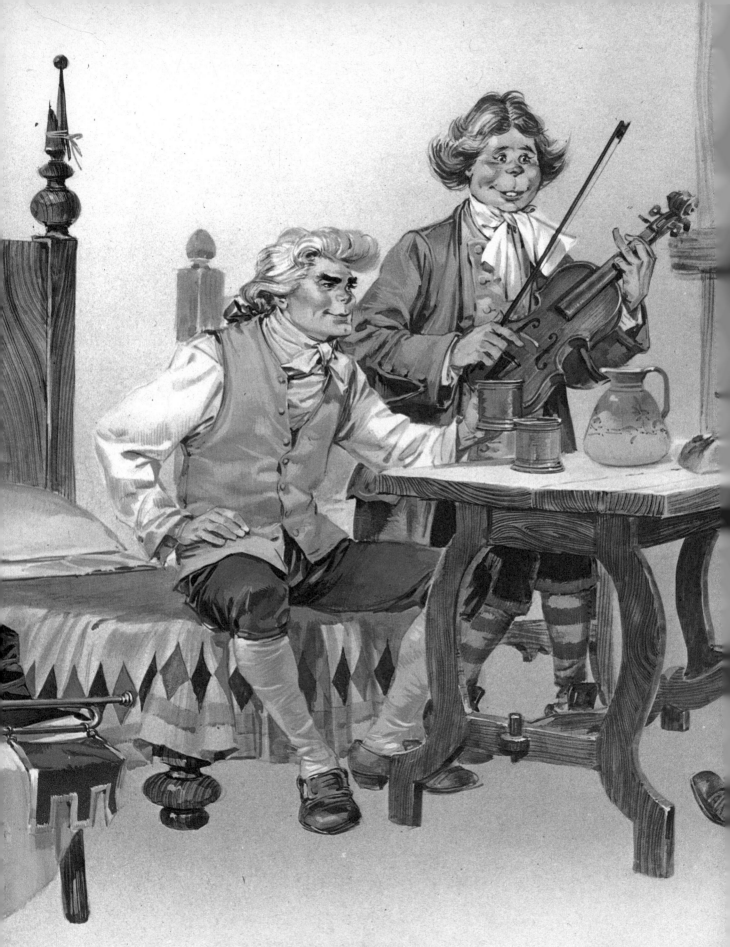

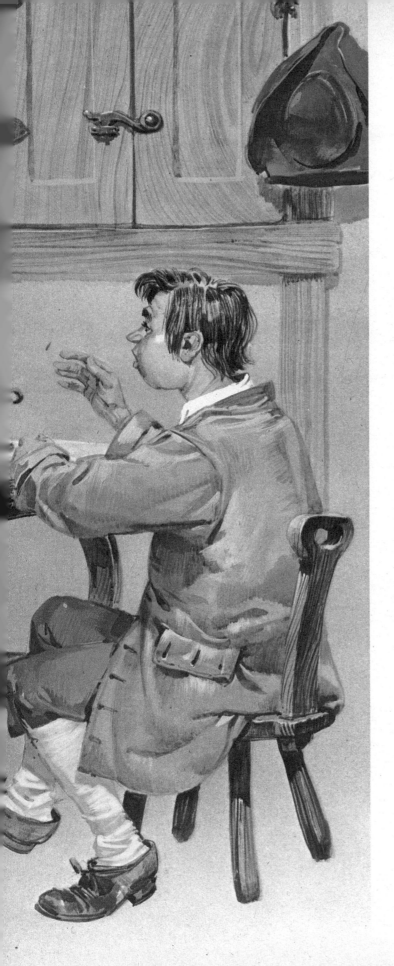

After one such occasion the three players hurried back to their room at the inn to talk over a curious tale they had heard during dinner. According to the townspeople, nearby was a mysterious castle that none of them had ever dared enter. It was said to be bewitched, but also overflowing with treasures belonging to an evil rich man, and strange happenings were sure to befall anyone daring enough to pass through its huge gates.

In order to avoid danger to all alike, the brothers agreed that they should proceed to the strange castle one at a time to try their luck at disclosing its secrets and perhaps enriching themselves. The violinist, the vain eldest brother who thought himself most intelligent, insisted that he be allowed to go first.

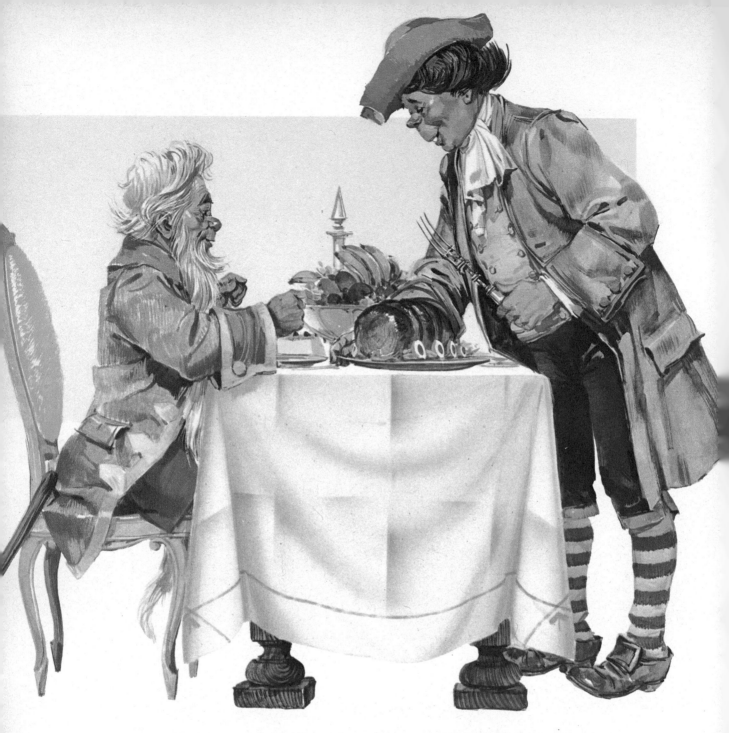

As soon as the violin player entered, the heavy gates
clanged shut behind him. At first he was terrified, but
after wandering through many treasure-laden
chambers he came to a magnificently set dining table,
covered with tasty food and drink. Just as he prepared to
gorge himself, a curious old dwarf with a long gray
beard came in and, without saying a word, sat down to
join him in his meal.

The violinist offered the silent dwarf some roast, but as the old man took it with his fork he let it drop to the floor. Then as the musician politely bent down to recover it for him, the smiling dwarf pounced on his back and began beating him vigorously with his rod. Finally, dodging blows all the while, the poor violinist managed to escape through the castle gates and ran all the way back to the inn.

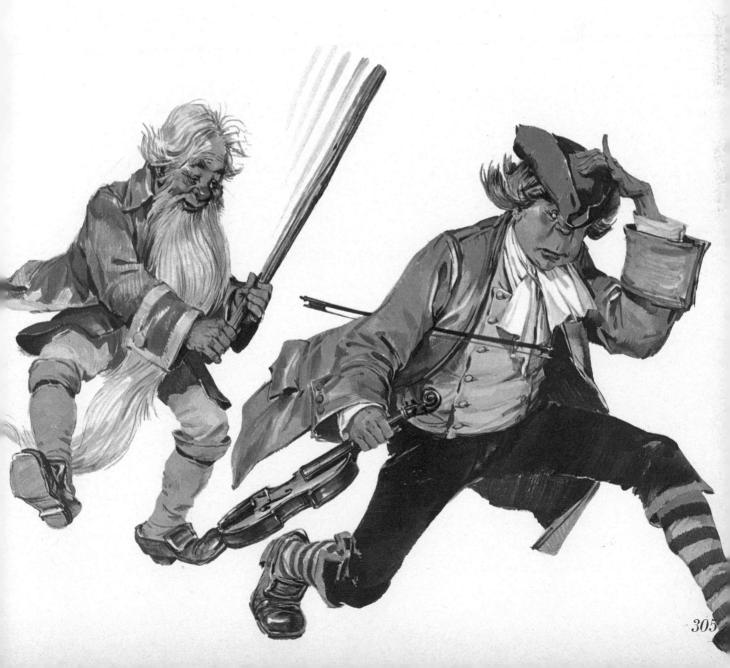

The next morning when his brothers awoke and saw the violinist lying there bruised and sore, they asked what had happened. He described his painful misadventure with the queer old dwarf and, when they seemed skeptical of his fantastic story, told them to go see for themselves.

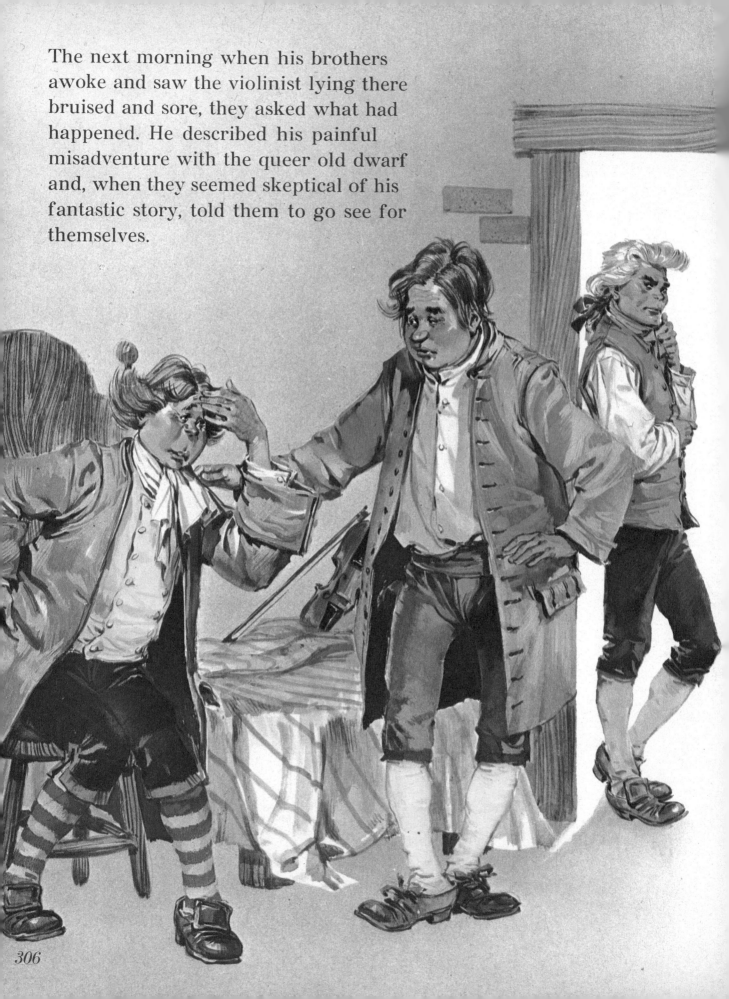

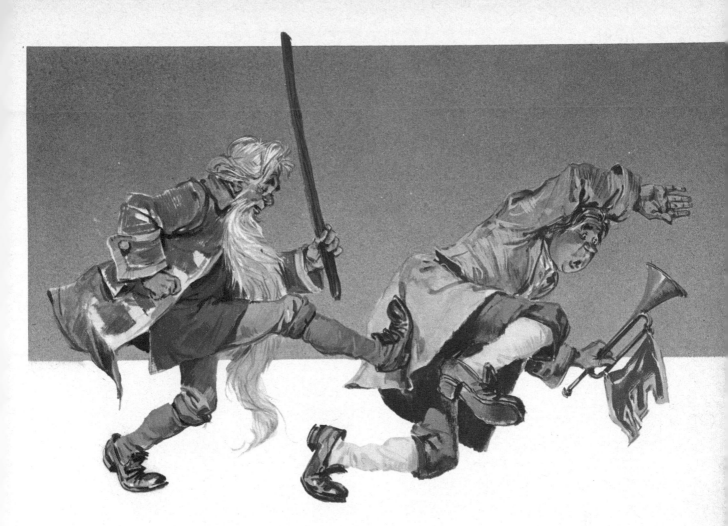

The trumpeter, the second oldest brother, then set off for
the mysterious castle on his own. With no trouble at all,
he entered the gates, wandered about the lavish halls,
and finally sat down at the richly set table. Then the
gray-bearded dwarf appeared, and everything happened
as before—dropping the meat, bending over, and then
the nasty pummeling. Glad to escape with his life, the
trumpeter scurried back to his brothers and related
what had occurred.

Next came the turn of the handsome youngest brother,
the flutist, who was much shrewder than the others.

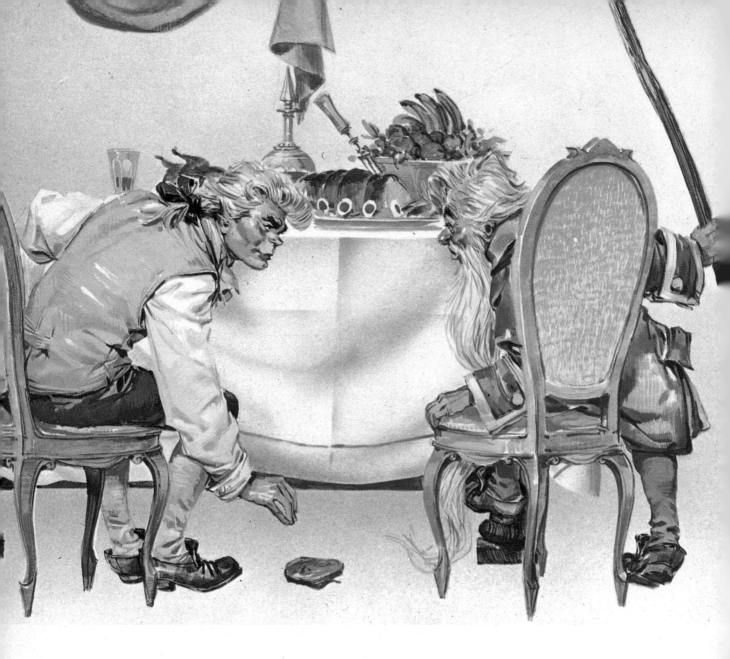

After arriving at the castle and wandering about, he sat down to the tempting feast laid out as usual. Again, the old dwarf entered and everything happened as before—except that this time the flutist never for a moment took his eyes off the little man. When he dropped his piece of roast, the youth bent over to pick it up but jumped upright as soon as he saw the sly dwarf raise his rod. The flutist then grabbed the old man's beard and tugged at it with all his might. And off it came in his hands! For the first time, the dwarf gave out with a great shriek.

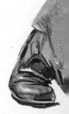

"I beg you, give me back my beard!" he groaned. "If you do, I will show you how to break the magic spell of the castle and will make you rich."

The young man, feeling the power of the beard as he held it, replied: "You may have your beard only when you have told me all the secrets."

Weakened without his beard, the crafty dwarf was forced to agree.

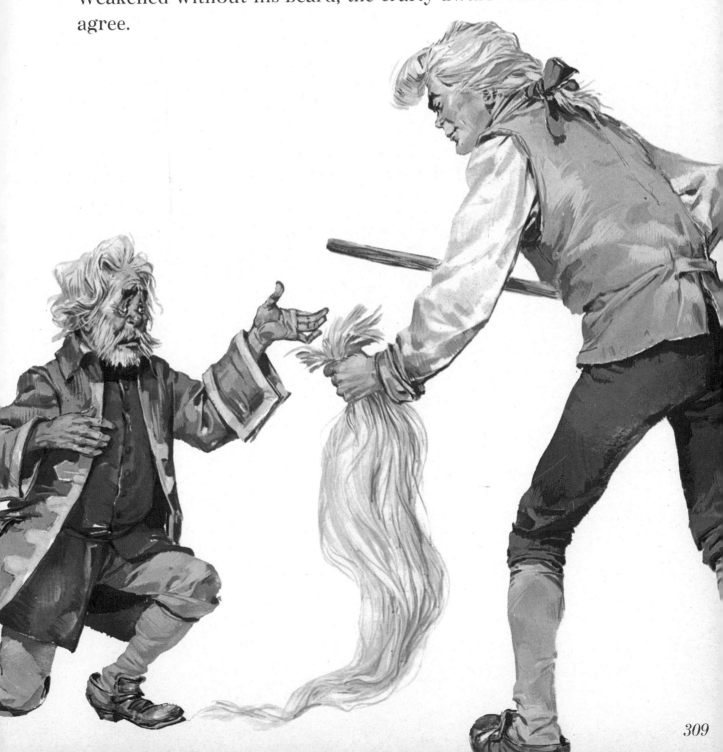

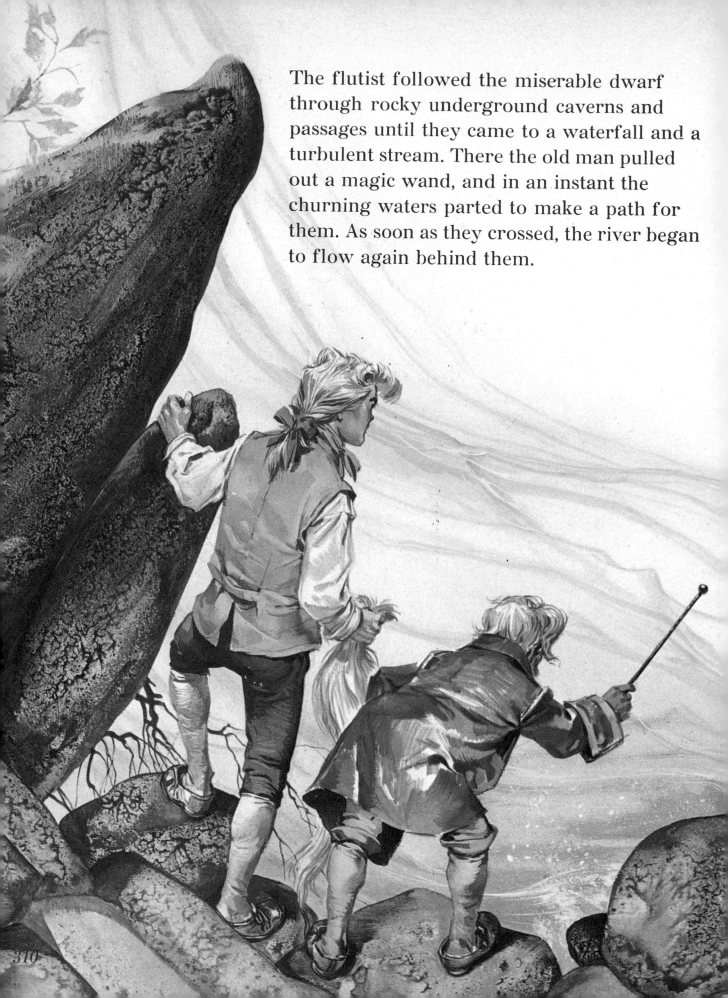

The flutist followed the miserable dwarf
through rocky underground caverns and
passages until they came to a waterfall and a
turbulent stream. There the old man pulled
out a magic wand, and in an instant the
churning waters parted to make a path for
them. As soon as they crossed, the river began
to flow again behind them.

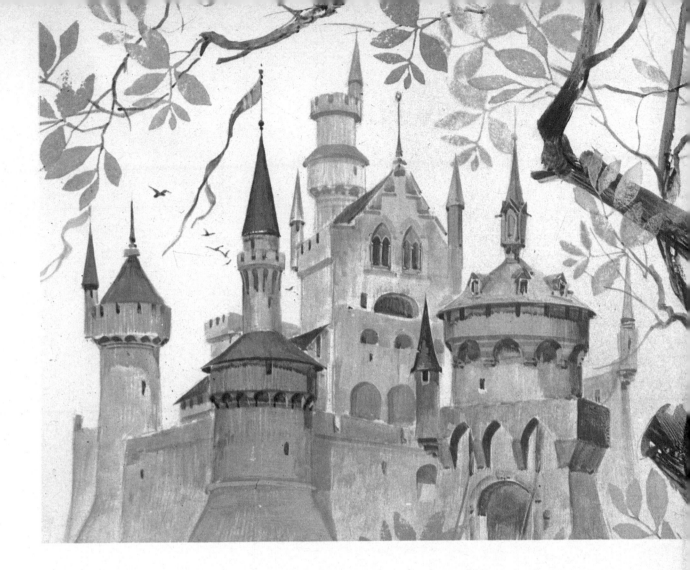

On the other side they found a lovely flowering meadow and in the distance another, more splendid castle. The youth asked the old dwarf who the owner of these rich holdings was.

"Their owner lies within," replied the dwarf. "She is a beautiful princess put to sleep many years ago by an evil sorcerer. No one has ever been able to get past me to break the spell and rescue her. Now, without my beard, I am powerless and must help you to gain your wishes. Come!"

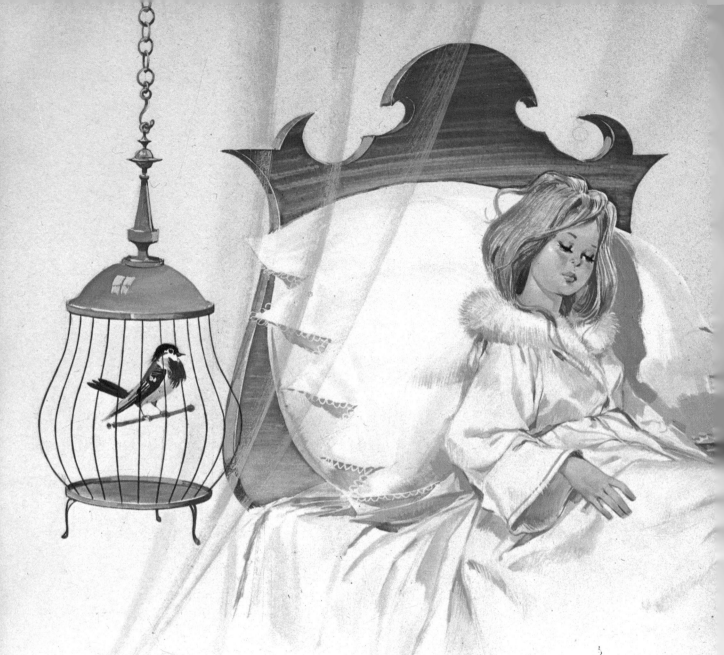

In one of the upper chambers of the silent castle they found a large curtained bed, and inside reclined the lovely sleeping princess. Alongside her bed was a birdcage, holding a pretty little chirping bird.

"Only you can awaken this enchanted creature from her long sleep and win her love," said the old dwarf, as he pointed out the bird to the young man.

Pluck out that bright red feather and hold it closely thus.
The legend says that it will burn and smolder into dust.
Place the ashes on her lips and shortly you will see
That she will soon be filled with life and once again be free.

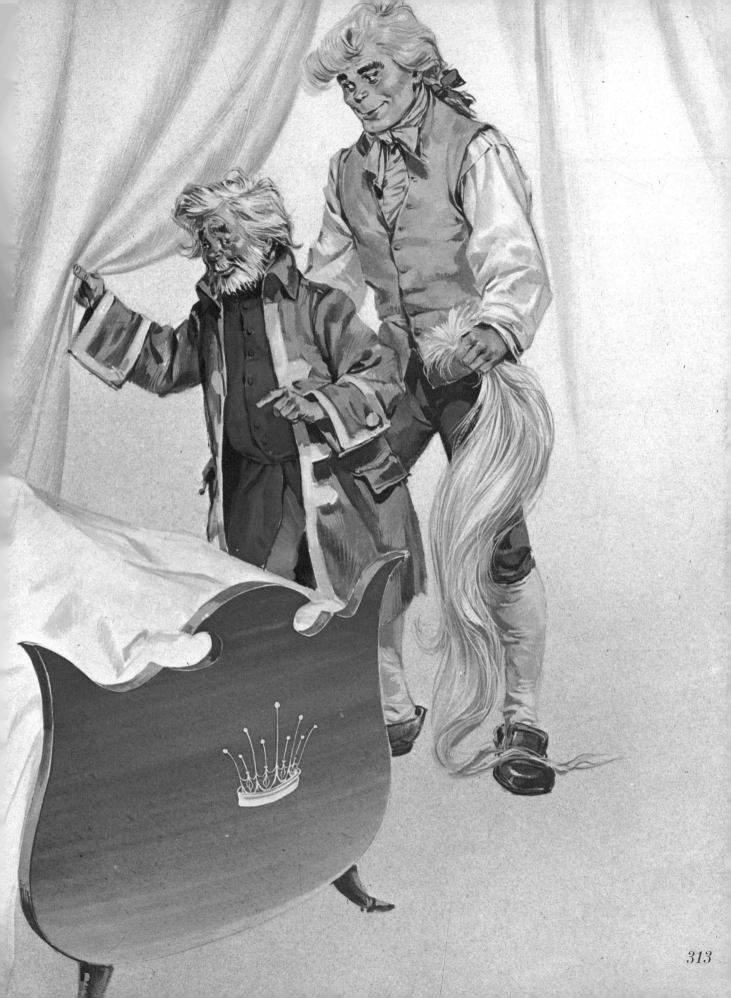

The flutist went to the cage and picked up the little bird with the red feather on his breast. He looked at the sleeping princess with great tenderness and then, very gently, plucked the bright red feather from the bird's breast and laid it on the princess' heart. Suddenly the feather began to smolder and turn a vivid red, and soon all that remained was powdery ashes. The young musician placed these on the princess' lips, and immediately the lovely girl opened her eyes and smiled at him, as she arose.

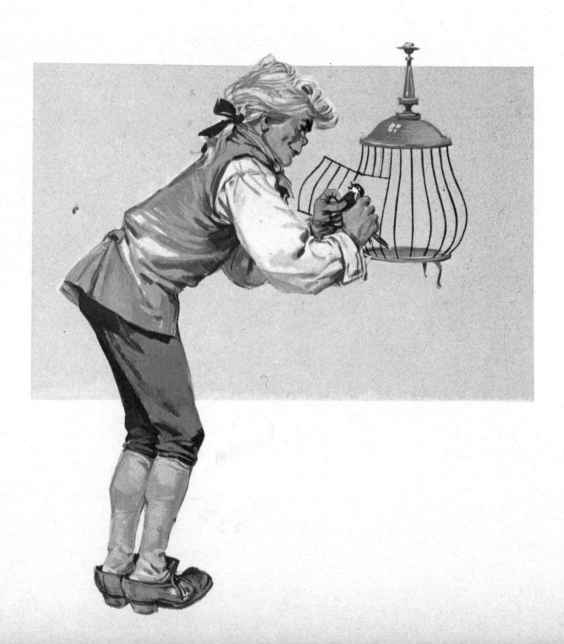

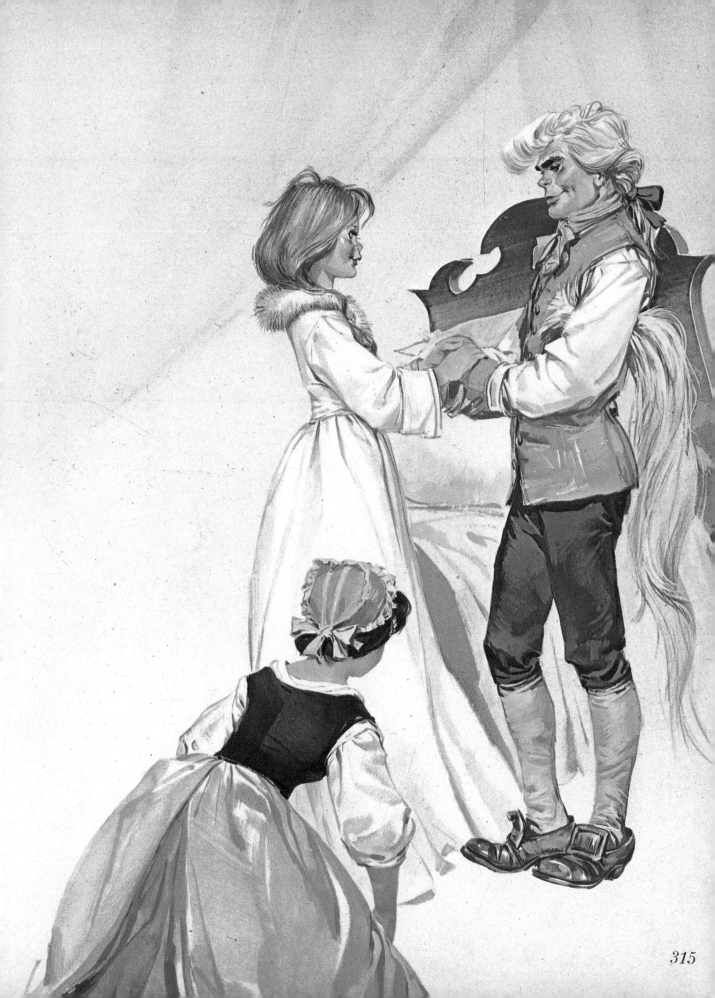

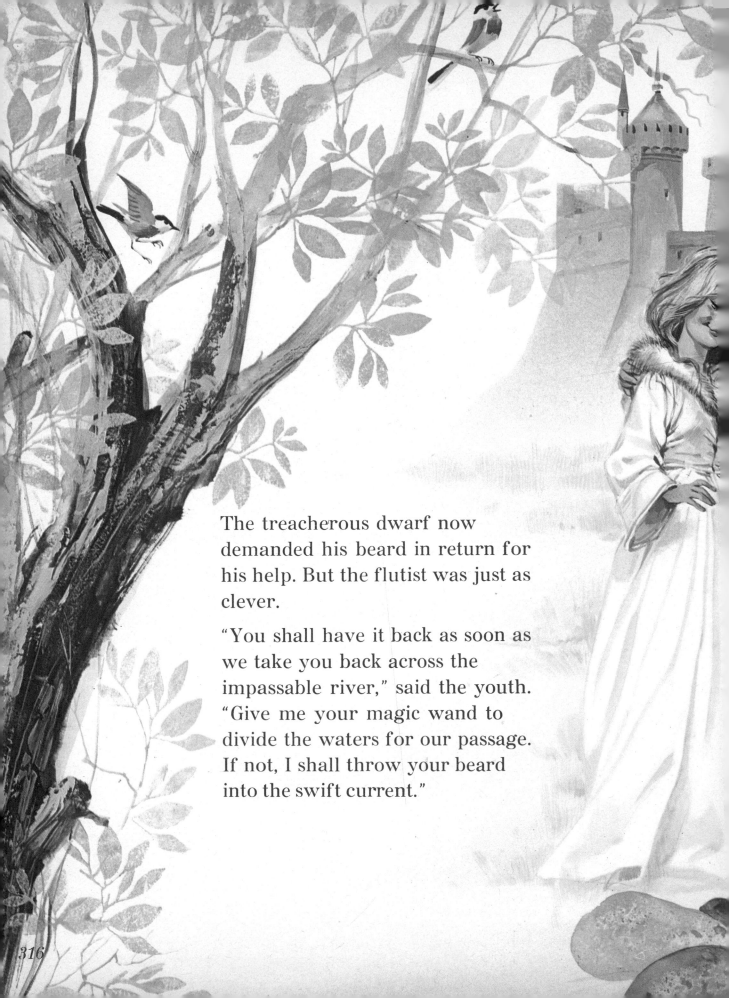

The treacherous dwarf now demanded his beard in return for his help. But the flutist was just as clever.

"You shall have it back as soon as we take you back across the impassable river," said the youth. "Give me your magic wand to divide the waters for our passage. If not, I shall throw your beard into the swift current."

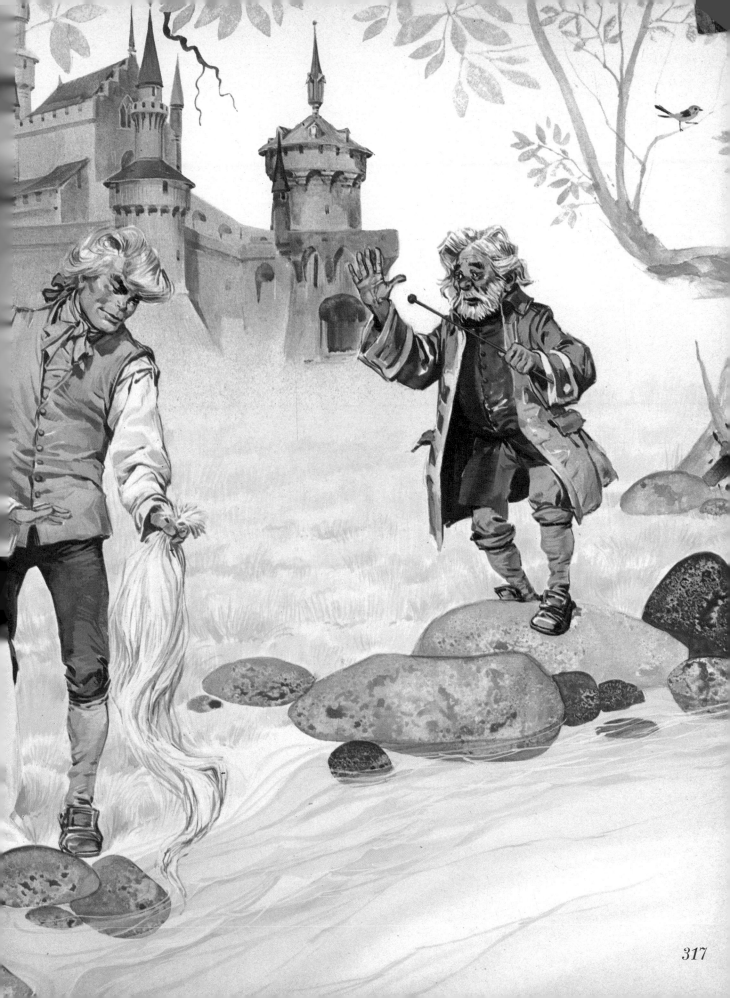

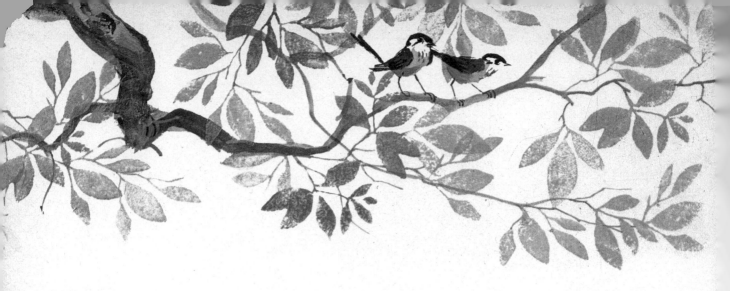

With a touch of the wand, the young man parted the waters and sent the dwarf across to the opposite bank first. The old man crossed without looking back, and only when he reached the other shore did he see how he had been tricked, for the flutist had released the torrent with another touch of the wand, and the furious dwarf was forever stranded on his side of the river. The youth threw his beard to the wily old man, who still begged for his magic wand—but to no avail. And so the young couple returned to their castle to reign together in peace and joy ever after.

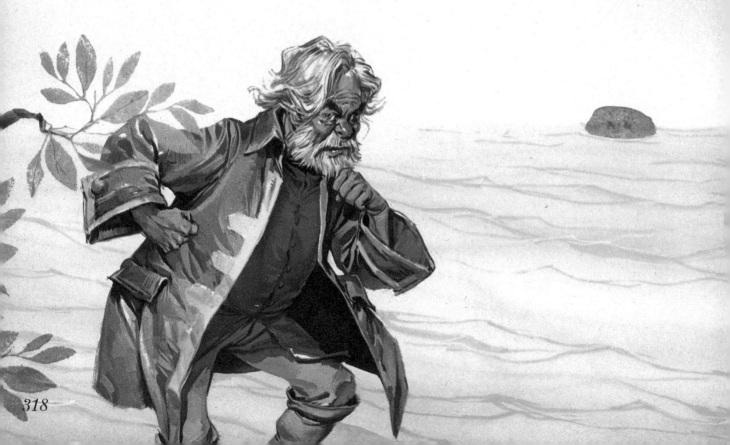

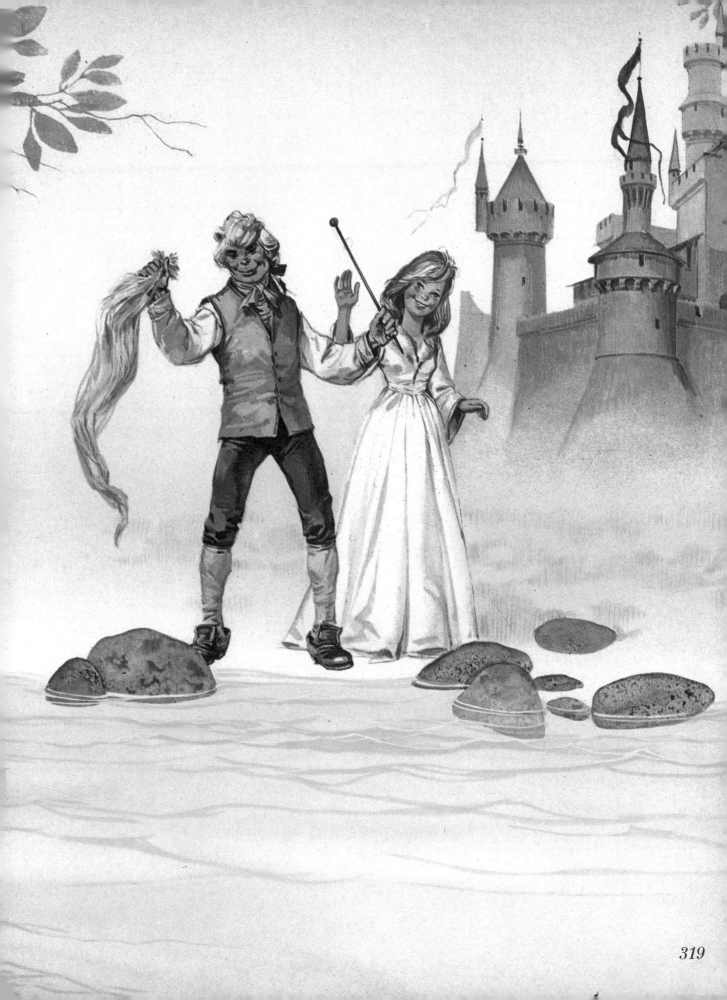